Advance praise for

Prescriptions for a Healthy House

Modern culture has many benefits but all too frequently convenience and costs are exchanged for health. It's true for food and it is every bit as true for our shelter. The authors have compiled the most authoritative reference in the field of how to build your home or office to maximize its benefit for your health. I have used this book in the construction of my home and office and highly recommend it.

— Dr. Mercola, Founder www.mercola.com,
world's most visited natural health site

Prescriptions for a Healthy House contains must-have information for those of us who wish to live safer, healthier, and more sustainable lives in our new or existing home environments. The authors offer a wealth of information, resources, and careful advice and specifications on a wide variety of helpful topics.

— Allison Friedman, cofounder, Rate It Green
www.rateitgreen.com

Living a truly healthy lifestyle involves more than eating well and exercising. It includes living that lifestyle in a healthy home. This revolutionary book explains why that's so important and how to make it happen. *Prescriptions for a Healthy House* is fascinating and practical, and gives you the life-changing, health-giving information you need in a clear, personable way. Deep bows to the authors.

— Marilynn Preston, creator and author of "Energy Express,"
the longest-running syndicated fitness column in the US

Wedding baubiologie with beauty, this book is the foremost authority on creating healthy, nurturing homes. I refer to *Prescriptions for a Healthy House* on an almost daily basis.

— Robyn Griggs Lawrence
Editor-in-Chief, *Natural Home* magazine

PRESCRIPTIONS for

A Healthy House

A PRACTICAL GUIDE FOR

Architects, Builders & Homeowners

Paula Baker-Laporte, FAIA
Erica Elliott, MD and John Banta, CAIH

THIRD REVISED EDITION

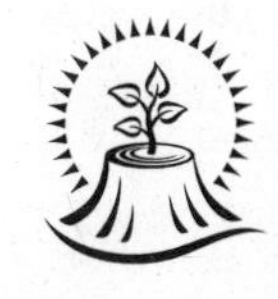

NEW SOCIETY PUBLISHERS

Cataloging in Publication Data:
A catalog record for this publication is available from
the National Library of Canada.

Cover design by Diane McIntosh. Images: iStock.

Printed in Canada.
First printing April 2008.

Paperback ISBN: 978-0-86571-604-9

To order directly from the publishers, please call toll-free (North America)
1-800-567-6772, or order online at www.newsociety.com

Any other inquiries can be directed by mail to:

New Society Publishers
P.O. Box 189, Gabriola Island, BC V0R 1X0, Canada
(250) 247-9737

New Society Publishers' mission is to publish books that contribute in fundamental ways to building an ecologically sustainable and just society, and to do so with the least possible impact on the environment, in a manner that models this vision. We are committed to doing this not just through education, but through action. This book is one step toward ending global deforestation and climate change. It is printed on Forest Stewardship Council-certified acid-free paper that is **100% post-consumer recycled** (100% old growth forest-free), processed chlorine free, and printed with vegetable-based, low-VOC inks, with covers produced using FSC-certified stock. Additionally, New Society purchases carbon offsets based on an annual audit, operating with a carbon-neutral footprint. For further information, or to browse our full list of books and purchase securely, visit our website at: www.newsociety.com

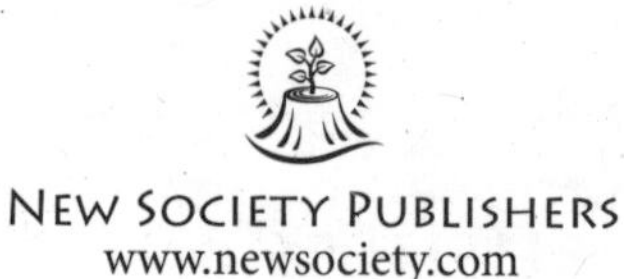

This book is dedicated
to the millions of people
who are chronically ill
from indoor environmental exposures.
May we be forewarned
and learn from your suffering.

Contents

Part II Specification

Acknowledgments

For this 3rd edition of *Prescriptions for a Healthy House* we would like to thank our readers, who over the years have used this book in search of a healthier way to build their homes. We thank the folks at New Society Publishers for keeping us in print and inviting us to update our information to make this work current in a rapidly growing field. We also want to take this opportunity to thank them for their exceptional vision in publishing a whole roster of books for creating a better world. We wish to acknowledge our editor, Diane Killou, for her thoughtful, skilled, and thorough work.

Many thanks to Jesus Bendezu and Liz Jan from the Baker-Laporte office for their research assistance, to Stephen Wiman for his review and additions regarding water purification, and to Toni and Paul Fuge for their review and updates regarding sustainable forestry.

We are grateful to the many Building Biologists who have taken time from their busy careers to enrich the 3rd edition with their informative essays about various aspects of the Building Biology approach to healthy building. Thank you, Warren Clough, Mary Cordaro, André Fauteux, Rowena Finegan, Larry Gust, Katharina Gustavs, Ernst Kiesling, David McAuley, Peter Sierck, Will Spates, Dan Stih, George Swanson, Athena Thompson, Vicki Warren, and last but not least Helmut Ziehe, founder of the International Institute for Bau-Biology & Ecology in Clearwater, Florida, teacher and mentor of many of us who are concerned about healthy homes.

The authors wish to thank the many people who offered their guidance, expertise, and encouragement in the completion of the original manuscript. Special thanks go to Pauline Kenny for her tireless efforts and computer wizardry, which helped transform the data into something that resembled a book. Our gratitude goes to Will and Louise Pape, who graciously offered their ranch as a working retreat center and gave practical advice and inspiration each step of the way.

Paula would like to acknowledge her husband, Robert Laporte, not only for his patience in living with a "writing" partner but also for the teaching and inspiration he has shared with her in the field of natural building.

John Banta wishes to thank his wife, Trisha, who has patiently endured her husband's authorship of two books in one year, and James Holland of Restoration Consultants, who has continued to be a personal mentor.

Paula Baker-Laporte, FAIA, BBP
John Banta, CAIH
Erica Elliott, MD

Foreword

By Helmut Ziehe

I am honored to be asked to write the foreword for this book, which I find extraordinarily suitable for practical use by architects, builders, and homeowners. Building professionals, who already understand the complexities of conventional construction, can now learn how to incorporate the principles of Bau-Biologie (Building Biology) into their buildings in order to make healthier places to live.

Bau-Biologie is a German word. "Bau" means building and "bio" comes from the Greek "bios," meaning life or mode of life. Combined, the words refer to how buildings influence life, or the relationship between buildings and life. Bau-Biologie has two aspects. One is the study of how building materials and construction methods impact human health and how this knowledge can be applied to the new construction and the modification of homes and workplaces. This is what we call basic Bau-Biologie. The other aspect is ecological and is concerned with the impact buildings have on the environment. The words Bau-Biologie and Building Biology are used interchangeably and are trademarked in the United States.

The Bau-Biologie movement began in Germany some 40 years ago. A number of concerned professionals from various disciplines noted a general decline in health following the post-World War II surge in construction. Hubert Palm coined the term Bau-Biologie and wrote a book about it. Gustav Freiherr von Pohl did some research on water veins and their influence on people's health. Anton Schneider, a wood specialist, and some colleagues formed a group and taught Bau-Biologie at a vocational school in Rosenheim, Bavaria. After a successful start, the program became the Institut für Baubiologie und Ökologie Neubeuern (IBN). Under Anton Schneider, the IBN flourished. Through courses, seminars, books, and a magazine entitled *Wohnung und Gesundheit,* it soon gained a reputation in Germany, Austria, Switzerland, and the Netherlands and throughout Northern Europe.

I first studied Building Biology after an "aha" experience in North Africa in 1980 that changed the course of my career and life. I was the resident engineer for a new city of 90,000 inhabitants. It was a nice design, but the building materials were wrong! Concrete was the basic material. They had sand in abundance, and everything else had to be imported. One- to three-story houses were built, but the mistake was that these concrete buildings heated up so much that even air conditioning could not bring substantial relief. The people were forced to live in these houses, but the majority refused, living in tents instead.

I found the solution by looking at houses dating back as much as 4,000 years that used clay as the basic building material and covered walkways for shading and ventilation.

Very simple! The new town designers and the local committee were unwilling to accept the truths in my observations about the genius of the indigenous architecture and the shortcomings of the modern buildings we were imposing on these people. This eye-opening experience led me to forsake my education and my career as a modernist architect and to embrace the precepts of Bau-Biologie. I had no intention of going back to a conventional architectural practice once my job in North Africa was finished.

After leaving North Africa, I lived in England, where I became aware that Bau-Biologie education was not available in English. I contacted Anton Schneider to study and eventually translate the Correspondence Course. This led me to found the International Institute for Bau-Biologie & Ecology (IBE), first in England and then in the United States. Eventually the knowledge of Bau-Biologie was disseminated to other English-speaking countries.

In England in 1984 I worked on the translation and began determining if there was indeed an interest in Bau-Biologie in the English-speaking world. The translation went well, even with a manual typewriter and freezing conditions, but over a period of two years I had only twelve students! However, one of the students was David Pearson, who promised to write a book on Bau-Biologie. *The Natural House Book* appeared some two years later.

In 1987, I relocated to the United States. In the beginning I worked alone in my new Florida residence and the Institute started slowly. At that time in North America there were very few people focusing on the built environment and its relationship to human health. Of note were the human ecologist and physician Theron G. Randolph, the architect Richard Crowther, and the writer Ken Kern (author of *The Owner-Built Home*).

When a reporter asked me in 1989 how many students I had, I answered: "Only eight." He replied: "Everyone has to start small." A big boost came shortly afterward as a result of an article in *East West Journal,* which initiated a surge of public awareness of and interest in Bau-Biologie. Another very important event was meeting Wolfgang Maes, a very successful Bau-Biologist from Germany and initiator of the Bau-Biologie Standards. He proposed seminars and came from Germany to help run the first three. They were a great success. John Banta was among the first graduating students.

With the computer age underway, the course material could be fine-tuned. I was no longer capable of doing all the work of the Institute alone. My staff and I refined the original Correspondence Course and created a Mini-Course, now called IBE 111 — Natural, Healthy Buildings: An Introductory Overview of Bau-Biologie Principles.

During the following years I was invited to numerous events in the US and abroad, including an invitation to speak in Quebec in 1993; the AIA Chicago annual conference; various exhibitions in Austin, New York, Seattle, Los Angeles, San Francisco, and Phoenix; and many feng shui conferences throughout the country. In the midst of all this were invitations to Indore and to Bogota, Mexico City, Rio de Janeiro, and Sao Paulo, leading to the dissemination of the Building Biology principles into the Latin American countries and the translation of the Mini-Course into Portuguese. Without my actually traveling there, IBE established a presence in Australia and New Zealand. In New Zealand, one of my students, Reinhard Kanuka, founded an institute and offered the American translation of the Correspondence Course to his students.

Sometimes I wonder where I found the strength to endure twenty-five years of Bau-Biologie development. Although the progress was at times discouragingly slow and the financial rewards less than supportive, much encouragement along the way reinforced my belief in this valuable body of knowledge. My commitment to it has been renewed again and again.

I am entirely aware that a single person cannot do it alone. To disseminate a relevant body of knowledge, there needs to be a collaboration of people who are captured by the same mission. I think we have begun to achieve this. Bau-Biologie, or Building Biology, has found its niche in society. This newest edition of *Prescriptions for a Healthy House,* which includes contributions from many of the continent's leading Bau-Biologists, is a milestone along the way.

Authors' note: Rather than have a conventional foreword written in praise of our book, we invited Helmut Ziehe, founder of the International Institute for Bau-Biology & Ecology, to write about the history of Bau-Biologie, where our inspiration for the book originated. In 2004, Helmut suffered a severe stroke. His students rallied to his side and carried on the work of the Institute with a renewed sense of commitment. Helmut continues to progress in his recovery with the same courage and perseverance with which he single-mindedly ran the Institute against all obstacles for so many years to the great benefit of his students. His language skills have had to be slowly and painfully relearned. Knowing the effort it has taken him to write this foreword, we are honored and touched.

Preface

It has been said that we shape our buildings and then our buildings shape us. When we consider that the average North American spends 90 percent or more of life indoors, the significance of this statement becomes apparent. In this era of unprecedented technological advancement, it stands to reason that we would use our knowledge to create indoor environments with exceptional vitality that would enhance our health and our sense of well-being. But this has not been the case.

Indoor air pollution is one of the top four environmental health risks identified by the US Environmental Protection Agency (EPA) and the Scientific Advisory Board authorized by Congress to consult with the EPA on technical matters.[1] Indoor pollution is estimated to cause thousands of cancer deaths and hundreds of thousands of respiratory health problems each year. Millions of children have experienced elevated blood levels of contaminants resulting from their exposure to indoor pollutants.[2]

How has this sad state of affairs developed? Since the oil embargo of 1973, we have placed a high priority on energy efficiency, creating buildings that are increasingly airtight. Concurrently, the building industry has promoted inexpensive synthetic building products and furnishings that are mass-produced and require little maintenance. Since little attention has been paid to the toxicity of these products until very recently, consumers have remained largely ignorant of the health threats they pose.

The average person has little background in chemistry and makes the false assumption that building products must be reasonably safe to be allowed on the market. The disturbing truth is that, according to the EPA, there are now more than 88,000 chemicals in common use.[3] Many of these have been associated with cancer, birth defects, reproductive disorders, and neurological and behavioral problems. Furthermore, "as amazing as it may seem, there are no mandatory pre-market health testing or approval requirements under any federal law for chemicals in cosmetics, toys, clothing, carpets, or construction materials, to name just a few obvious sources of chemical exposure in everyday life."[4]

The limited testing that has been implemented rarely takes into consideration the ongoing, low-level exposure to the hundreds of chemicals we inhale or absorb simultaneously throughout our daily lives. The toll on human health resulting from exposure to the chemical soup surrounding us is finally becoming clear. In 1986, the National Academy of Sciences estimated that 15 percent of the population suffered from chemical sensitivities.[5] Based on current unofficial reports by physicians specializing in environmental medicine, that number is rising rapidly. These figures do not include people who unknowingly suffer from problems either directly or indirectly related to chronic, low-level toxic exposure. All too often symptoms are falsely attributed to the normal aging process.

Exposure to toxins in the indoor environment, even at low levels, has been linked to a vast spectrum of illnesses ranging from chronic sinus infections, headaches, insomnia, anxiety, and joint pain to full-blown multiple chemical sensitivity and other immune system disorders.

In spite of overwhelming evidence of the health risks, the majority of new construction in the United States continues to create environments that harm human health. There is, in fact, nothing complicated about creating a healthy building. The solution is composed of many simple but important steps. Many safer alternative materials and methods of design and building are becoming readily available. Nevertheless, the homeowner who desires to create a healthy building or remodel an existing building is still a pioneer facing the following major obstacles:

- Building for health is not the current standard of the construction industry. Although most architects and builders are now aware that health problems are associated with standard building practices, the industry in general has not responded with appropriate changes. There are no set and sanctioned prescriptions to follow for healthy building. In the nine years since the publication of the first edition of *Prescriptions for a Healthy House*, several organizations have emerged with the purpose of demonstrating and rewarding the creation of healthier, more energy efficient, and more ecologically friendly homes. The American Lung Association has built exemplary model homes. Several voluntary rating and certification programs, such as LEED-R, Green Seal, and the National Association of Home Builders' Green Rating System, and various county and state guidelines have emerged to promote the creation of healthier homes. The California Air Resources Board has defined stringent environmental codes that have been adopted throughout the US and have influenced manufacturers of building products. As encouraging as these advances are, there is still no guarantee that a new home built today will support the health of its occupants.
- The homeowner receives false information. Most building professionals are uninformed about the details of healthful design and building. The prospective client who has heard about healthful building is often advised by professionals either that there is no need for concern or that healthful building is cost prohibitive.
- There is a dearth of concise information. If homeowners are still committed to creating a healthy house and have managed to find an architect and builder who are receptive to working with them, then they must undertake together the daunting task of educating themselves and others. Distilling enough information to create a set of specifications for a project is an undertaking requiring extensive time and dedication.
- Even if healthy materials and practices are

specified, a lack of quality control may result in a major degradation of the building, which in turn can lead to occupant health problems, decline in energy efficiency, and structural damages. These damages may be especially difficult to discover and costly to repair when they are hidden in wall cavities or other inaccessible spaces.

The purpose of this book is to take the mystery out of healthy house building by walking the owner/architect/builder team through the construction process. We explain where and why standard building practices are not healthful, what to do differently, and how to obtain alternative materials and expertise. The Resource List in Appendix B provides sources for all products and services printed in bold type in the text.

We hope you will find this 3rd revised and updated edition of *Prescriptions for a Healthy House* to be a useful tool in your quest for healthier living.

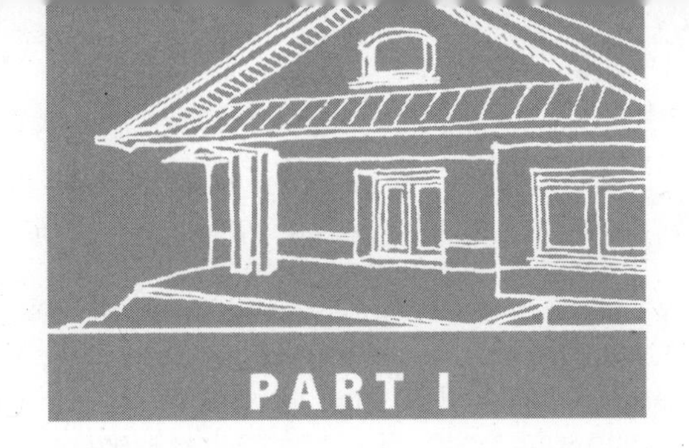

Overview

Introduction

Until about 35 years ago, indoor air pollution was a very limited phenomenon. Since that time, two basic things have changed in the way buildings are constructed. First, thousands of synthetic chemicals have been incorporated into building materials. Second, building envelopes are sealed so tightly that chemicals and occupant-generated pollutants remain trapped inside homes, where they are inhaled into the lungs and absorbed through the skin. Prior to the energy crisis, the typical home averaged approximately one air exchange per hour. Now, in a well-sealed home, the air is often exchanged as infrequently as once every five hours, and that is not enough to ensure healthful air quality. Furthermore, the synthetic building materials used to seal out air and water often result in the trapping and condensation of water vapor in the walls, leading to mold and structural deterioration.

There are two basic approaches to solving the indoor pollution problem and creating healthier living environments. The first and more mainstream approach in North America involves eliminating as many pollutants as possible from within the building envelope and ensuring an airtight barrier on the inside so there is less need to worry about the chemical composition of the structure and insulation. This approach addresses for the most part conventional frame construction and the prevention of water intrusion. Filtered or clean outside air is then mechanically pumped in, keeping the house under a slightly positive pressure so that air infiltration is controlled. If one does not have the luxury of clean, vital, and refreshing natural surroundings, then a certain amount of isolation and filtering may be essential.

The second approach involves building the structure of natural or nontoxic materials that are vapor diffusible or "breathable." Building materials are chosen for their capacity (hygric capacity) to reach a state of equilibrium with the natural surroundings on one side and the indoor environment on the other, creating a comfortable interior climate by moderating natural conditions without distorting their nurturing aspects. This approach is based on the precepts of Bau-Biologie, or Building Biology, which views the natural environment as the gold standard against which built environments should be measured. Our home is considered to be a third skin, with our clothes being the second. By Building Biology standards, a home that nurtures health is not only free of toxins and synthetic materials. It also achieves a natural balance of ionization, reduces the influence of human-caused electromagnetic fields, avoids building over naturally occurring geopathic disturbances, and much more. Building Biology recognizes the genius of nature and the failure of industrialized building to fully understand natural laws in our attempts to create vital environments with the synthetic materials that are prevalent in conventional construction today.

Although little known in this country, the term "Building Biology" was translated from the German and introduced into the English language in 1987 by the founder of the International Institute for Bau-Biologie & Ecology, Helmut Ziehe. The institute has since fostered a dedicated and multidisciplinary following of practitioners who have used these principles to create healthier living environments for their clients. Paula Baker-Laporte and John Banta are both students and practitioners of Building Biology.

In this 3rd edition of *Prescriptions for a Healthy House* we have invited some of our Building Biology colleagues to contribute in their areas of expertise. Among these writers are experts in the fields of inspecting, diagnosing, repairing, and furnishing homes. Many of them focus on the work they do to remedy buildings that have, over time, become unhealthy environments for the people who live in them. With the inclusion of these essays we hope to extend the usefulness of the book to those wishing to turn their existing homes into healthier living environments.

Dispersed throughout the book are relevant medical and building case studies, the stories of real people from different walks of life with whom the authors have personally come into contact over the past few years. What they all have in common is firsthand experience of the consequences of living in unhealthy environments. They have agreed to share their stories with you.

Building or renovating a home involves making thousands of choices. Whether you are working with conventional building methods and materials or with natural, "alternative" ones, this book has been designed to walk you through the construction process and help you to make choices that will promote your health and well-being and the optimum serviceability of your home.

How Much More Will It Cost to Build a Healthy Home?

Assume for a moment that you are house hunting. Your real estate agent contacts you and is very excited about a real bargain, a house going for 20 percent less than market value. Upon further inquiry, you learn that the house contains lead paint and asbestos insulation and sits on a bed of radon-emitting granite. It is located in a flood plain, has poor drainage, and smells a little moldy. The previous owners have died of cancer. With this new information, the home now seems to be less than a bargain.

Our health is priceless and when buying, renovating, or building a new home its ability to nurture health should be our top priority. Unfortunately we are faced with a building/real estate industry that does not make health a top priority. Builders often include many amenities such as three-car garages, whirlpool baths, extra rooms, and fancy fixtures, faucets, and appliances while ignoring even simple health safeguards such as nontoxic paints, floor drains, and carbon monoxide monitors. Appraisers focus primarily on size rather than quality, and real estate agents often promote the visual cosmetics of the home. However, much of what makes a home healthy is not visible to the naked eye. This book is about how to avoid substances and building practices that are as harmful to your health as lead, asbestos, mold, or radon but are commonly used in construction today. It is for the homeowner, builder, and home designer who wish to make health a priority in creating homes that are responsive and nurturing for all who live in them.

How much more will it cost to build a healthy home? This is frequently the first question posed to Paula by her clients. The answer usually lies somewhere between zero and 25 percent more than standard construction. In some cases, little or no extra money is required to build and maintain a healthy home. A few examples are listed below:

- Additive-free concrete costs no more than concrete with toxic admixtures, provided that climatic conditions are appropriate for the project.
- Zero-VOC paints are now readily available through most paint manufacturers.
- Shortening wiring runs with careful planning not only will reduce exposure to electromagnetic fields but also will save money.
- Unscented and nonchlorinated cleaning products cost no more and can be just as effective as compounds containing harsh chemicals.

In other cases, healthier alternatives are more expensive initially but more economical in the long run. For example:

- The most inexpensive types of roofing to install are comprised of tar and gravel or asphalt shingles, but the useful life of these products is much shorter than that of many of the less toxic roofing systems discussed in Division 7.
- Although forced-air heating is less expensive to install, a properly designed gas-fired, hydronic radiant floor heating system is not only more comfortable and healthier but also virtually maintenance-free. Higher initial installation costs will be outweighed over time by lower heating bills and more comfort.

In some areas your decision to "go healthy" will cost more, and you will be faced with some difficult choices. We will try to offer you facts and a range of alternatives so that your choices can be well informed. In many instances there is no right answer. Sometimes your decision will come down to a trade-off between luxury and health. But then, what is luxury without health? You could ultimately spend a fortune on medical bills and lose your quality of life, as have the people who have shared their stories with us in the case studies throughout the book.

Furthermore, as responsible citizens of the world we must weigh our building choices from an environmental perspective. The cost to the environment of many current building practices is astronomical. Our children and grandchildren will ultimately pay for our excesses and waste. To weigh the environmental cost of our choices, we must consider their lifecycle impacts:

- We can choose products that are locally produced from renewable resources.
- We can choose to build less by building with well-designed and efficient plans.
- We can build-in energy efficiency and longevity.
- We can make solar heating, solar electricity, water catchment, and ecological waste management our budgeting priorities.

Sources of Indoor Pollution

Indoor air pollutants can be classified into five main categories: volatile organic compounds, toxic byproducts of combustion, pesticides, electromagnetic fields, and naturally occurring pollutants. Each category of pollutant is described in a following section.

Volatile Organic Compounds

Organic compounds are chemicals containing carbon-hydrogen bonds at the molecular level. They are both naturally occurring and

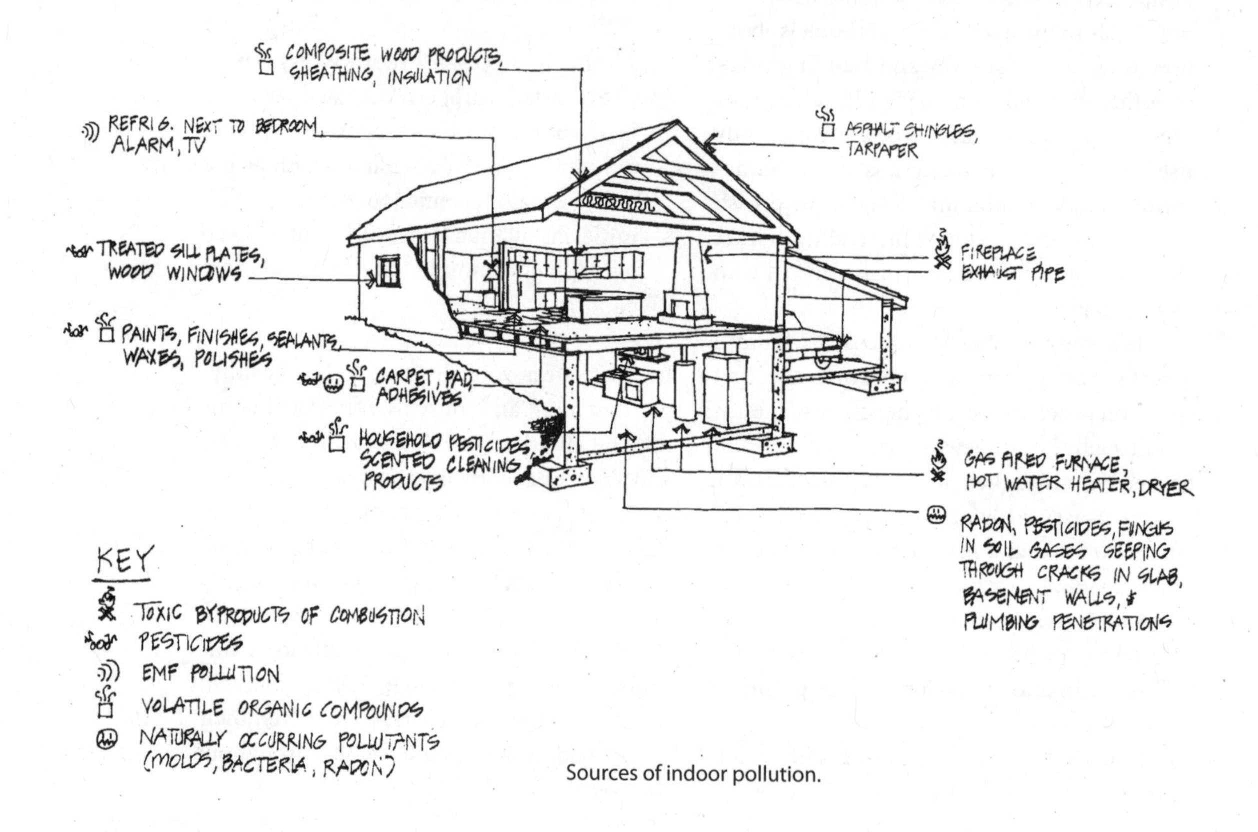

Sources of indoor pollution.

manufactured. Most synthetic organic compounds are petrochemicals derived from oil, gas, and coal. Organic compounds can exist in the form of a gas, a liquid, or solid particles. Substances that readily release vapors at room temperature are called volatile organic compounds (VOCs). This outgassing is a form of evaporation of volatile compounds contained in solid material and results in a slow release of chemicals into the air.

VOCs constitute a major source of toxic overload and can threaten individual health. Any organ of the body can be affected. Some of the more common symptoms include rashes, headaches, eye irritation, chronic cough, chronic sinus infections, joint and muscle pain, memory loss, inability to concentrate, irritability, fatigue, anxiety, depression, and an increasing number of allergies.

Organic compounds can be classified into three categories based on derivation from petroleum products. The primary organic compounds include components directly derived from gas, oil, and coal and include propane, butane, benzene, xylene, paraffins, toluene, and styrene. These products are then used to derive the intermediate substances such as formaldehyde, phenols, acetone, isopropanol, and acetaldehyde. The end products produced include solvents, waxes, lacquers, synthetic detergents, synthetic fibers, and paints. Common sources of volatile organic compounds occurring in the indoor environment include:

- plywood
- particleboard
- wood paneling
- carpets and carpet pads
- insulation
- paints
- finishes
- solvents
- adhesives
- synthetic fabrics
- cleaning products
- body care products
- mothballs
- insecticides
- aerosol products
- art and hobby materials
- dry cleaned garments
- air fresheners

VOCs can also be generated from natural substances. These include terpenes, which outgas from wood, and aromatics from natural oils. Some more chemically sensitive individuals react to naturally occurring VOCs. These individuals are urged to test their reactions to each product before making a major purchase, even if the product is derived from a natural source.

You are undoubtedly familiar with the distinctive smell of a new house. The odor is composed primarily of outgassing chemicals from toxic volatile organic compounds. Some building products now report the parts per million of VOCs on their labels, but this information can be misleading. Yes, it is true that the fewer parts per million the better, but certain chemicals such as dioxin are not safe in any detectable amount.[1] One of the goals in constructing a healthy house is to reduce the use of toxic VOCs.

Toxic Byproducts of Combustion

Gas, oil, coal, wood, and other fuels burned indoors consume valuable indoor oxygen unless air for combustion is supplied from the outdoors. In tight, energy efficient buildings, these fumes can cause serious health consequences.

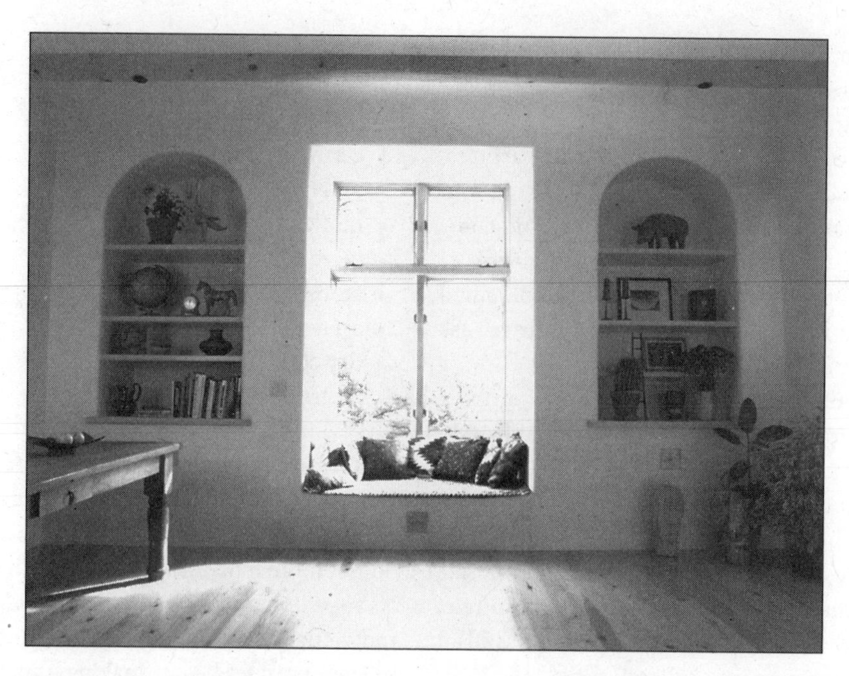

Plastered walls, recycled wood flooring over radiant floor heating and specialty finishes are used in this straw bale home in New Mexico. Interior view shows deep window seat in the country kitchen. Architect: Baker-Laporte and Associates; Builder: Prull and Associates; Photo: Julie Dean.

Indoor combustion is found in fireplaces; woodstoves; gas-fired appliances such as ranges, clothes dryers, and water heaters; furnaces; gas- and kerosene-fired space heaters; and oil and kerosene lamps. Some of the potentially harmful emissions include nitrogen dioxide, nitrous oxide, sulfur oxides, hydrogen cyanide, carbon monoxide, carbon dioxide, formaldehyde, particulate matter, and hydrocarbons from natural gas fumes such as butane, propane, pentane, methyl pentane, benzene, and xylene. The indoor levels of these pollutants are determined by the amount of fuel burned and the rate of exchange with outdoor air.

What are some of the potential health effects of combustion byproduct gases? In a study of 47,000 chemically sensitive patients, the most important sources of indoor air pollution responsible for generating illness were the gas stove, the improperly vented hot water heater, and the furnace.[2] Hazardous fumes can leak at the pipe joints and remain undetected, especially if they occur under flooring. In addition, every pilot light adds fumes, and the burning process itself releases fumes into the air. The primary effects of exposure to gas fumes are on the cardiovascular and nervous systems, but they can affect any organ of the body. Some of the earliest symptoms from exposure to gas fumes include depression, fatigue, irritability, and inability to concentrate.

Carbon monoxide is commonly produced during incomplete combustion, especially from gas-fueled appliances. Carbon monoxide quickly diffuses throughout the entire house. Typically, these appliances must be removed from the homes of chemically sensitive patients to restore their health. Chronic exposure can result in multiple chemical sensitivities because carbon monoxide has the ability to interfere with the detoxification pathways in the liver, allowing the accumulation of toxic substances. Other effects of chronic carbon monoxide exposure include heart arrhythmia, decreased cognitive abilities, confusion, and fatigue.

Carbon dioxide is produced from burning natural gas. Elevated levels result in decreased mental acuity, loss of vigor, and fatigue. Nitrogen oxides are also released from gas appliances. A major source of contamination is the gas stove, particularly older models with pilot lights. These gases are known to impact the nervous and reproductive systems.

Coal, gas, and woodburning fireplaces that are not equipped with sealed doors emit particulate matter as well as toxic fumes. They also consume indoor oxygen unless fresh outdoor air is supplied to them. Particles not expelled by blowing or sneezing can find their way into the lungs, where they can remain for years.

It is important to mention that when an automobile is parked or operated in an attached garage, gas, oil, and other volatile organic compounds diffuse into the structure and will affect air quality in the home. Garages therefore must be properly isolated from the main structure.

Well-ventilated and well-sealed sources of combustion can be operated with very little degradation of the indoor air. However, even sources of minimal exposure must often be removed from the homes of chemically sensitive patients to restore their health.

Pesticides

Although some pesticides may technically be considered VOCs, these often odorless and invisible substances have become such a health threat that they warrant a separate discussion. Pesticides, or biocides, are poisons designed to kill a variety of plants and animals such as insects (insecticides), weeds (herbicides), mold (mildewcides), and fungus (fungicides). They were first developed as offshoots of nerve gas used during World War II. Most pesticides are synthetic chemicals made from petroleum. They are composed of active ingredients — the chemical compounds designed to kill the target organism — and inert ingredients — chemicals that deliver the active ingredients to the target, preserve them, or make them easier to apply.

Many people believe that the pesticides they buy, or those used by lawn and pest control companies, are "safe." They assume that the government is protecting them; that pesticides are scientifically tested; that if used according to the instructions on the label they will do no harm; and that the products would not be on the market if they were unsafe. All of these assumptions are incorrect.

EPA registration does not signify pesticide safety.[3] The EPA approves pesticides based on efficacy, not safety. Efficacy means the pesticide will kill the targeted pest. Out of the hundreds of active ingredients registered with the EPA, fewer than a dozen have been adequately tested for safety.[4] In fact, it is a violation of federal law to state or imply that the use of a pesticide is "safe when used as directed." When the

CASE STUDY 1

Acute Exposure to Pesticides with Long-Term Consequences

Louise Pape's life changed drastically in 1993. On a warm spring day, she and her husband were slowly driving home with the windows rolled down to enjoy the cool breeze. At the roadside she spotted a man from a tree care company wearing a gas mask and spraying pesticides on the trees with a large hose. Louise suddenly felt a shower of chemicals on her face, in her eyes, nose, and mouth, as the sprayer overshot his target. She later learned that the pesticide was a mixture of malathion and carbaryl (Sevin).

That incident was the beginning of a nightmare illness for Louise, an environmental planner who, ironically, had just finished developing a safe pesticide plan for her employer, a transnational corporation. She was disabled for several months with flu-like symptoms, aching joints and muscles, severe headaches, dizziness, thyroid problems, insomnia, and shortness of breath. She was often bedridden and sometimes lapsed into a near comatose state upon reexposure to even minute amounts of pesticides. Louise eventually developed full-blown multiple chemical sensitivity disorder. For four years, she was virtually homebound, still unable to tolerate the trace amounts of pesticide and other chemical exposures that occur during routine activities out in the world. Despite her illness, Louise and her husband have become articulate spokespersons in educating the public about the hazards of pesticides and other chemicals. The ranch home they built in 1995 has become a model for nontoxic living.

Discussion

Many of the most harmful pesticides fall into three categories: organochlorines, organophosphates, and carbamates. In the above case, the onset of illness was associated with a single large exposure to an organophosphate and carbamate mixture. The cause of the prolonged illness was obvious. In most cases, however, the cause is not so obvious. Many people are exposed to repeated low-dose applications of pesticides, which can result in general malaise with flu-like symptoms, chronic fatigue, and subtle neurological deficits. When patients complain of such symptoms to their doctors, they are rarely questioned about exposures to pesticides or other chemicals. Most emergency room doctors are familiar with acute pesticide poisoning, but few physicians have knowledge of the long-term, chronic effects of pesticide exposure.

EPA, in the face of overwhelming evidence of negative human health effects, does decide to ban a pesticide, the process is slow and fraught with compromise. For example, on June 8, 2000 the EPA agreed to phase out home and garden uses of chlorpyrifos,[5] a known neurotoxin that is the active ingredient in Dursban and Lorsban. Between 1991 and 1996, more than 17,000 cases of unintentional chlorpyrifos exposure were reported to poison control centers. Although less toxic and nontoxic alternatives are available for all chlorpyrifos applications, more than 11 million pounds of the ingredient were being applied annually. The phase out allowed:

- home and garden use sales to continue through December 31, 2001
- existing stock to be sold in retail outlets until depleted
- continued use on food crops (except to-

CASE STUDY 2

Chronic Illness from "Harmless" Pesticide

Barbara Adler was in good health until March 1996, when she experienced the sudden onset of severe migraine headaches, loss of energy, frequent dizzy spells, and difficulty concentrating. She consulted with a neurologist and many other health care practitioners over the ensuing months, but none was able to help relieve her symptoms or shed light on the cause of her deteriorating health.

At some point in her search for wellness, she reviewed the journal she had been keeping in which she recorded significant events in her life. She noted that, around the time of the onset of her symptoms, her husband had purchased a bug spray from one of the local nurseries. He was told that the insecticide would be appropriate for the bugs on his houseplants. Barbara remembers that the bug spray smelled noxious to her, and she put some of the sprayed plants in the garage. She looked at the label on the bottle and saw that it contained Diazinon, a potent organophosphate known to have toxic effects on the nervous system. Barbara returned to the nursery to register a complaint and was told that Diazinon was not harmful.

Discussion

Although it is illegal for manufacturers to claim their pesticides are "safe," Dr. Elliott notes that in her experience local nurseries and other establishments selling pesticides frequently tell customers that organophosphates such as Sevin, Dursban, and Diazinon are harmless when applied according to instructions. In fact, many people with multiple chemical sensitivity disorder attribute the onset of their illness to pesticide exposure. While the patient in the above case became ill after an acute exposure to which she reacted immediately, the majority of cases occur when repeated, low-level exposures cause a gradual decline in health and vitality.

matoes), on golf courses, and for mosquito and fire ant control
- continued spot and local use for termite control until December 31, 2002
- use in new home pretreatment until December 31, 2005
- unrestricted export

Inert ingredients, which can account for up to 99 percent of a pesticide, are not usually identified on the label. The Trade Secrets Act protects manufacturers from being required to fully disclose them even if the ingredients are potentially hazardous to human health. No studies of any kind are required on the inert ingredients. Many inert ingredients can be more toxic than the active ingredients, yet warning labels apply only to active ingredients. In a Freedom of Information Act lawsuit, the Northwest Coalition for Alternatives to Pesticides (NCAP) obtained from the EPA a list of 1,400 of the 2,000 substances being used as inert ingredients in pesticides. These ingredients included Chicago sludge and other hazardous waste, asbestos, and some banned chemicals such as DDT.[6]

A recent study found that combining pesticides can make them up to 1,600 times more potent.[7] A good illustration of this synergy is found in a class of pesticides called

Pesticide Facts

- A National Cancer Institute study indicated that the likelihood of a child contracting leukemia was more than six times greater in households where herbicides were used for lawn care.[9]
- According to a report in the *American Journal of Epidemiology,* more children with brain tumors and other cancers were found to have had exposure to insecticides than children without cancer.[10]
- According to the New York State Attorney General's office, 95 percent of the pesticides used on residential lawns are considered probable carcinogens by the EPA.[11]
- 2,4-D was a component of Agent Orange and is used in about 1,500 lawn care products.[12]
- Pesticides have been linked to the alarming rise in the rate of breast cancer.[13]
- Besides causing cancer, pesticides have the potential to cause infertility, birth defects, learning disorders, neurological disorders, allergies, multiple chemical sensitivities, and other disorders of the immune system.

pyrethroids, which are mistakenly thought to be harmless because they are plant-derived. The unlabeled inert ingredient commonly mixed with the pyrethroids is PBO (piperonyl butoxide). Alone, each substance has limited toxicity to insect species; when they are combined, the mixture is extremely effective. PBO potentiates the pyrethroid by destroying one of the enzymes in the detoxification pathway that deactivates the pesticide in the insect. Humans exposed to this mixture suffer impaired ability of the liver to metabolize toxins in the environment.

Biocides can be absorbed through the skin, inhaled, or swallowed. Many building products and household furnishings such as carpets, paints, and wood products are treated with biocides. Infants and small children are more likely to be harmed by biocides because their developing organs and nervous systems are more easily damaged and because they are more likely to come into direct contact with treated carpets and lawns.

Pesticides can drift a long distance from the site of application, leaving residues throughout the surrounding community. Pesticides contaminate everything and everyone they contact. Residues are found in rain, fog, snow, food, water, livestock, wildlife, newborn babies, and even in the Arctic ice pack. People and pets may track pesticide residues into the house. An EPA study in Florida found the highest household pesticide residues in carpet dust.[8]

Pesticides may cause both acute and chronic health effects. Acute health effects appear shortly after exposure. Chronic health effects may not be apparent until months or years later. Chronic effects generally result from long-term exposure to low levels of toxic chemicals but may also arise from short-term exposure. A tragic misconception about pesticides is that the potential for harm is primarily the result of acute or immediate poisoning. In fact, delayed effects pose the greatest problems to human health. Many pesticides are fat soluble and bioaccumulate in tissues, where they can exert prolonged effects on the immune, endocrine, and nervous systems.

When building or remodeling a healthy home, you can lower your pesticide exposure by not treating the soil under the building and by eliminating or sealing standard building products that contain biocides. Division

CASE STUDY 3

Chronic Illness from Repeated Low-Level Pesticide Exposure

E. Merriam is a 59-year-old woman who complained of frequent flu-like symptoms after beginning employment at a new location. Symptoms seemed to recur every month and were especially severe over the winter. Conventional medications were of no benefit. After two years of watching her health decline, she discovered that the building in which she worked was being treated prophylactically one weekend a month with a pesticide that contained an organophosphate called Dursban. Associating her flu-like symptoms with the monthly pesticide applications, she felt she could no longer continue to jeopardize her health and left her job. Three years later, she finally regained her health but she remains sensitive to petrochemicals.

Discussion

In December 2001, the EPA partially banned the organophosphate Dursban for indoor use because of overwhelming evidence of harm to humans and wildlife. But, in spite of its acknowledged extreme toxicity, it can legally be used until stockpiles run out. Outdoor use, including agricultural applications, is still permitted.

Chlorpyrifos is the active ingredient in many pesticide products, including Dursban. Organophosphates are known to be neurotoxic and can cause damage to the brain and central nervous system, resulting in learning, memory, and behavior problems. They can also damage the immune system, increasing the risk of severe allergies, chemical sensitivities, and cancer.

10 includes a discussion of pest management that emphasizes preventing pest invasions through the use of physical barriers and the control of moisture, which eliminates potential food sources.

Electromagnetic Fields

Electromagnetic energy is ubiquitous. Some electromagnetic waves, such as sunlight, are natural. Other fields, such as radio and television waves, microwaves, and power line frequencies, are generated by human activity. Scientists classify electromagnetic waves according to frequency, which corresponds to the wavelength. At one end of the spectrum are the infinitesimally short, high-frequency gamma rays. At the other end are long, extremely low-frequency vibrating waves that may stretch for thousands of miles and are used by submarines for underwater communication.

The magnetic field that envelops the Earth produces a steady, nonoscillating direct current at 7.83 cycles per second, or 7.83 hertz, similar to that of the human body. This current pulsates on and off, but the electrons producing the electricity always move in a single direction. Each cell in the body has a pulsating vibration with an associated electromagnetic field (EMF). Communication between cells in the body is a function of electrical charges. These charges generate electrical currents that govern many of the body's major functions, such as heartbeat, nerve conduction, and transport across cell membranes. These natural fields pulse on and off but do not oscillate.

Manufactured fields oscillate back and forth. Unlike natural current, the electrons

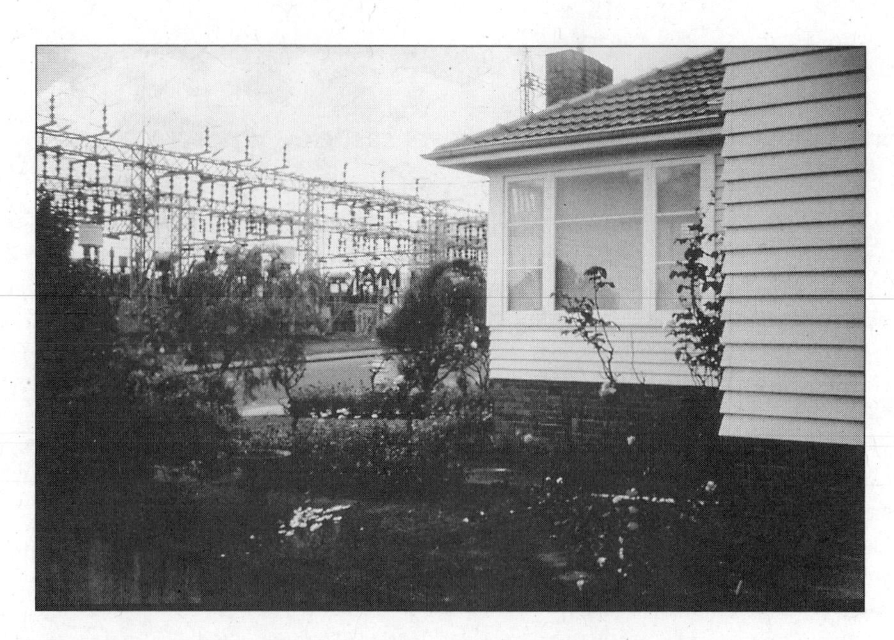

A poor choice for a home site in an area of elevated electromagnetic fields.
Photo: Reinhart, Kanuka, Fuchs.

creating the fields change direction and thus are called alternating current (AC). The electrical power grid operates at 60 hertz and simultaneously produces an electric and a magnetic field. Each field has distinct properties and is measured separately using different meters. Common sources of 60 hertz electromagnetic fields include power lines, electrical wires, electric blankets, fluorescent lights, televisions, and other household appliances.

Radio waves are a form of electromagnetic field. On a typical radio receiver set you will find a dial, known as a frequency tuner, used to change stations. As you move the dial to the higher numbers, you are increasing the frequency of the radio electromagnetic field you are seeking; when you move the dial to lower numbers, you are reducing the frequency. AM radio stations are found between 550 and 1600 kilohertz (550,000 and 1,600,000 hertz). If the radio could be tuned all the way down the dial to 60 hertz, you would be listening to the (very noisy) sound of electrical equipment.

There are major differences between radio waves and the electrical waves used to power equipment. One difference is that radio waves are broadcast through the air; they are wireless and can travel for extended distances. Electricity, on the other hand, is transported through wires. It would be ideal if the fields from wiring systems stayed in the wires while the electricity is transported from one place to another. The problem is that wires "leak." They broadcast electromagnetic fields, with the distance dependent on amperage. Amperage is analogous to the volume at which electric fields are being transmitted through the wires.

Assume that a radio receiver could be tuned to radio stations operating between 40 and 80 hertz. As mentioned previously, if you were to tune the dial to 60 hertz, you would hear a lot of noise because electricity in the United States operates at 60 hertz. Next, assume that you take the same radio receiver to Europe. Upon tuning the radio to 60 hertz, you would hear nothing because the European power system operates at 50 hertz.

To experiment with the sound of electricity, take a cheap AM transistor radio and tune it between stations at the low end of the dial. By holding the radio near an operating electrical appliance or a dimmer switch, you will pick up static. The buzzing noise you hear is not the 60 hertz frequency but rather higher frequency interference created by the 60 hertz frequency. Before meters for measuring elevated electromagnetic fields were readily available, some people would use an AM radio to obtain a rough idea of whether an area contained elevated manufactured electromagnetic fields. The method is far from foolproof, but it was certainly better than nothing. Several models of inexpensive meters are available today that provide more accurate assessments.

Many scientists agree that electromagnetic fields have biological effects, but they disagree on the exact effects and whether they are harmful. Research has indicated that magnetic fields can induce a small electrical field inside the body, which in turn creates an electric current in and around the cells.[14] This current has been thought to alter the function of cell chemistry and to inhibit or enhance cell growth. Although there is no consistent dose/response relationship between magnetic fields and cancer, experiments on laboratory animals have shown that magnetic fields cause changes in protein synthesis and hormone levels.

Studies in Europe have indicated that exposure to varying levels of electric fields can contribute to nervous disorders such as insomnia, depression, and anxiety. One US study found an increase in aggressive behavior among baboons exposed to electric fields.[15] Other studies have indicated that there may be a synergistic influence between magnetic and electric field exposures, making the combination more harmful than exposure to either field alone.

Over the past 50 years, people have been exposed to ever increasing amounts of manufactured radiation. The long-term consequences of this exposure are not clearly understood. Millions of Americans are now unwittingly engaged in long-term experiments on themselves. Whereas Sweden and Switzerland have set national limits for certain types of electric and magnetic field exposure, the US government has not. From time to time our government has officially recommended "prudent avoidance" (without defining the levels it would be prudent to avoid). Yet epidemiological studies have linked elevated child leukemia risks to exposures as low as 4 milligauss.[16] Given the potentially dangerous (albeit controversial) consequences of EMF exposures, coupled with the ease of reducing these exposures in new construction, it may make sense to explore strategies for EMF reduction when planning and building a new home. Several simple and inexpensive measures to reduce EMF exposures are explained in Division 11 (in the sections on appliances and electric and magnetic fields) and in Division 16.

Curiously, the magnetic portion of the electromagnetic field is indirectly prohibited by the National Electrical Code. The code specifically prohibits net current, or current that is uncanceled, because it creates heat and is a potential fire hazard. Net current is also what creates magnetic fields, although most electricians are not aware of this. When magnetic fields are found in wiring, this usually is the result of a wiring error that violates code. Preventing magnetic fields caused by wiring is simply a matter of introducing protocol on the jobsite that ensures a building has been wired to code.

Naturally Occurring Pollutants

Not all toxins are manufactured. Some naturally occurring substances in homes can have harmful effects on humans. Some of these pollutants include radon and radioactive contaminants, trace metals, house dust, molds, and pollens.

Radioactive Contaminants

Radioactive contaminants such as radium and uranium occur naturally within the Earth's crust. During the decay or breakdown of uranium, radon is produced. Radon is an invisible, odorless radioactive gas that seeps from the ground into homes, commonly through cracks in the foundation or basement slab or through mechanical openings. Radon can also enter the groundwater and affect water supplies.

Closed spaces present a hazard because radon levels can build up to values thousands of times higher than outdoor levels. High radon levels can cause radiation exposure equivalent to thousands of chest x-rays per person on an annual basis. Information on detecting and preventing radon contamination in homes is provided in Division 7.

Heavy Metals

Heavy metals are natural components of the Earth's crust. They cannot be degraded or destroyed. Heavy metals are trace elements with a density at least five times that of water. Living organisms require trace amounts of some heavy metals, including iron, copper, manganese, molybdenum, and zinc, but even these beneficial trace minerals can cause toxic reactions in excessive amounts.

Other heavy metals, such as mercury, lead, aluminum, and cadmium, have no known beneficial effect on living organisms, and their accumulation over time can cause serious illnesses. Each metal targets different areas of the body. An area commonly affected is the brain and nervous system, resulting in learning, behavior, and memory problems, mood disorders, tremors, and early dementia. But any organ of the body can be targeted and symptoms can be as wide ranging as high blood pressure, anemia, rashes, and cancer.

Heavy metals are present in the air, food, water, and countless human-made chemicals and products.

Heavy metals in trace amounts can often be found in drinking water. Metals such as aluminum, copper, and lead can accumulate over time in human tissues and are known to cause damage to the brain, liver, and kidneys. Having drinking water tested for contaminants is advisable in order to determine if a water purification device will be necessary. Refer to Division 11 for further information.

Other sources of heavy-metal exposure in the indoor environment include insecticides and herbicides, fungicides and rat poison (arsenic and cadmium), cigarette smoke, paint pigments (cadmium and lead), contaminated air and soil around the home, dust particles, cookware (aluminum), pipes (lead and copper), and flame retardants (antimony).

Biological Pollutants

Biological pollutants include pollen, house dust, and mold spores. Pollens from weeds, grasses, flowers, bushes, and trees enter the house through the doors and windows. They can be problematic for people with allergies. Air filtration methods are addressed in Division 15.

House dust is composed of much more than simply soil. It is a complex mixture of dust mites, animal dander, mold spores, textile particles, heavy metals from car exhaust, skin cells, and more. Mites are a major culprit in causing allergies from house dust. They feed on skin cells and breed in mattresses, pillows, carpets, and upholstered furniture. Although generally harmless, their skeletal parts and fecal matter, which stick to dust, can elicit allergic reactions in sensitive people. Dust mites require humidity ranges greater than 50 percent to thrive.

Mold plays a significant role in triggering allergies, asthma, and chemical sensitivities. Mold can produce byproducts as toxic as some of the most hazardous manufactured chemicals that affect the nervous and immune systems. Though commonly assumed

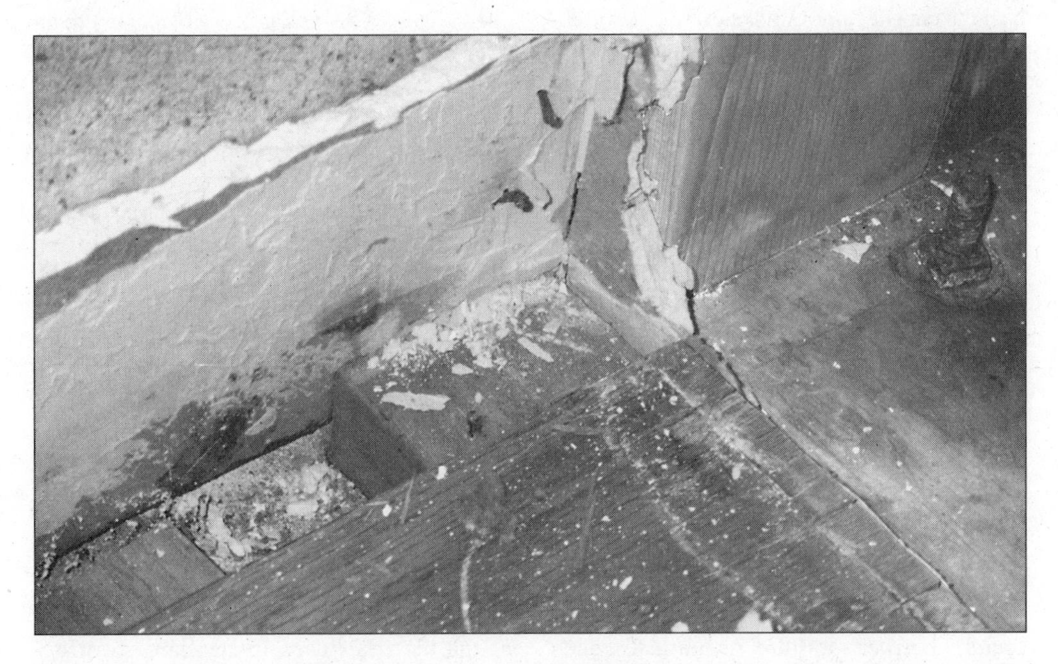

The Problem: Gypsum board was glued directly to concrete block below floor level. Ground moisture passing through the block wall and condensation has resulted in mold growth on the gypsum board. Recommendation: Proper drainage design would have prevented moisture movement through the wall. Gypsum board is particularly vulnerable to mold growth when damp. If the block had been furred out prior to installation of gypboard then there would have been more opportunity for drying to occur.
Photo: Restoration Consultants.

CASE STUDY 4

Chronic Illness from Acute Exposure to Virulent Mold Species

In 1993 when Tomasita Gallegos was 37 years old she first consulted Dr. Elliott. At that time she was frightened, in a state of severe agitation, and somewhat disoriented. Her face was bright red; her mouth showed increased salivation; her eyes were watery with constricted pupils; and her skin was warm to the touch. She was referred to Dr. Elliott by another physician, who felt she might have experienced a pesticide exposure.

Ms. Gallegos was employed as a housekeeper in a private home. The morning of the day she became ill, she was instructed to clean the guest house, which had been recently occupied. Shortly after the patient entered the guest house, she became acutely ill with the above-mentioned symptoms. After the acute symptoms subsided, she was left with multiple problems, including chronic fatigue, panic attacks, chest pains, headaches, memory loss, and extreme chemical sensitivity. Her constellation of symptoms was baffling since it was determined that no harmful chemicals had been used on the premises.

An environmental engineering company was consulted to evaluate the guest house. Upon removing the furnace and cooling coils to allow access for a thorough cleaning of the ductwork system, the consultant found approximately two inches of water with green slime at the bottom of the supply plenum. Because the area was dark and cool and in the direct airstream of the house ductwork, the spread of microorganisms was very likely. Close inspection revealed that a defective humidification system was the source of the leaking water. Most of the microbial agents were fungi that, although found widely in nature, were highly concentrated in the interior environment. Many fungi produce toxic compounds called mycotoxins. The intense microbial exposure had the effect of sensitizing the patient, leaving her with an overreactive immune system, commonly known as environmental illness. At present, with diligent avoidance of molds, toxic chemicals, and allergens, Ms. Gallegos is slowly beginning to regain her health.

Discussion

Why was this patient so severely affected from such a brief exposure? The type of mold was a particularly virulent species. In addition, some individuals are more susceptible to fungal contaminants than others. If the detoxification pathway in the liver is already at maximum capacity, it might take only a relatively small exposure to overwhelm the system. This theory is called the rain barrel effect and refers to total toxic load. When more toxins enter the "barrel" than the body can excrete, the barrel overflows and symptoms develop.

to be found only in older homes, mold can be found wherever moisture accumulates, such as basements, bathrooms, windowsills, laundry rooms, or wherever leaks and flooding occur. Moist building materials, including new materials, can become breeding grounds for mold and bacteria within a few days. Many of the materials used in standard construction of new homes are susceptible to water damage and fungal growth. A moldy home is frequently a sign of a home with deteriorating building materials. Even when molds are

CASE STUDY 5

Asthma Related to Mold Exposure

When Dori Bennett was 46 she consulted with Dr. Elliott for the sudden onset of severe asthma. She had apparently been in good health until she moved into a new home. A leak in the home was repaired prior to the move, and the house had passed inspection. After her asthma progressed to the point of requiring hospitalization, it was suspected that the source of her problem was in her home. An environmental consulting firm noted heavy growth of mold in the crawl space. Molds found included *Aspergillus, Actinomycetes, Bacillus, Cladosporium, Fusarium, Mucor, Penicillium, Phoma,* and *Ulocladium.* Several strains of virulent molds, some of which are known to cause asthma, pneumonia, hypersensitivity pneumonitis, and immune dysfunction, grew on culture plates.

Her family hired an environmental cleanup crew to rid the house of the mold in order to prepare it for resale. An outdoor unit was constructed to house a large heater fan to blow air under the house, while a unit on the opposite side of the house removed moisture-laden air. It took six weeks to dry out the earth under the house. A detailed mold remediation of the house and contents followed. The cost of the cleanup was $40,000. When further testing showed that the house was fully remediated, it was sold. Ms. Bennett now lives in a home free of mold growth and her health is slowly improving.

Discussion

Mold and mycotoxin exposure can affect any organ in the body, including the respiratory, nervous, and immune systems. Homeowners, building managers, and health care professionals need to be much more aware of this potential problem.

contained inside walls or other building cavities such as attics and crawl spaces, the slightest air current can send spores swirling through the air, where they can be easily inhaled.

Carpets act as large reservoirs for dust, bacteria, and mold. Microbes commonly grow within the ductwork of forced-air heating systems, which can spread mold and dust throughout the house. Unless kept spotlessly clean, toilets and many modern appliances that use water reservoirs, such as vaporizers and humidifiers, can breed microbes. Methods for preventing and controlling mold infestation are discussed throughout the specifications.

Strategies for Creating a Healthy Home

The use of toxic substances in construction is standard. Furthermore, certain prevalent construction practices lead to destructive moisture conditions, pest invasions, or unsafe combustion, all of which can cause even the most chemically inert home to become unhealthy over time. The occupants too will greatly influence the longevity and healthfulness of any home through the day-to-day interaction they have with it.

We have organized the information in Part II of this book to correspond to the standard 16-division format commonly used by residential contractors. In Part II we will explain the many instances, some obvious and others less so, where undesirable materials and practices may be found in standard construction. Healthier options for materials are listed and quality control measures for the construction phase are specified. Following is a brief overview of the strategies behind the specifications found in Part II of this book. These five strategies are:

- Designing for health
- Employing a climate-based understanding for construction detailing
- Reducing toxic emissions through choice of building materials
- Introducing quality control measures during construction
- Providing for an ongoing healthy home environment through occupant education

Designing for Health

Although all homes should be designed to support health, healthy housing is unfortunately considered to be a specialized field of residential design. There are basic design features that should be included in all homes, but they are often overlooked. These features, essential to our health, safety, and sense of well-being, include:

Something in My Home is Making Me Sick: General Testing Protocols

WILL SPATES

The process of performing a building inspection to address a client's concerns is much more than taking instrument readings and reporting on the findings. A good building inspector should be part building scientist, part investigative journalist, part psychologist, and part building contractor. A nickname for the home inspector is "house doctor," which makes sense since the process of diagnosing and curing a sick home has many parallels to diagnosing and curing an ailing person.

The homeowner perceives a need and contacts the inspector to help address it. The building inspector's job is to understand how a building is affecting the client or how environmental conditions are affecting the building. It is critical to ask the right questions. There is a pollutant affecting the client or the building; this pollutant has a reservoir within the building or an adjacent area of influence; and there is a pathway and a driving force allowing the pollutant to come in contact with the person or building. This is true for everything from electromagnetic fields to moisture and mold to pesticides, a whole range of building pollutants that can be investigated and measured if one has the necessary tools and skills to make this invisible world visible.

Typically your first contact with the inspector will be a phone interview during which you explain in detail the history of your home, any changes you have made to it, and any changes you have observed in its feel, smell, and appearance over time. A seasoned inspector, like a doctor, will be able to take a good case history, ask you the right questions, and offer insights based on your experience and your concerns. This interview is critical to laying the foundation for the inspection. Has remodeling, a recent pesticide application, or the installation of a new wireless phone or internet

Design for Responsiveness to the Natural Climate

In all but the most hostile environments, a home that is designed to be responsive to its surroundings will provide a wide range of opportunities for its residents to reap the health benefits of nature while reducing dependency on energy-consuming mechanical space conditioning.

- Good window design can greatly reduce dependence on mechanical heating and cooling. Placing windows to prevent overheating and to facilitate cross ventilation and solar gain when needed can result in both energy savings and a higher level of comfort. Proper window placement, the right type of window design, and glass coating, used in conjunction with overhangs and trellises, can contribute to a successful home design.
- Proper room layout and window placement can also provide good natural lighting and a sense of well-being while reducing dependence on electrical lighting.
- Screened porches, overhangs, trellises, and patios can provide opportunities for extended outdoor living while acting as climatic buffer zones around the home.
- A paved entry path, covered entry porch, and foyer will reduce the amount of tracked-in dirt and provide a convenient place for shoe removal or cleaning, resulting in a cleaner home.
- An extension of the design process to

service occurred? All these conditions and more can affect sensitive individuals.

Even the most obscure building symptoms can be reduced by improving the environment.

An inspector is trained to treat buildings, not diagnose people, but improvements in the environment often lead to the improved well-being of a building's occupants. Many autoimmune-type diseases find their beginnings in a sensitizing event. The focus of the inspector's investigation will be attempting to discover the onset of this event and, based on the inspection and test results, recommending a means to minimize your exposure to whatever has made you ill and/or is making your building deteriorate.

Nature is the measuring stick for a Building Biologist's inspection. The baseline for elevated levels will be the natural surroundings. The interior of your home should have lower levels of dust, particulate matter, and mold than the surrounding outdoors. Your electromagnetic fields, especially in your sleeping area, should be minimal. During the course of the investigation the inspector may uncover other conditions of which you had no previous awareness but that can affect your health.

In my work as an inspector, my intention is to understand what is happening in the home or office and be able to present this information to my client in a supportive way. In other words, I cultivate a good "bedside manner." This is a critical aspect of the client/inspector relationship. The last thing I want is for the information I present to overwhelm my client or leave them feeling that conditions are outside their control. Remember, there is a natural or least toxic alternative to all our building challenges. Little changes built up over time can lead to big improvements. You can start by simply removing all the plug-in air fresheners and

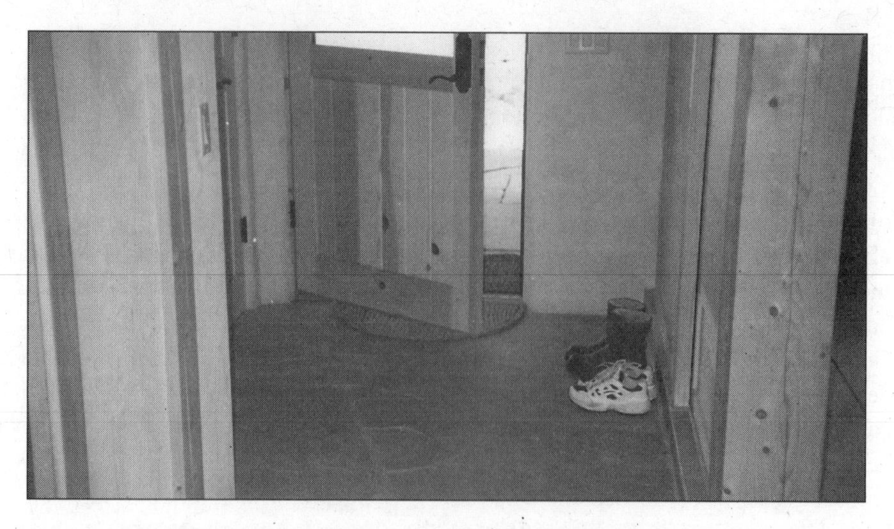

This entryway is designed for "tracking off" dirt and for shoe removal. It features a covered paved entry way and a sunken vestibule with easily mopped stone floors, that effectively keeps outside mud and dirt from finding its way into the home.
Photo: Paula Baker-Laporte.

installing pleated filters on the air conditioning system or letting more fresh air into your home.

After the client interview and building history, it is time to begin the physical investigation. The inspector will have formed a hypothesis of what is occurring within the building and will attempt to prove or disprove this hypothesis by taking the appropriate measurements with the appropriate instruments and testing devices. A typical baseline investigation targets a building's systems and measures the operational conditions for a number of parameters, depending on the focus. Just as the doctor will take your vital signs during a general checkup, the building inspector will begin the general investigation with measurements for temperature, humidity, moisture content, mold, airborne particulates, air exchange, chemical components, and electromagnetic fields, the building's "vital signs." Further testing can be expensive and is indicated only when the building inspector has cause for concern based on the results of the case history and initial inspection.

A Building Biology inspector will use Building Biology standards, which are based closely on a natural and healthy environment. Deviations from these standards indicate a departure from a healthy environment. The farther we progress away from a natural baseline, the unhealthier a building becomes. Building health is a measurable phenomenon when your inspector has the skills and tools.

Making positive changes to unhealthy building conditions will result in an improvement and a move toward the goal of a healthy building. Reductions in moisture intrusion will result in a drier building and prevent damage to building materials and also possible mold growth. Improvements in the temperature and humidity performance

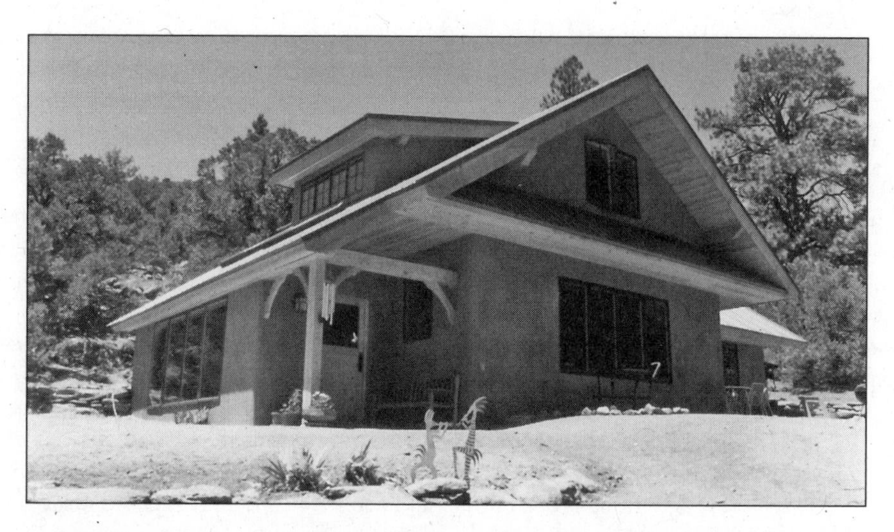

Deep roof overhangs and a covered entry help protect the natural wall elements of this straw-clay timber frame home. Architect: Paula Baker-Laporte; Builder: Econest Building Co. Photo: Paula Baker-Laporte.

and filtration of an air conditioning system can be the difference needed to prevent a proliferation of dust mites (a prime allergen for asthmatics). Eliminating chemical pesticides and using commonsense natural pest control in their place will reduce exposure to neurotoxins that challenge immune systems. In short, Building Biologists are looking for ways to make buildings as healthy as possible. Build tight, ventilate right, and make conscious decisions about the materials you bring into your home. This is the house doctor's equivalent of "eat right and get plenty of exercise and good rest."

Maintaining a healthy home, like maintaining a healthy body, requires preventive "medicine." It is the homeowner's job to become knowledgeable about and perform the necessary maintenance for the systems that keep the home healthy. This includes regular mechanical system maintenance, regular home cleaning with a good HEPA vacuum, periodic changing of water and air filters, and minimizing exposure to electromagnetic fields and chemicals through prudent avoidance.

Will Spates has been practicing Building Biology for over 15 years and has been involved in the design, construction, and maintenance of environmental systems for over 30 years. He is the founder and president of Indoor Environmental Technologies, a testing and consulting firm that has performed over 4,000 inspections. He can be reached at wspates@IETbuildinghealth.com and at IETbuildinghealth.com.

CASE STUDY 6

The Relationship Between Allergies and Chemical Exposure

In the 1950s it was estimated that about 14 percent of the population suffered from allergies. According to some estimates, this proportion at present is estimated at between 40 and 75 percent. Why the dramatic increase? Allergists in Japan pondered the same question. A hypothesis was put forth that certain chemicals act as sensitizing agents. To test the hypothesis, two groups of mice were exposed to high levels of the Japanese equivalent of juniper pollen, and then tested for an allergic response. In both the study and the control groups about 5 percent of the mice developed allergies to the pollen. The study group was then exposed to benzene fumes from car exhaust. Upon retesting, there was a significant increase in the study group's allergic response to the pollen, while the control group remained at 5 percent.[a]

Discussion

Although there is clearly a link between chemical exposures and allergies, the exact mechanism has not yet been elucidated. Most people who have acquired multiple chemical sensitivities also suffer from traditional allergies to pollens, dust, dander, and mold. Benzene is only one of many pollutants known to damage the immune system. Since these chemicals are found in thousands of modern products for home and industrial use, millions of people are constantly exposed to low levels at home and at work.

a. M. Muranaka et al. "Adjutant Activity of Diesel Exhaust Particulates for the Production of IgE antibody in mice." *Journal of Allergy and Clinical Immunology.* Vol. 77 (April 1996), pp. 616-623.

include surrounding landscaping can incorporate vegetation to help shade, allow in sun, block harsh winds, or funnel helpful breezes. Edible vegetation can also double as an organic food source.

Design for Combustion Source Management and Safety

The introduction of harmful combustion byproducts into the home poses a serious health threat that can be entirely avoided through proper design and equipment specification. The measures we describe are neither code-required nor commonly found in standard construction.

- The mechanical room and mechanical equipment should be designed so that no exchange of air takes place between them and the living space.
- All gas appliances should be properly vented to the outside.
- The garage should be separated from the living space so that air exchange does not occur between the two.
- Any home with gas or other combustion appliances should be equipped with carbon monoxide monitors.
- A source of fresh air intake should be provided to make up for air consumed in combustion and air exhaust processes.

Design for Water Management

Many health problems begin when buildings become moldy. Throughout this book we

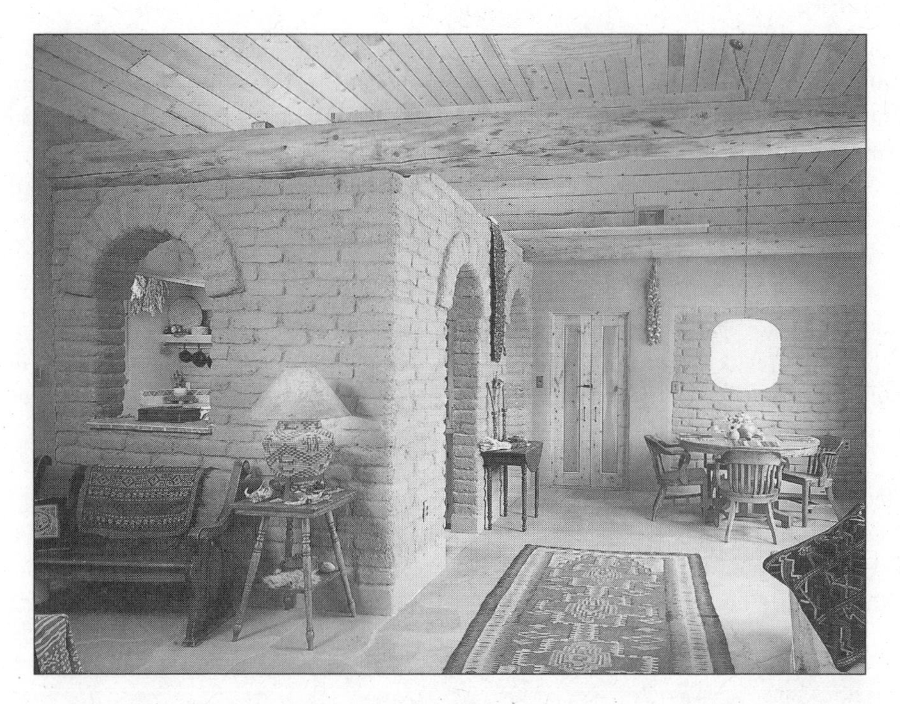

Adobe interior walls and stone flooring store heat in the winter and remain cool in the summer while the straw bale walls of this home (not shown) provide a high degree of insulation. These natural materials provide an energy efficient solution for the cold winters and hot summers of Northern New Mexico. Architect: Baker-Laporte and Associates; Builder: Living Structures; Photo: Eric Swanson.

suggest strategies for the proper control of water and water vapor. Moisture control begins with good design that includes:

- sufficient roof overhangs and protection over door and window openings that will help keep rain and melting snow away from the building and its penetrations
- a well-designed and detailed perimeter drainage system that will keep basements, crawl spaces, and floor slabs dry
- sufficient means for evacuating moisture generated from within the building by human activity
- placement of floor drains and detailing so that a water discharge resulting from equipment failure (and equipment often eventually fails!) will not have costly and health threatening consequences

Design for Durability and Serviceability

- A large part of home design involves issues of cost and quality. If the owner is informed about lifecycle costs and not just the initial costs of materials and systems, he or she will be much more likely to make choices favoring durable and easily maintained materials. For example, a tar-and-gravel roof is less expensive than a single-ply membrane roof, but the first roof may come with only a two-year warranty while the second one may have a ten-year warranty. The first roof will outgas for several weeks each time it is replaced and the home will become filled with carcinogenic tar fumes. The second roof may be a "torched down" application that causes little pollution when patched or replaced. If the owner plans to stay in the home for more than five years, the second roof, although more expensive initially, will in the long run be a healthier and more cost-effective choice.

- Every homeowner has specific needs that will affect the indoor environmental quality and should be fully considered in the design phase. For example, there may be a need for extra ventilation in hobby areas or a locked closet to keep inappropriate materials away from small children.
- Family sizes grow and shrink. As people age, they require greater ease of accessibility. Small children require constant surveillance. As children grow they require more autonomy. More and more people are choosing to work at home. A flexible design can more easily accommodate these lifestyle changes and allow a family to stay in the home as changes occur. A desire for stability can promote initial choices based on quality and longevity. Anyone who has ever moved can relate to the extreme stress caused by the process of relocation.

My Air Smells Bad! What Can I Do?

LARRY GUST

Identifying the cause of smelly indoor air can be a complex process. The English language is not a good tool for describing smells and there is often little agreement about what an odor smells like, making it difficult for a professional to identify the offending substance from a description of the smell. To make identification even more difficult, there are tens of thousands of synthetic compounds and thousands of naturally created compounds that produce odors. Complicating matters still further, many compounds in the air are broken down by the natural process of oxidation to form new compounds. The new material may smell when the old one did not, or the new material may smell completely different from the original. Identification can be simpler with more common odors such as mold, gasoline, natural gas, or alcohol.

There are sophisticated approaches and instruments for identifying the chemical composition of an odor. Once the chemical is identified, potential sources can then be determined and the building can be searched for these sources. However, this approach uses expensive equipment in a lab, costs hundreds of dollars per air sample, and may require multiple types of samples.

Luckily, most of us come equipped with an exquisitely sensitive instrument — the nose! The human nose is incredibly effective for tracking smells. The olfactory sensitivity of most people is at a part per million level. In other words, people can smell one part of the offending substance in a million parts of air. A few individuals can detect odors at a part per billion level, the level normally reserved for animals such as dogs. So tracking the odor back to its source can be done by using your nose.

Employing a Climate-Based Understanding for Construction Detailing

The building industry in the United States, a country with vast climatic variations, is primarily regulated by a handful of building codes. These codes do not sufficiently address the fact that in each climatic zone there are particular concerns about how moisture, temperature, wind, vegetation, and wildlife will impact the building envelope. Historically, regional building types throughout the world evolved over time as local materials were fashioned into a perfect response for the surrounding climatic conditions. Much of this indigenous wisdom has been cast aside in our lifetime. Residential building techniques have undergone sweeping experimentation since World War II. With the introduction of mass produced and transported building components and the increased dependence on mechanized heating and cooling, our homes are for the most part constructed in the same manner regardless of location. The need for energy conservation has led to tight, highly insulated envelope construction.

As a result of these factors, we have placed greater performance demands on the building envelope than ever before. A new suburban home in Cincinnati may look identical to one built in Los Angeles. In spite of vastly different climatic conditions, the two buildings will be mechanically equipped to provide the occupant with an interior temperature of 70 degrees Fahrenheit 24 hours a day, 365 days a year.

A word of caution: some strong chemical vapors can be a health threat. People who are already sensitive or allergic to smells should not be involved in this type of investigation. Other people should not continue tracking odors that become too strong to be comfortably tolerated. You should stop following solvent fumes, gasoline fumes, or natural gas odors when they become uncomfortably strong. If this happens, it would be a good idea to call for help and air the space out. Note that natural gas, propane, and other household fuel sources contain odorants to alert you if they are leaking. These gases are an explosion hazard, so if you suspect that a dangerous gas leak may be the cause of the odor, call for help immediately. The gas company will provide a free leak detection service.

If the entire house smells, it may be helpful to air it out first and then close it up again to see if the formerly pervasive smell can be detected closer to the point of origin. Because people experience what is called olfactory fatigue, becoming less and less sensitive to the smell with prolonged exposure, you may need to give your nose a rest from time to time.

Moldy smells are common. The source of these smells can sometimes be located by looking for places where water intrusion has dampened building materials, decorative items, or other household goods. Water intrusion can be located by looking for water stains on drywall, baseboard, carpets, or corrugated boxes stacked on a concrete floor. In homes built on a concrete slab, problems with water movement through the slab can cause mold growth in the carpet and pad, particularly along outside walls or under furniture with skirting that

However, the interaction between the climate and the building envelope in these cities will be very different. Professionals in the building industry are now discovering that certain assumptions made 30 years ago about how the new products would interact with climate and mechanized space conditioning were shortsighted. As a result, we are experiencing widespread envelope failure. To further complicate matters, similar buildings will fail in different ways in different climates. These failures affect not only the longevity of buildings but also their ability to support human health.

Architects, builders, and homeowners must become familiar with the localized conditions of the potential homesite. An inquiry into the kinds of problems that have developed in local buildings because of the natural environment would be beneficial. The local building lore can potentially be a rich source of information. Listed below are a few examples (by no means inclusive) of differing regional conditions and respective challenges:

- The air of coastal locations is typically characterized by high salt content, resulting in metal corrosion.
- Areas experiencing alternating freeze/thaw conditions will be subject to ice damming problems. Buildings will also be much more susceptible to deterioration caused by water seeping into cracks and then expanding as it turns to ice.
- Wood products exposed to the elements in southwestern deserts will suffer from accelerated drying due to extreme UV exposure and low humidity.
- Moisture and mold problems associated with condensation caused by air condi-

prevents air circulation. You may be able to smell this mold by getting close to the carpet.

Mold growth inside the walls that results from water intrusion can sometimes be located by removing the electrical wall outlet faceplates and smelling the air in the outlet boxes, particularly those mounted in the outside-facing walls. The smell from a moldy basement or crawl space will move upstairs because rising warm air exiting at the top of the house draws replacement air from the basement and through other holes in the building such as outlet and switch boxes and heating/air conditioning ducts. Also look for water leakage in cabinets under sinks. It is always prudent to call in a mold specialist in cases of suspected mold and I do not advise a homeowner to open wall cavities or baseboards. You can, however, lead the inspector to places where you have noticed moldy smells.

Less common but sometimes problematic are bacterial smells. An example is the odor of dirty socks, or locker-room odor. Wet building materials and fabrics in a home can create a problem with bacterial as well as mold growth.

Another approach to tracing an odor is to think about everything that happened prior to its detection. When did you first notice it? Did this coincide with something being brought into the house or a precipitating event? This might include one or more of the following:

- painting and decorating
- new clothing or household goods
- pest control treatments
- new furniture, carpeting, or drapes
- a change in cleaning products or housekeeping services
- new asphalt-type roofing, yours or neighbor's

tioning are typical in climates with high temperatures and humidity.

- Fire safety is a major concern in wooded areas.
- Nearly every region has specific insect and vermin problems.

Certain conditions unique to your building location will not be remedied or addressed by building codes, standard building practices, or materials manufacturers. Architects and builders must be jointly responsible for investigating specificities. To this end, we highly recommend the *Builder's Guides* by Joseph Lstiburek (see Further Reading at the end of this chapter).

Furthermore, there is undeniable evidence that global warming is changing our climate and increasing the incidence of extreme weather events. Building designs and practices that were once considered adequate for a given region may now need to be more stringent as the incidence of floods, hurricanes, tornados, ice damming, and other destructive events increases. For more information on measures to be taken to adapt to increased climatic impact, refer to John Banta's book *Extreme Weather Hits Home: Protecting Your Buildings from Climate Change* (see Further Reading).

Reducing Toxic Emissions Through Choice of Building Materials

As we explained previously, modern building techniques have created sick buildings in part by using building materials that outgas toxic emissions. It stands to reason that to create healthy buildings we must find ways to reduce

- significant rain, with or without high winds, causing building leakage
- house painting, yours or neighbor's
- lawn treatments, yours or neighbor's
- long periods of non-use for sinks, bathtubs, or showers, leading to drying of water in the drain trap
- spills or leaks that could enter your basement from nearby industries or gasoline stations
- septic tank wastewater system failure

The "house detective" process can be time consuming and lengthy, but you know your home better than anyone else. You can save time and money by giving the situation careful attention and thought before your professional arrives. If all else fails, you can call a specialist to help identify the source by collecting a sample of the offending air for lab identification of its chemical components. Good sniffing!

Larry Gust is a Building Biology Environmental Consultant (BBEC) certified by the International Institute for Building Biology & Ecology (building biology.net). He holds a degree in electrical engineering and is a Certified Mold Remediator through the Indoor Air Quality Association (iaqa .org) and a Certified Electromagnetic Radiation Safety Advisor through the Science and Public Policy Institute Safe Wireless Initiative. Since achieving the BBEC certification in 1992, he has been operating an indoor environmental consultancy covering all aspects of the built environment, including mold, chemical, and electromagnetic pollution (healbuildings.com). He lives in Southern California and practices nationwide.

the sources of pollution generated by these materials.

The following products and materials are common sources of indoor pollution in standard construction:

- insecticides, mildewcides, herbicides, and other biocides found in building materials or applied onsite
- composite wood products that are bound with formaldehyde-emitting glues, including particleboard, chipboard, plywood, and manufactured sheathing
- building products, finishes, cleaning products, and additives that emit harmful VOCs, including solvent-based paints, sealants, finishes, and adhesives
- asphalt and products containing asphalt, including impregnated sheathing, roofing tars, and asphalt driveways
- building materials containing mold
- materials that are absorbent, are hard to clean and maintain, and require frequent replacement (such as carpeting)

There are several strategies for reducing the chemical load introduced into a home. In order of effectiveness, these strategies are:

1. Eliminate sources of pollution.
2. Substitute healthier materials.
3. Exercise prudence when using unavoidable toxic substances.
4. Cure materials before they are installed within the building envelope.
5. Seal materials so that they outgas less.

Elimination

If all toxins could simply be eliminated from buildings, we would have the basis for an ideal environment. In many instances, this is not only possible but also cost-effective. For example, countertop materials can often be attached to cabinets with mechanical fasteners, thereby eliminating the need for toxic adhesives, and exposed woods may be left unsealed in locations where sealing is unnecessary.

Substitution

Where chemicals must be used, it is almost always possible to substitute a less toxic substance in place of a standard one. For example, paint with no harmful emissions, VOCs, or preservatives can be specified in substitution for a standard paint that contains harmful chemicals such as formaldehyde. Since the first writing of this book, awareness of and demand for healthier building materials have increased and there are many more healthy alternatives on the market to choose from.

Prudent Use

In a few cases, the use of a toxic substance is unavoidable. For example, there is no acceptable substitute for the solvent-based glues used to join plastic plumbing lines. However, the specifications outlined in this book provide guidelines for reducing the amount of exposure to these products.

Curing

In cases where toxic substances are chosen for reasons such as cost or durability, the impact of the product will be reduced if it is properly cured. For example, in the specifications we explain how to cure plywood before it is applied. Many materials can be purchased with factory-applied finishes that have been heat-cured. Such finishes, which may have been quite noxious in their liquid state, are safely applied and cured under controlled conditions. Many factory applied finishes will have

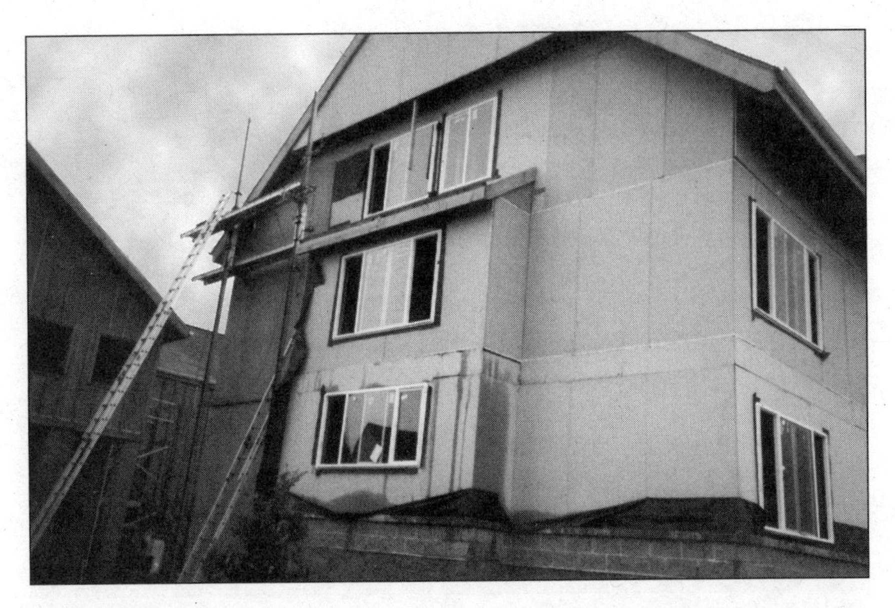

The Problem: Exterior gypsum board sheathing has been installed on this home during the rain. Building paper is now being installed over the wet sheathing. This will trap the moisture and is likely to result in a moldy wall. Recommendation: Building materials should be protected from the elements and rapidly dried if they do become wet.
Photo: Restoration Consultants.

little or no impact on air quality by the time they are installed in the home.

Sealing

If a toxic building component cannot be eliminated or substituted, then sealing it will help to reduce the rate of outgassing. Although this approach is far from perfect, there are cases where we recommend vapor sealants or barriers for this purpose. For example, premanufactured wood windows are routinely dipped in fungicides. As it is almost always cost-prohibitive to have custom windows made, sealing the windows with a special clear sealer or primer will help limit pesticide exposure.

Throughout the planning of a healthy home, you will be weighing the health risks, costs, time, and aesthetics of the above five strategies to find the solutions that are best for you.

Introducing Quality Control Measures During Construction

Even a home with the finest design and most careful materials selection can become a home that does not support health if quality control is lacking on the jobsite. Typically, the quality control measures that a homeowner might expect or wish to have performed will not be carried out unless they are clearly specified and included as part of the building contract. To ensure that the design intent and the written and drawn instructions are properly executed, certain procedures and tests should be agreed upon and required. Quality control

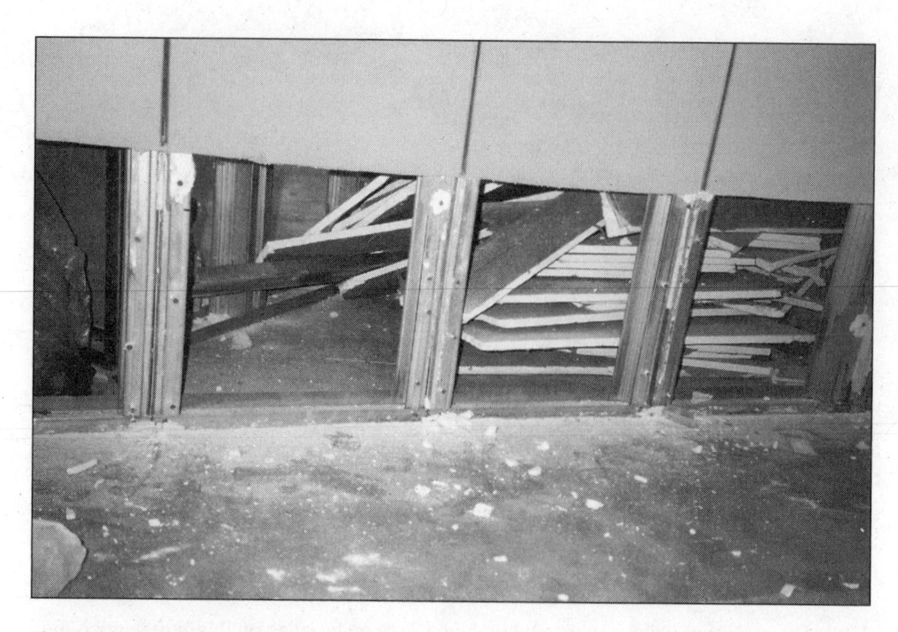

The Problem: Construction debris was not properly removed from this site. A wall cavity was used for debris disposal and then covered over. When there was an accidental flood in this building the hidden material became wet and could not dry out quickly. A serious mold problem resulted. Recommendation: Building cavities should be left clean and free of debris. Photo: Restoration Consultants.

measures are discussed throughout this book (particularly in Division 1 and in the environmental testing section in Division 13) and include:

- clear contractual agreements between the owner and the builder regarding both standard and special project procedures, protocols, materials, and contract close-out
- procedures, inspections, and tests to be performed during construction and upon commissioning of the building to assure that the building will perform as intended

Providing Occupant Education

A home that is well conceived and well built as described above will provide a healthy environment initially. However, the home will continue to nurture the optimum health of its occupants only if they are fully educated about the healthy maintenance of their home.

Owner's Manual

The contractor should provide the owner with a manual that contains the following information:

- a description of the building construction materials and components, including updated drawings and specifications with any "as built" changes clearly marked
- maintenance schedules and manuals for household and mechanical appliances
- a checklist outlining the owner's responsibilities in overseeing the regular and periodic maintenance and inspection of the

CASE STUDY 7

Fragrant Fumes

In 1996 E. B. was a 58-year-old man with a ten-year history of chronic sinus congestion, hoarseness, and headaches. By the time he consulted with Dr. Elliott, he had tried many forms of treatment, including nasal surgery, frequent courses of antibiotics, decongestants, and steroid nasal drops. After removing dairy products from his diet, he noticed only a partial improvement in the congestion. Dr. Elliott then suggested that he try eliminating all scented products from his body, including detergents, soaps, and colognes. Through a process of trial and error, E. B. discovered that his aftershave lotion was a significant cause of his symptoms. His voice has now returned to its former resonance and he is without headaches and sinus congestion.

Discussion

Manufacturers of fragranced products need list only "fragrance" on the label, not the actual chemicals. The perfume industry is self-regulated and is not required to provide formulations, test results, safety data, or consumer complaints to the Food and Drug Administration. Millions of people are made ill by artificial fragrances, which are now used in almost every cleaning, laundry, and personal care product on the market. Most people are unaware that fragrances can cause or contribute to health problems. The most common symptoms related to fragrances include asthma, headaches, dizziness, fatigue, mental confusion, memory loss, nausea, irritability, depression, rashes, and muscle and joint pains. With increasing awareness and growing demand, products are now becoming available that are fragrance-free or scented with purely plant-derived substances.

building exterior, including drainage, roof gutters, roofing, painting, and staining
- a checklist of regular maintenance requirements for which outside services may be called upon, such as chimney sweeping and ductwork cleaning
- warranties and contact numbers of appropriate subcontractors

Proper Use of Exhaust Fans, Smoke Detectors, and CO Monitors

Smoke detectors and CO (carbon monoxide) monitors will warn occupants only when functional. Exhaust fans will prevent excess moisture or remove pollutants from cooking only if the occupant remembers to use them. When exhaust fans are in operation, the owner may need to provide make-up air by opening a window or manually turning on a supply switch. Understanding and maintaining such devices is an important part of maintaining a healthy home.

Avoiding Artificial Fragrance in the Home

The use of toxic fragrances is so prevalent in our culture that many chemically sensitive individuals have a hard time finding a home to rent or buy that is free of acquired odors from scented products. In fact, these common synthetic fragrances pose a health threat to any occupant and should not be used in a healthy home. As Dr. Elliott explains, artificial fragrances are found throughout most homes and workplaces in body and hair care products, household cleaners, detergents, fabric softeners, air fresheners, and even some magazines. Fragrance is cited as an indoor irritant and pollutant in several major studies.[17]

In the days before "better living through chemistry," fragrances were made from flowers. Now approximately 95 percent of all ingredients used by the fragrance industry are synthetic.[18] According to the US Food and Drug Administration, about 4,000 petroleum derived chemicals are used in fragrances.[19] These include toluene, formaldehyde, acetone, benzene derivatives, methylene chloride, phenyl ethyl alcohol, methyl ethyl ketone, and benzyl acetate. A single fragrance can contain as many as 600 different chemicals.

In a 1988 study, the National Institute of Occupational Safety and Health identified 884 toxic substances in a partial list of 2,983 chemicals now being used by the fragrance industry.[20] Many of these substances are capable of causing cancer, birth defects, central nervous system disorders, reproductive disorders, and skin irritation. According to the National Academy of Sciences, there is minimal or no data on toxicity for 84 percent of the ingredients found in fragrances.[21]

Currently there is no agency regulating the fragrance industry. The FDA is aware of the serious nature of the problem but is unable to undertake the astronomical expense of testing each of the chemicals found in fragrances. Without such testing, the FDA would be subject to lawsuits by manufacturers if fragrances were banned. Thus, as is often the case, the onus falls on the consumer to make informed choices. At the end of this chapter you will find the names of some companies that supply fragrance-free products or products with fragrances derived from natural sources.

Avoiding Biocide Use in the Home and Garden

Pesticide use should be unnecessary in a well-built home. Similarly, a well-planned and healthy garden with site-appropriate plant selections and careful gardening practices should not require the use of any toxic herbicides. There are almost always effective benign methods for dealing with house and garden pests. Because of the potentially devastating health consequences of pesticide use, more benign solutions should be rigorously pursued when a pest problem arises. The principals of integrated pest management are discussed at greater length in Division 10.

Healthful Home Cleaning

Cleaning substances with a skull and crossbones abound in our grocery stores for use in home care, but these highly toxic and caustic substances should not be used for the maintenance of a healthy home. Fortunately, safe and environmentally friendly cleaning products are readily available. Please refer to the list at the end of this chapter and to the general cleanup section in Division 1 for healthy suggestions for every cleaning need.

A Healthy Home Must Be a Smoke-Free Home

Almost everyone knows of the threat caused to personal health by smoking tobacco. Most people are also well aware of the threat caused by inhaling passive smoke. Once smoke is absorbed into the surfaces of a home, it takes extensive renovation to eliminate it. A no-smoking policy along with the careful design and use of fireplaces is essential to the maintenance of good air quality.

Further Reading

Anderson, Nina et al. *Your Health and Your House.* Keats Publishing, 1995. A resource guide to health symptoms and the indoor air pollutants that aggravate them.

Banta, John. *Extreme Weather Hits Home: Protecting Your Buildings from Climate Change.* New Society Publishers, 2007. Discusses measures that can be taken to prevent or lessen the effects of climate change on your home.

Bower, John. *Healthy House Building: A Design and Construction Guide.* Healthy House Institute, 1993. Step-by-step guide illustrating the author's construction of a model healthy house.

Bower, John. *The Healthy House: How to Buy One, How to Build One, How to Cure a Sick One.* 4th ed., Healthy House Institute, 2000. Describes in great depth a three-step approach consisting of elimination, isolation, and ventilation. As many toxins as possible are identified and eliminated; a tight air barrier isolates occupants from infiltration; and air is exchanged and purified by means of mechanical ventilation. The author speaks from firsthand experience in successfully creating a chemical-free sanctuary for his spouse.

Breecher, Maury M. and Shirley Linde. *Healthy Homes in a Toxic World.* John Wiley and Sons, 1992. The authors identify household health hazards, the human health conditions associated with them, and solutions for healthier environments.

Colburn, Theo et al. *Our Stolen Future.* Plume, 1997. A gripping account of the scientific research linking reproductive failures, birth defects, and sexual abnormalities to synthetic chemicals that mimic natural hormones, causing disruption of the endocrine system.

Dadd, Debra. *Nontoxic, Natural and Earthwise.* J. P. Tarcher, 1990. A practical, easy-to-use guide to nontoxic alternatives for cleaning products, personal care products, lawn and garden supplies, baby care items, pet care products, and household furnishings.

The Green Guide. Available from Mothers and Others for a Livable Planet, 40 West 20th St., New York, NY 10011, 888-ECO-INFO. This newsletter discusses various relevant topics and promotes safe and ecologically sound consumer choices.

Green, Nancy Sokol. *Poisoning Our Children.* The Noble Press, 1991. The contemporary pesticide problem comes alive as the author relates the nightmare she endured after unwittingly poisoning herself in her own home with repeated pesticide exposures.

International Institute for Bau-Biologie & Ecology Correspondence Course. Available through Helmut Ziehe, IBE, Box 387, Clearwater FL 33757, 727-461-4371, buildingbiology.net. This certified home-study course has been translated into English from the original work of Anton Schneider, the driving force behind the Bau-Biologie movement in Europe. The course provides a comprehensive discussion of the interrelationship of the built environment, human health, and planetary ecology.

Lawson, Lynn. *Staying Well in a Toxic World: Understanding Environmental Illness, Multiple Chemical Sensitivities, Chemical Injuries, and Sick Building Syndrome.* Lynnword Press, 1994. A highly readable, informative, and comprehensive overview of the devastating effects of toxic surroundings by a former medical writer with a thorough understanding of the contemporary chemical problem.

Leclair, Kim and David Rousseau. *Environmental by Design.* Hartley and Marks, 1993. Provides a "cradle to grave" environmental analysis of common building materials.

Lstiburek, Joseph. *Builder's Guides.* Available through The Energy & Environmental Building Association, 10740 Lyndale Avenue South, Suite 10W, Bloomington, MN 55420, 952-881-1098, eeba.org. A series of climate-based field guides with explanations, details, and techniques to effectively implement energy- and resource-efficient residential construction.

Our Toxic Times. Published by the Chemical Injury Information Network, PO Box 301, White Sulphur Springs, MT 59645, 406-547-2255. A useful newsletter for people interested in understanding how chemicals impact human health.

Pearson, David. *The Natural House Book: Creating a Healthy, Harmonious, and Ecologically Sound Home Environment.* Fireside, 1989. The author gives a thoughtful explanation of the human health and environmental impacts associated with standard building practices. He then shows an inspiring array of natural building materials and systems from around the world.

Rea, William J. *Optimum Environments for Optimum Health and Creativity.* Crown Press, 2002. Rea is the founder of the Environmental Health Center in Dallas. He has extensive experience working with patients who have extreme multiple chemical sensitivities. His book is a guide for healthier homebuilding practices. It has broad general application and a special emphasis on strategies for creating clean homes for chemically sensitive individuals.

Rogers, Sherry A. *Tired or Toxic? A Blueprint for Health.* Prestige Publishing, 1990. Detailed and comprehensive medical explanations of how chemicals are impacting human health.

Roodman, David Malin and Nicholas Lenssen. *A Building Revolution: How Ecology and Health Concerns Are Transforming Construction.* Worldwatch Paper 124, 1995.

Schoemaker, Joyce and Charity Vitale. *Healthy Homes, Healthy Kids.* Island Press, 1991. The authors discuss ways to protect children from everyday environmental hazards found in the home.

Stih, Daniel. *Healthy Living Spaces: Top 10 Hazards Affecting Your Health.* Healthy Living Spaces, 2007. Stih speaks from his experience as a home inspector about common causes of sick buildings and what you can do to prevent and remedy these hazards.

Thompson, Athena. *Homes That Heal and Those That Don't: How Your Home Could Be Harming Your Family's Health.* New Society Publishers, 2004. A thorough guide that takes the homeowner on a room-by-room tour of the home, identifying sources of pollution and offering healthy solutions for each potential problem.

Thrasher, Jack and Alan Broughton. *The Poisoning of Our Homes and Workplaces: The Indoor Formaldehyde Crisis.* Seadora, 1989. Detailed analysis of the indoor formaldehyde crisis in the United States.

Venolia, Carol. *Healing Environments: Your Guide to Indoor Well-being.* Celestial Arts, 1988. The author takes the reader through a series of environmental awareness-raising exercises, expanding a holistic approach to health and the built environment that includes the wellness of body, mind, and spirit.

Venolia, Carol and Kelly Lerner. *Natural Remodeling for the Not-So-Green House.* Lark Books, 2006. This practical and inspiring book, written by two architects, is a guide to remodeling with planetary and personal health in mind.

Wilson, Cynthia. *Chemical Exposure and Human Health.* McFarland, 1993. A reference guide to 314 chemicals, with a list of symptoms they can produce and a directory of organizations.

Zamm, Alfred and Robert Gannon. *Why Your House May Endanger Your Health.* Simon and Schuster, 1982. Based on a ten-year scientific study, this book explains how millions of Americans may be suffering ill health because their homes have become toxic chambers. The authors discuss remedies for many of the major health hazards found in the home.

Retail Outlets and Catalog Distributors

Allergy Relief Store, 250 Watson Glen, Franklin, TN 37064, 800-866-7464, 615-790-3525, allergyrelief store.com. Mail order catalog offering supplies and building products for the allergy-free home.

Allergy Resources, 557 Burbank St., Suite K, Broomfield, CO 80020, 800-873-3529. Nontoxic cleaning compounds and body care products.

American Environmental Health Foundation, 8345 Walnut Hill Lane, Suite 225, Dallas, TX 75231, 800-428-2343, 214-361-9515, aehf.com. Sells a wide range of household, building, personal care, and medical products as well as organic clothing, books, and vitamins.

Aubrey Organics, 4419 N. Manhattan Ave., Tampa, FL 33614, 800-282-7394, aubrey-organics.com. Over 200 hair, skin, and body care products made from herbs and vitamins, without synthetic chemicals.

Building for Health — Materials Center, PO Box 113, Carbondale, CO 81623, 800-292-4838 (orders only), 970-963-0437, buildingforhealth.com. Distributor of a wide variety of healthy building products. The owner, Cedar Rose, is also a building contractor who has practical experience with most products sold by the Center.

The Cutting Edge Catalog, PO Box 4158, Santa Fe, NM 87502, 800-497-9516, cutcat.com. Full-line catalog with state of the art products for immune system protection.

Dasun Company, PO Box 668, Escondido, CA 92033, 800-433-8929. Catalog sales of air and water purification products.

Eco Design/Natural Choice, 1365 Rufina Circle, Santa Fe, NM 87505, 800-621-2591. Catalog sales of natural paints, stains, and healthy home products.

Eco Home Center, 3101 Main Ave., Suite 2, Durango, CO 81301, 970-259-8326, ecohomecenter.com. Ecological building and home supplies.

Eco-Products, 3655 Frontier Ave., Boulder, CO 80301, 303-449-1876, ecoproducts.com. Ecologically sound building products.

Environmental Home Center (ecohaus), 4121 1st Ave. South, Seattle, WA 98134, 800-281-9785, 206-682-7332, environmentalhomecenter.com. Green building supplies and household products.

Green Nest, 18662 MacArthur Blvd., Suite 200, Irvine, CA 92612, (888) 473-6466, GreenNest.com. This on-line store is owned and operated by Lisa and Ron Beres, certified Baubiologists. The site is a source for a wide diversity of products and information for the healthy home.

Healthy Interiors (Casa Natura), 328 Sandoval St., Santa Fe, NM 87501, 877-650-1600, 505-820-7634, casanaturainc.com. Organic mattresses, bedding, and clothing, wool carpeting, and wood furniture.

Janice's, 30 Arbor St. South, Hartford, CT 06106, 800-526-4237 (orders), 860-523-4479 (information), janices.com. Supplier for natural and organic bedding and linens and hypoallergenic and unscented personal care products.

The Living Source, PO Box 20155, Waco, TX 76702, 254-776-4878 (customer service/orders), 800-662-8787 (voice mail orders), livingsource .com. Catalog sales of "products for the environmentally aware and chemically sensitive."

NEEDS, 6010 Drott Dr., East Syracuse, NY 13057, 800-634-1380, needs.com. Mail order service offering a wide array of personal care products for the chemically sensitive.

Nirvana Safe Haven (formerly the Nontoxic Hotline), 3441 Golden Rain Rd., Suite 3, Walnut Creek, CA 94595, 800-968-9355, nontoxic.com. Catalog sales of products for achieving and maintaining indoor air quality and safety for homes, offices, and automobiles.

Planetary Solutions, 2030 17th St., Boulder, CO 80302, 303-442-6228, planetearth.com. Environmentally sound materials for interiors.

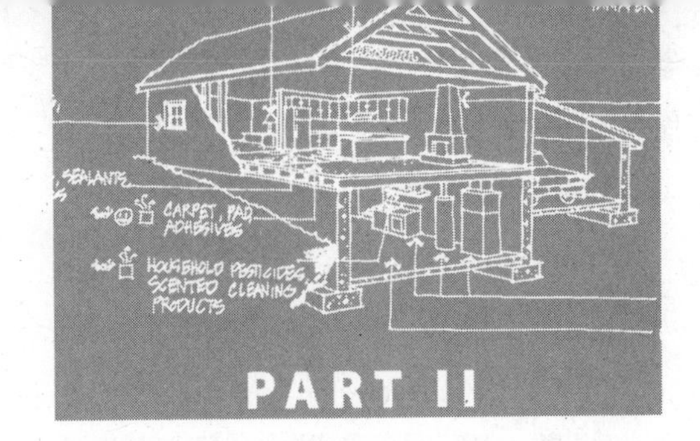

Specification

Introduction

Construction specifications are the detailed written instructions that support architectural drawings. Together, the "specs" and the drawings comprise the construction documents. The drawings explain the physical layout and appearance of the building, how it will be structured, and the choice of general construction materials. Specifications contain instructions that cannot be shown easily on the drawings. They indicate how materials are to be handled and installed, and prescribe brand names of products and performance requirements. Detailed specifications are not often included in the documents for residential construction. However, if you want to build a healthy home, detailed specifications are essential because many standard practices and materials are unacceptable.

The specifications in this book are designed as a guideline for homeowners, architects, and builders to use in building a healthy home. To organize the specifications, we use the 16-division Master Format list, developed by the Construction Specification Institute and widely recognized as the standard for construction specifications. The Master Format covers all aspects of construction in a sequence familiar to architects and builders. Part II is therefore comprised of divisions rather than standard chapters. Although in 2004 CSI changed over to a 50-division format, we have kept the original 16 divisions in this new edition for the sake of simplicity.

Construction specifications contain information about performance standards that ensure the structural integrity and quality of construction. Our guidelines are not intended as a substitute for standard specifications but as an addition to them. For example, standard concrete specifications will specify the strength of concrete to be used, how it is to be mixed and poured, and procedures for testing its strength. The specifications in this book do not include such basic information. Instead, the information appearing in the following

16 divisions focuses on the health of home occupants as well as the health of home builders and subcontractors.

Where appropriate, the differences between healthy and standard construction are explained. Products, manufacturers, tradespeople, and consultants involved in healthy building are specified. Telephone numbers and websites are included in the Resource List in Appendix B so that you may conveniently locate the closest distributors.

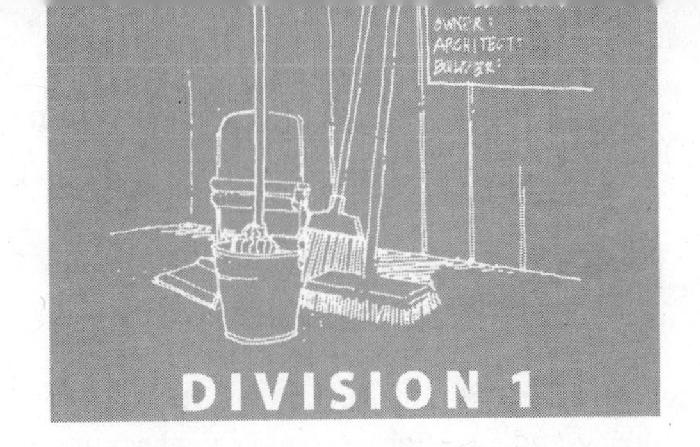

General Requirements

Statement of Intent

Clear communication among contractor, owner, and architect is a key factor in the success of any building project. When creating a healthy home, there are many special project procedures that must be communicated with even greater clarity than in standard construction. The owner's intentions and instructions for special procedures can be formally transmitted in the statement of intent, thus making them part of the construction contract.

Here is a sample of specifications language that succinctly states the owner's wish to create a special project:

This house is being constructed as a healthy house. The following specifications outline special project procedures and acceptable building products. The products specified herein are intended to be as free of harmful chemicals as is presently possible and reasonably attainable. In using these products and following these procedures, we are safeguarding to the best of our ability the health of future inhabitants and of the workers involved in this construction. Our concern extends also to the workers involved in the manufacture of these products.

Coordination

Building a healthy home can be a pioneering endeavor. Choosing the right architect and contractor is of paramount importance. Creativity, intelligence, common sense, and commitment to the ideals of healthy house building are essential qualities for each of the participants. At times you and your team will be experimenting with products that have not been on the market long enough to have a performance history or wide distribution. At other times you may find yourself participating in a revival of materials and techniques that were used successfully for centuries but have been replaced in standard construction by commercialized products containing harmful chemicals.

The contractor will need to allow more time for locating special materials, scheduling their use, and supervising their installation. You may encounter initial resistance from subcontractors who are reluctant to do things that are unfamiliar to them. Some of the healthier products might be harder to work with because they do not contain certain harmful additives that make application easier. For these reasons, the general contractor will need to supervise the project more closely than in standard construction.

During the construction of a healthy building, the owner may wish to hire subcontractors to carry out specific environmentally related testing, quality control inspections, procedures, or installations. Included in standard contracts from the American Institute for Architecture (AIA) is document A201, "General Conditions for Construction," which acknowledges the owner's right to hire his or her own subcontractors. Careful coordination with the contractor is necessary, however, because any delays and expenses incurred by the contractor because of this work will be the responsibility of the owner. Some of the additional testing and inspections are described in Division 13. Other quality control procedures will be outlined where appropriate throughout the text. If you do not use a standard AIA contract, you may need to add language to your contract to outline the parameters for specialty subcontractors to be hired by the owners.

In summary, a healthy home can take more time and effort to build, which may be reflected in the contractor's scheduling and pricing. Once committed to the project, however, the contractor is like the symphony conductor, who must lead all players to a successful performance regardless of the difficulty of the piece. You will wish to clearly state this expectation in your specification document. An example of such language follows:

- **The contractor shall be responsible for obtaining all specified materials or approved substitutes and for performing all special project procedures within the contract time, as stated within the construction contract.**
- **The contractor shall be responsible for the general performance of the subcontractors and tradespeople and for any necessary training, specifically with regards to the special project procedures, materials, and prohibitions as outlined in these specifications.**

Special Project Procedures

Healthy home building does not permit many behaviors and practices that are commonly accepted at standard jobsites. The procedural expectations must be clearly stated by the owner and upheld by the contractor. Some basic rules that you may wish to include and expand upon in your specifications are:

The following special project procedures must be obeyed at all times:

- **Smoking is prohibited within or near any structure on the jobsite.**
- **The use of gas-generated machinery and gas- or kerosene-fired heaters is prohibited within or near the building.**
- **No insecticides, herbicides, or chemicals other than those specified may be used on the jobsite without prior approval by the architect or owner.**
- **All materials are to be protected from**

contamination and moisture damage during storage and after installation.

Procedures to Prevent Insect and Rodent Infestation

Some simple measures can be applied from the outset of construction that will prevent infestation of rodents and insects. Consider adding the following requirements to the above list:

- **All foodstuffs shall be disposed of in containers that will be removed from the jobsite and emptied at the end of each workday.**
- **All debris shall be removed from under and around the building premises and properly disposed of in a Dumpster. The Dumpster shall be removed when full on a regular basis so that piles of debris do not accumulate on the ground around it.**

Quality Control

There may be some instances where you will be asked by your contractor to share in the responsibility for application of an experimental material. You may choose to accept this responsibility on a case-by-case basis. However, aside from any agreed-upon exceptions, the contractor must be willing to provide the same warranty for your finished home as would be provided if standard products were being used. The contractor should have no problem doing so as long as the manufacturer's instructions are carefully followed.

Manufacturers will specify the conditions required for the proper application of their products, such as proper curing times, acceptable temperature ranges, or specific preparation of substrates. Because the materials contain fewer chemical additives, the manufacturer's specifications may be both different from and less forgiving than what tradespeople are accustomed to. Consequently, workers may require close supervision by the contractor to maintain a high standard.

Another area requiring special vigilance on the contractor's part lies in the careful screening of materials as they arrive onsite to ensure that no spoilage, adsorption of odors, mold, or other forms of contamination have occurred.

We know of a case where batt insulation was shipped to the jobsite in a truck that had been used to transport fertilizer. Once the installation was installed, the home took on a distinctly unpleasant odor because of the adsorbent nature of the batt insulation. In another case, a painter who was unfamiliar with milk-based paints did not realize that the products he was using had spoiled. The finished home smelled like sour milk.

Subcontractors may be unfamiliar with some of the healthier products we recommend and may not recognize a problem when it arises. These products typically have little odor, and a strong odor may be an indication for concern. The contractor's nose becomes an important quality control mechanism. Exceptions include products such as silicone caulks and vapor barrier sealants, whose strong odor upon application quickly dissipates and becomes neutral. A call to the architect or manufacturer may be helpful for reassurance when questions arise.

It is important to have a clear agreement from the outset about your expectations concerning quality. This agreement can be formalized in the specifications using language similar to the following:

CASE STUDY 1.1

A Mishandled Spill

Early in his career as an environmental consultant, John Banta received a frantic call from a woman with chemical sensitivities who was in the process of having a home built. The client had painstakingly detailed plans and specifications with the help of John and her architect. The project had proceeded virtually without problems, and was entering the final interior painting and sealing process when a worker for the subcontracting painter accidentally kicked over a bucket of nontoxic paint, spilling it on the unfinished floor. The worker ran to his truck and grabbed a can of mineral spirits, which he used to clean up the spill. The solvent soaked into the floor and the fumes filled the house. John's client became distraught because her new house was making her feel sick.

Discussion

In spite of all the best efforts, accidents still happen. The subcontractor failed to educate his worker. The spilled paint was water-based, which meant that the use of mineral spirits was unnecessary and inappropriate. The painter should have wiped up as much as possible using clean rags and then scrubbed the rest with water. Since the floor was unfinished, any remaining paint could have been removed with sanding.

Many attempts were made to remove the noxious mineral spirit odor from the home, but the solvent had been absorbed by the construction materials. Even pulling up the contaminated portion of the floor was insufficient to fix the problem. The cleaning substance used by the painter was clearly in violation of the job contract and it appeared that a lawsuit was imminent. Fortunately, the house was quickly sold to a less sensitive person who wanted an ecologically constructed home and who was not affected by the residual odor of mineral spirits.

- **The contractor shall perform and maintain the special project procedures with the same quality of workmanship as would be expected with standard materials and methods.**
- **The contractor shall maintain a quality control program that ensures full protection of workers against exposure to prohibited materials and practices.**
- **Except as otherwise approved by the architect or owner, the contractor shall determine and comply with the manufacturer's recommendations on product handling, storage, installation, and protection.**
- **The contractor shall verify that all materials are undamaged, uncontaminated, and free of acquired odors prior to installation. Any products found to be defective shall not be used unless approved by the owner or architect.**

Signage

Even if your contractor is well aware of your intentions, he or she will probably not have the chance to personally speak to every person who will work at your site during the course of construction. It is important that the special rules that apply to your home be posted

This is a Healthy House
ONLY SPECIFIED PRODUCTS & PROCEDURES ALLOWED
Toxic substances including pesticides, fungicides,
noxious cleaning products are prohibited.
Gasoline-generated machines or open combustion heaters
shall not be used inside the house.
SMOKING PROHIBITED
Spills of fuels, solvents, or chemicals must be avoided
(If a spill occurs, report it to construction supervisor or Architect immediately)
Alternatives to specified materials must be approved in writing
prior to use by Owner and/or Architect

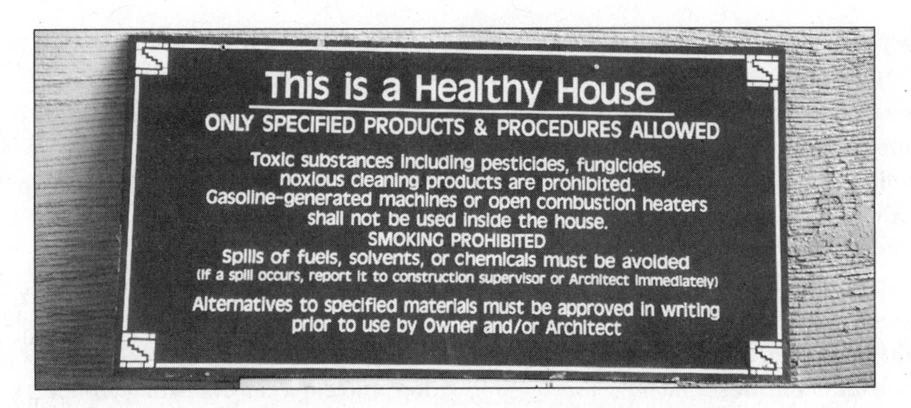

A sign, posted in a prominent place on the job site, alerts everyone as to the special project procedures. Photo: Paula Baker-Laporte

in a prominent spot where all who enter will read them. You can specify that a job sign be made and posted. Sample wording that can be placed in your specifications follows:

The following sign is to be made and prominently posted on the jobsite. It is the responsibility of the general contractor to ensure that the labor force, all subcontractors and their labor forces, all suppliers, and all other visitors are made aware of these rules and follow them at all times.

SIGN TO BE POSTED:

This house is being constructed as a healthy home. Only specified products and procedures may be used. If in doubt, contact the general contractor.

The use of any toxic substances such as insecticides, fungicides, or noxious cleaning products is prohibited anywhere on this site.

Smoking within or near the building and its garage or outbuildings is strictly prohibited.

No gasoline-generated machines or open combustion heaters shall be used inside or near the house after the foundation is completed.

Spills of fuels, solvents, or chemicals must be avoided. If a spill occurs, report it to the general contractor immediately.

Alternatives to specified materials must be approved in writing by the owner and/or architect prior to use.

Prohibited Products

Because it is difficult to foresee every single product application that will be required in a project, it is prudent to list the major categories of prohibited materials that are the worst health offenders. This gives the general contractor and subcontractors the "big picture" in terms of materials. Sample language containing such a list follows:

The use of substances listed below is prohibited:

- **herbicides, fungicides, insecticides, and other pesticides, except as specified**
- **composite wood products containing urea/formaldehyde binders**

- **asphalt or products containing asphalt or bitumen**
- **commercial cleaning products other than those specified**
- **adhesives, paints, sealers, stains, and other finishes except as specified**
- **any building materials contaminated by mold or mildew**
- **any building materials or components that have been contaminated while in storage or during shipment**

Contact the architect for further instructions about any application where these substances would normally be used if information for a substitution is not in this document.

Product Substitution Procedure

Contractors will often ask if they can substitute a product that is different from the one you have specified. The specified product may be unavailable, too expensive, or too difficult to apply, or contractors may have one that they have used before and prefer. New and healthier products continue to be developed; it may be worth your while to consider certain substitutions. The first step in researching alternatives is to examine the Material Safety Data Sheet (MSDS). (Refer to the section on MSDS that follows.) You may also request a physical sample. To ensure that no substitutions are made without your consent or that of your architect, you may wish to add the following language to your agreement:

- **No products may be substituted for the specified product unless agreed upon in writing by the owner or architect.**
- **An MSDS and product literature must be provided on any substitution for it to be considered.**
- **Submit a physical sample to the owner or architect whenever possible.**

Product Evaluation

Since the last edition of this book, the availability of products considered acceptable for a healthy house has skyrocketed. An emerging problem when evaluating products for use in your healthy home is determining just how healthy a product will be. Some manufacturers have deliberately sought to capitalize on the burgeoning green market by engaging in what is being termed "green washing," making claims that are not necessarily borne out by evidence. Others have created acceptable products to satisfy regulatory compliance. Not all products that are promoted as green are acceptable for a healthy home and some are more acceptable than others. Some products are considered green because they use recycled materials; others may be labeled green because they come from a sustainable resource or conserve energy. Chemical formulations may be "safe for the environment" but when confined in an indoor area may still cause adverse reactions for people. Very few products will be universally acceptable for people with multiple chemical sensitivities. Consumers interested in healthy construction need to remain vigilant and do their homework. Chemically sensitive individuals will need to be the most vigilant.

Several resources have emerged to help consumers do their own research to find safer and more environmentally sound products. In 1986, California voters passed Proposition 65, the Safe Drinking Water and Toxic

Enforcement Act.[1] It was intended by its authors to help protect Californians by informing them about chemicals known to cause cancer, birth defects, and other kinds of harm. The law states that "no person in the course of doing business shall knowingly and intentionally expose any individual to a chemical known to the state to cause cancer or reproductive toxicity without first giving clear and reasonable warning...." The governor is required to publish annually a list of chemicals that are considered problematic. The current list contains several hundred chemicals.

In 2003, the law was amended by the legislature to set aside a sizable amount of any penalties collected under this law to help pay for future enforcement. The results have been far-reaching. The law's requirement that products with any of the hazardous ingredients listed have a warning on the label has served as an inducement for manufacturers to create healthier products for the California market, which are then often distributed nationwide. Since the list is updated annually, it is in a manufacturer's best interest to develop products that are safe so they do not have to be reformulated later.

Other incentive certification programs have been developed to help promote products that meet low-emissions criterion. One of these is the **GreenGuard** Certification Program for Low Emitting Products, founded in 2001. The certification is a voluntary program available to manufacturers who choose to submit their products for regular evaluation. The program is supported by fees paid by the manufacturers. Product criteria vary with the type of product, but in general a product must be tested to release less than the preestablished levels of volatile organic compounds, aldehydes, formaldehyde, and styrene. Adhesive and sealant products also have limits on the amount of 4-Phenylcyclohexene (4-PC) they can emit.

While GreenGuard certified products may be better than many of the conventional products available, certification doesn't guarantee that the products are free of all emissions. Therefore, because products are tested individually, the total impact of several low-emissions products used together may affect sensitive individuals. Furthermore, the tests reflect levels at seven days after installation, and levels of emissions will be higher when first installed, before the rooms are flushed out. Ingredients that are listed under California's Proposition 65, the US National Toxicology Program, and the International Agency on Research on Cancer are not prohibited for certification but must be listed. Primary or secondary outdoor pollutants cannot exceed concentrations permitted by National Air Quality Standards. Volatile organic compounds must be less than one-tenth of the Threshold Limit Value set for industrial exposure by the American Conference of Government Industrial Hygienists. Products are tested in a chamber following a set protocol and not under actual use conditions. Because the tests use an amount of material with the same "exposed surface area to room volume" found in a typical indoor environment, the results are intended to approximate an accurate picture of emissions in real-life situations.

While GreenGuard provides some level of independent certification of emission levels, it does not provide an evaluation of the products themselves and how well they work or other considerations for usage. The McDonough Braungart Design Chemistry firm offers a certification based on the principles popularized by their book *Cradle to Cradle: Remaking the Way We Make Things*. Throughout their lifecycle, products certified by **Cradle to Cradle** must satisfy established criteria for both human and environmental health. To qualify, materials need to be sustainable and able to be recycled or broken down to form beneficial nutrients. Products must identify their ingredients down to a level of 100 parts per million, meet other toxicity requirements, have a plan for using solar energy for their manufacture, conserve water, not pollute water, and be socially responsible. Cradle to Cradle certification is offered at various levels. Because at the lowest level it can be used by products that have not been evaluated for emissions, being certified does not necessarily demonstrate acceptability from a health standpoint. Even being rated at the highest level does not ensure that a product will be suitable for all chemically sensitive individuals.

Green Seal is an independent nonprofit organization dedicated to safeguarding the environment. It is continually establishing new standards and certification programs for various product and service categories. Once a product category standard is developed by Green Seal, manufacturers can submit their products for evaluation. After they become listed, products are reviewed each year to ensure they continue to comply. The Green Seal program is discussed further in the section on commercial cleaning products later in this chapter. Other product categories include adhesives and floor care products. The reader should review the standards for products of interest to determine acceptability. For example, the standard for compact fluorescent lighting allows up to 10 milligrams of mercury per lamp, although lower-level compacts are available.

Scientific Certification Systems offers an Environmental Certification Program for products meeting voluntary indoor air quality goals. The company has participated in creating independent third-party standard verifications for a number of programs. Their Indoor Advantage Gold program sets limits for formaldehyde, aldehydes, and 4-PC in paints and other household maintenance products. Requirements for products vary and should be checked on the Scientific Certification Systems website.

Although certifications provide information that products meet certain minimum criteria, the actual test results for products are kept confidential, so it is not possible for the consumer to compare the various certified products to one another to see which have the lowest emissions. Forums are beginning to emerge that provide a platform for consumers to post their experiences with a product. The potential of these venues is tremendous, especially for chemically sensitive individuals, but only time will tell which will emerge as having the greatest value. One resource for consumer review and comment on green building products is **Rate It Green**, which lists many of the products we recommend and will hopefully emerge as a strong companion to our book for the consumer interested in constructing a healthy house.

The Material Safety Data Sheet (MSDS)

The Material Safety Data Sheet (MSDS) provides information about the chemical substances in a product, its handling precautions, and its known health effects. The responsibility for preparing the MSDS lies with the chemical manufacturer. All manufacturers are required to create an MSDS for every chemical compound they offer. The following information must be included:

- with the exception of trade secrets, the specific chemical name and common names for hazardous ingredients
- physical and chemical characteristics
- physical hazards
- health hazards
- primary routes of entry to the body
- OSHA permissible exposure limit (PEL) and any other recommended exposure limit
- whether the chemical is a confirmed or potential carcinogen
- precautions for safe handling and use
- emergency and first aid procedures
- name, address, and telephone number of the manufacturer or other responsible party.

MSDSs can be obtained from either the distributor or the manufacturer of the product in question.

What an MSDS Will Not Tell You

There is important information that an MSDS does not reveal. Thanks to the Trade Secrets Act, companies are not required to list ingredients they define as trade secrets. Although the OSHA Hazard Communication Standard requires that an MSDS list all health effects, the health effects of trade secret ingredients can be exempted.[2] Furthermore, hazardous ingredients that are present in amounts of less than 1 percent and carcinogens present in amounts less than 0.1 percent need not be listed. Another significant omission is the lack of disclosure of "inert" ingredients, which can account for up to 90 percent or more of product volume. Some of these so-called inert ingredients are more hazardous than the active ingredients.[3]

Although the consumer is not allowed access to the unlisted information, one of the codes under the same law (OSHA Hazard Communication Standard 29, Code of Federal Regulation 1910.1200) permits physicians and other health care providers to access all product ingredient information for diagnostic and treatment purposes. Most doctors are unaware of their right to know.

The permissible exposure levels (PELs) set by OSHA and the threshold limit values (TLVs) established by the American Conference of Governmental Industrial Hygienists (ACGIH) are misleading. Industry interests have played a major role in establishing these exposure limits, most of which were set without prior testing.[4] The small amount of testing that has been carried out was based on exposing rats to a single dose of a single chemical, with cancer or death as the end point. In reality, people are exposed to hundreds of chemicals at a time. These chemicals can accumulate in the body tissues over time and their effects can be synergistic. Monitoring for cancer or death does not take into account the many noncarcinogenic effects of chemicals, such as damage to the nervous, endocrine, and immune systems. It is important to recognize that workplace standards are not set for the safety of the worker but rather for what is considered feasible for industry.

Health effects listed in an MSDS are often vague and misleading. They are most accurate when listing the acute, short-term effects, such as eye and nose irritation, rashes, and asthma. The data on chronic, long-term exposure are often lacking and do not take into account cumulative or synergistic effects.

How an MSDS Can Be a Useful Tool

Although the MSDS has shortcomings, it is still an important tool for people involved in construction. If you are not working with a physician/architect team knowledgeable about chemicals, the MSDS can be confusing to interpret. However, the MSDS may provide useful information when used in conjunction with other tools. The National Institutes of Health's National Library of Medicine has developed a searchable database for a wide variety of household product information.[5] The database can be searched by product, ingredients, and MSDS. By comparing MSDS chemical lists with the information available through the library, it is possible to gain a better understanding of recognized potential hazards for the listed chemicals.

Certain rules of thumb can also be used to evaluate a chemical listed in the MSDS. For example, if no special precautions are required when using the chemical, if there are no listed health effects, and if cleanup involves only water, you might assume that the chemical in question has relatively low toxicity. On the other hand, if it is recommended that you wear gloves and goggles and use a respirator in a well-ventilated area, the product is likely a health hazard at least while being applied, though it may not have detrimental health effects once fully cured. Certain chemicals should pique your concern, such as chlorinated or fluorinated compounds and chemicals that contain toxins such as toluene, phenol, benzene, xylene, styrene, formaldehyde, and the heavy metals, to name just a few.

With more than 88,000 chemicals in common use and no toxicity data on most of them, our evaluation can be only partial at best. The US Environmental Protection Agency has published a list of 53 chemicals that ranked highest as persistent, bioaccumulative, and toxic compounds, or PBTs.[6] The California Office of Environmental Health Hazard Assessment has published a list of chronic exposure levels for 80 common chemicals.[7] Lists such as these are far from comprehensive and they cannot help us choose products with certainty. They can, however, help us to identify known hazardous chemicals and exposure levels and to reject products that contain these.

In summary, although you cannot base your decisions solely on information from the MSDS, it is nevertheless useful. Below are two MSDS examples, with product and manufacturer names omitted. Because MSDSs do not always follow a consistent format, comparisons can be difficult. Section numbers will vary, but the information covered remains the same. While the MSDS for Product #1 is indicative of a product that may be safe to use and in fact is one we recommend to our clients, Product #2 has an MSDS that provides cause for concern.

Product Identification

This section includes the name of the product, the manufacturer, the date the MSDS was prepared, and the preparer's name. In the first sample MSDS, the product is a wood preservative. The second sample involves a foam insulation material. As seen in the examples, product information may range from very little to substantial.

Product # 1

TABLE 1.1

Material Safety Data Sheet	
Section I — Product Identity	**Manufacturer's Name:**
Date Prepared:	
Preparer's Name:	
Chemical Name: Water-based wood preservative	**Product:**
Chemical Formula: N/A (product is a mixture)	**Product Identification No.:**
DOT Shipping Class: Not regulated	
Emergency Telephone Number:	

Product # 2

TABLE 1.2

Material Safety Data Sheet	
Manufacturer:	**Date Prepared:**
Telephone Numbers:	
Emergency Number:	
Technical Information:	
Regular Business Hours:	

Material Identification and Hazardous Components

This section lists the chemical names of all product ingredients found to be reportable health hazards. Exposure limits in some instances are established by government agencies. As discussed earlier, OSHA PEL refers to the permissible exposure limits set by OSHA and ACGIH TLV refers to the threshold limit values set by the American Conference of Governmental Industrial Hygienists. These values are updated on a regular basis.

If you are not familiar with the toxicity of the chemicals listed and you have no references available on the subject, you can infer this information by examining the limits set by the government. When the limit is in parts per million, you can be sure that the product is highly toxic. NE stands for no established limit, and could mean either that adequate testing has not been performed or that the product is not considered highly toxic.

With a health rating of 1, flammability and reactivity levels of 0, and no established exposure limits, we can assume that the ingredients in this product are relatively safe.

In the second sample MSDS, the chemicals 4,4-diphenylmethane diisocyanate and chlorodifluoromethane (HCFC-22) are limited to parts per million. Both chemicals are in fact known to be extremely toxic. With prolonged or repeated exposure, diisocyanates and halogenated hydrocarbons can damage

Product # 1

TABLE 1.3

Section II — Hazardous Ingredients				
Hazardous Components (Special Chemical Identity/Common Names)*	CAS #	Wt. %	OSHA PEL	ACGIH TLV
Propylene glycol	57-55-6	30–50	None established	None established
Polyethylene glycol	25322-68-3	30–50	None established	None established
Disodium octaborate tetrahydrate	12008-91-2	20–30	15 mg/m^3 (dust)	10 mg/m^3 (dust)

* Denotes a toxic chemical reportable under SARA Title 111 Section 313, Supplier Notification provision

HMIS Information: Health: 1; Flammability: 0; Reactivity: 0

Product # 2

TABLE 1.4

Section II — Hazardous Ingredients/Identity Information				
CHEMICAL NAME	CAS NO.	OSHA PEL	ACGIH TLV	PERCENTAGE
Polyurethane resin	NE*	NE*	NE*	50–85
4,4-diphenylmethane diisocyanate	101-68-8	0.02 ppm CEIL	0.005 ppm TWA**	5–15
Chlorodifluoromethane (HCFC-22)	75-45-8	1,000 ppm TWA**	1,000 ppm TWA**	15–25

*Not established **Time-weighted average Hazard Rating: Health: 3; Flammability: 0; Reactivity: 1

the nervous, immune, and endocrine systems. Note that the health hazard rating is 3 out of a possible 4.

Physical and Chemical Characteristics

This section describes how the material behaves. The information is useful for the design of ventilation systems and for providing adequate equipment and procedures for fire and spill containment.

- Vapor pressure tells you how much vapor the material may give off. A high vapor pressure indicates that a liquid will easily evaporate.
- Vapor density refers to the weight of the pure gaseous form of the material in relation to air. The weight of a given volume of a vapor (with no air present) is compared with the weight of an equal volume of air.
- Specific gravity tells you how heavy the material is compared to water and whether it will float or sink.
- Evaporation rate refers to the rate at which a material changes from a liquid or solid state to its gaseous form.
- Volatile organic compounds (VOCs) provide you with an idea of the degree to which the substance will outgas. If the material is toxic, the degree of volatility would be important to consider.
- Water reactivity indicates whether the chemical reacts with water to release a gas that is flammable or presents a health hazard.
- Appearance and odor indicate how a product is supposed to look and smell. For example, if the product is supposed to be clear and odorless but arrives onsite with

Product # 1

TABLE 1.5

Section III — Physical Characteristics			
Boiling Range:	>369° F	**Vapor Pressure (mm Hg.):**	125mm Hg @ 100° F
Specific Gravity (H_20=1):	1.1 – 1.3	**Vapor Density (Air = 1):**	> 1
% Volatile (Volume):	< 1%	**Evaporation Rate (BuAc = 1):**	> 1
Volatile Organic Content (VOC):	3.8 lb./gal.		
Solubility (specify solvents):	Miscible in water, alcohol, acetone, some glycol ethers; insoluble in petroleum hydrocarbons		
Appearance and Odor:	Clear, odorless liquid		

NOTE: In the above MSDS, the evaporation rate is compared with the evaporation rate for butyl acetate. With this particular product, the evaporation rate is less than that for butyl acetate.

Product # 2

TABLE 1.6

Section III — Physical/Chemical Characteristics		
Boiling Point:	HCFC-22	-41.4° F at 1 ATM
	Polyurethane resin	NE
Vapor Pressure:	HCFC-22	136 psia at 70° F
Vapor Density (AIR = 1):	HCFC-22	2.98 at 1 ATM
Specific Gravity (H_20=1):	Polyurethane resin	1.1
Solubility in Water:	Insoluble, reacts with water	
Appearance and Odor:	Gel under pressure. Faint ether-like odor.	

NOTE: Hydrochlorofluorocarbons, or HCFCs, are fluorinated carbons that are harmful to the ozone layer.

Product # 1

TABLE 1.7

Section IV — Fire and Explosion Hazard Data			
Flash Point (Method Used):	Nonflammable	**Flammable Limits (% in air):**	Nonflammable
Extinguishing Media:	Nonflammable		
Special Fire Fighting Procedures:	Nonflammable		
Unusual Fire and Explosion Hazards:	None known		
Reactivity:	Stable	**Conditions to Avoid:**	Avoid extreme heat
Hazardous Polymerization:	May Not Occur	**Conditions to Avoid:**	None known
Incompatibility (Materials to Avoid):	None known		
Hazardous Decomposition or Byproducts:	None known		

Product # 2

TABLE 1.8

Section IV — Fire and Explosion Hazard Data	
Flash Point:	Polyurethane Resin >400° F
Extinguishing Media:	Water fog, foam, CO_2, or dry chemical
Fire Fighting Procedure:	Wear self-contained breathing apparatus and turnout gear. Hazardous decomposition products include CO, CO_2, NO, and traces of HCl. Cured foam: Wear self-contained breathing apparatus. Hazardous decomposition products include CO, CO_2, NO, and traces of HCl.
Usual Hazards:	Temperatures above 120° F will increase the pressure in the can, which may lead to rupturing. Cured foam: This product will burn. Do not expose to heat, sparks, or open flame. This product is not intended for use in applications above 250° F (121° C). Always protect foam with approved facings. This product is not a FIRE STOP or FIRE BARRIER penetration sealant.
Section V — Reactivity Data	
Stability:	Stable under normal storage and handling conditions. Do not store above 120° F. Cured foam will deteriorate when exposed to UV light.
Incompatibility:	Water, alcohols, strong bases, finely powdered metal such as aluminum, magnesium, or zinc, and strong oxidizers.
Conditions/Hazards to Avoid:	Contamination with water may form CO_2. Avoid high heat, i.e., flames, extremely hot metal surfaces, heating elements, combustion engines, etc. Do not store in auto or direct sunlight.

an acrid smell and/or appears cloudy, the product may be contaminated.

Fire and Explosion Hazard Data

The flash point tells you the minimum temperature at which a liquid will give off enough flammable vapor to ignite. Obviously, the more stable the product, the safer it will be.

Reactivity Hazard Data

This section can provide you with clues regarding the toxicity of a product.

Product #1 is stable (not reactive), with no incompatibility with other products and without hazardous decomposition or byproducts.

Product #2 is unstable when exposed to ultraviolet light and high heat and is incompatible with many substances.

Health Hazard Data

This section provides useful information that will help you determine the toxicity of the product in question.

Examining the health hazard section for Product # 1 would provide reassurance. The product appears to be only an irritant, with no known long-term health effects. (Of course, an edible product would be the ultimate assurance of product safety!) In contrast, the information below on Product #2 is not at all reassuring. This product is known to be carcinogenic, mutagenic, and teratogenic. It also may cause irreversible asthma, allergies, and other damage to the immune system. Although this product volatilizes quickly, workers who install it are exposed to extreme health hazards.

Safe Handling Precautions and Leak Procedures

This section offers more clues regarding the safety of the product. The fewer the precautions given, the more reassuring the information.

Control and Preventive Measures

This section lists the personal protective equipment that must be used, the type of ventilation to be used, and precautions to be taken when using the material for its intended purpose.

Product #1 requires no special protective clothing or equipment, which is an indication of product safety.

For Product #2, good ventilation and protective clothing over the entire body, including a face shield or goggles, are necessary.

The above MSDS examples demonstrate that the information supplied in the MSDS, although incomplete, is nevertheless useful. An MSDS allows you to obtain a general impression about the level of toxicity of many products you may consider using in home construction.

Product # 1

TABLE 1.9

Section V — Health Hazard Data	
Route(s) of Entry:	Eye contact, inhalation, ingestion
Acute Health Effects:	Eye contact: May cause redness or irritation
Inhalation:	N/A In sufficient doses may cause gastrointestinal irritation
Skin contact:	N/A
Chronic Health Effects:	Not listed as a carcinogen by the NTP, IARC, or OSHA; no adverse long-term effects are known.
Medical Conditions Generally Aggravated by Exposure:	No adverse long-term effects are known.
Emergency & First Aid:	Eye contact: Wash with clean water for at least 15 minutes. If irritation persists, get medical attention.
Inhalation:	N/A
Ingestion:	If irritation persists, get medical attention.
Skin contact:	N/A

Product # 2

TABLE 1.10

Section VI — Health Hazard Data		
Toxicology Test Data:	MDI:	Rat, 4 hr inhalation LC 50 — Aerosol 490 mg/m^3 — highly toxic
		Rat, 4 hr inhalation LC 50 — Vapor 11 mg/l — toxic
		Rat, oral LD 50 — > 10,000 mg/kg — practically nontoxic
		Rat, inhalation oncogenicity study — @ ~0.2, 1, 6 mg/m^3; URT irritant; carcinogenic @ 6 mg/m^3
	HCFC-22:	Rat, 2 hr inhalation LC 50 — 200,000 ppm

Product # 2

TABLE 1.10 (cont'd.)

Section VI — Health Hazard Data	
Acute Overexposure Effects:	Eye contact with MDI may result in conjunctival irritation and mild corneal opacity. Skin contact may result in dermatitis, either irritative or allergic. Inhalation of MDI vapors may cause irritation of the mucous membranes of the nose, throat, or trachea, breathlessness, chest discomfort, difficult breathing, and reduced pulmonary function. Airborne overexposure well above the PEL may result additionally in eye irritation, headache, chemical bronchitis, asthma-like findings, or pulmonary edema. Isocyanates have also been reported to cause hypersensitivity pneumonitis, which is characterized by flu-like symptoms, the onset of which may be delayed. Gastrointestinal symptoms include nausea, vomiting, and abdominal pain. HCFC-22 vapor is irritating to eyes. Liquid is irritating to eyes and may cause tissues to freeze. Contact of liquid with skin may cause tissue to freeze (frostbite). Dense vapor displaces breathing air in confined or unventilated areas. Inhaling concentrated vapors can cause drowsiness, unconsciousness, respiratory depression, and death due to asphyxiation. This compound also increases the sensitivity of the heart to adrenalin, possibly resulting in rapid heartbeat (tachycardia), irregular heartbeat (cardiac arrhythmias), and depression of cardiac function. Persons with preexisting heart disease may be at increased risk from exposure. Polyurethane resin forms a quick bond with skin. Cured foam is hard to remove from skin. May cause eye damage.
Chronic Overexposure Effects:	Acute or chronic overexposure to isocyanates may cause sensitization in some individuals, resulting in allergic symptoms of the lower respiratory tract (asthma-like), including wheezing, shortness of breath, and difficulty breathing. Subsequent reactions may occur at or substantially below the PEL and TLV. Asthma caused by isocyanates, including MDI, may persist in some individuals after removal from exposure and may be irreversible. Some isocyanate-sensitized persons may experience asthma reactions upon exposure to nonisocyanate-containing dusts or irritants. Cross-sensitization to different isocyanates may occur. Long-term overexposure to isocyanates has also been reported to cause lung damage, including reduced lung function, which may be permanent. An animal study indicated that MDI may induce respiratory hypersensitivity following dermal exposure.
Carcinogenicity:	Results from a lifetime inhalation study in rats indicate that MDI aerosol was carcinogenic at 6 mg/m^3, the highest dose tested. This is well above the recommended TLV of 5 ppb (0.05 mg/m^3). Only irritation was noted at the lower concentration of 0.2 and 1 mg/m^3. Lifetime exposure of rats to 5% HCFC-22 in air resulted in a slightly higher incidence of fibrosarcomas (a malignant connective tissue tumor) in male rats compared to controls. Some of these tumors involved the salivary glands. This effect was not seen in female rats at the same dose level or in rats of either sex at the lower dose level of 1%. Rats given HCFC-22 orally also showed no increased incidence of tumors. In addition, mice exposed to 5 and 1% HCFC-22 in a similar fashion showed no increased incidence of tumors. Spontaneously occurring fibrosarcomas are not uncommon in aging rats and the increase seen in male rats may have been due to a weak tumor-promoting effect or other nonspecific effect (stress, etc.) of HCFC-22.

Product # 2

TABLE 1.10 (cont'd.)

Section VI — Health Hazard Data	
Mutagenicity:	HCFC-22 has been shown to cause mutations in the bacterium *Salmonella*. This may be due to the unusual metabolic capabilities of this organism. HCFC-22 is not mutagenic in yeast cell, hamster cell, or in vivo mouse and rat cell assays (dominant lethal and bone marrow cytogenic toxicity tests).
Teratogenicity:	Offspring born to rats exposed to 5% of HCFC-22 for six hours per day during pregnancy showed stunted growth and a small, but statistically significant, incidence of absent eyes. However, this dose level also caused maternal toxicity. An increased incidence of absent eyes did not occur in rabbits exposed at 5% of HCFC-22 and below or in rats at 1% of HCFC-22 and below where maternal toxicity was not observed.
Medical Conditions Generally Aggravated by Exposure:	Breathing difficulties, chest discomfort, headache, eye and nose membrane irritation.
Emergency and First Aid Procedures:	**Inhalation:** Remove to fresh air. Give oxygen. If not breathing, give artificial respiration. Keep victim quiet. Do not give stimulants. Get immediate medical attention. **Skin:** If frostbitten, warm skin slowly with water; otherwise, wash affected areas with soap and water. Remove contaminated clothing and launder before reuse. Remove wet foam immediately from skin with acetone or nail polish remover. Dried foam is hard to remove from skin. If foam dries on skin, apply generous amounts of petroleum jelly or lanolin, leave on for one hour, wash thoroughly, and repeat process until foam is removed. Do not attempt to remove dried foam with solvents. **Eye:** In case of eye contact, flush with water for 15 minutes. Get immediate medical attention. **Ingestion:** In case of ingestion, get immediate medical attention.

Product # 1

TABLE 1.11

Section VI — Spill or Leak Procedures	
In case material is released or spilled:	Soak up spill with absorbent material.
Waste Disposal Method:	Dispose of in accordance with all local, state, and federal regulations.

Product # 2

TABLE 1.12

Section VII — Precautions for Safe Handling and Use	
	Allow foam to cure (harden).
Waste Disposal:	Dispose according to federal, state, and local regulations.
Container Disposal:	Dispose of according to federal, state, and local regulations.
Storage:	Store in cool, dry place. Ideal storage temperature is 60 to 80° F. Storage above 90° F will shorten the shelf life. Do not store above 120° F (49° C). Protect containers from physical abuse. Do not store in auto or in direct sunlight. Store upright.

Product # 1

TABLE 1.13

Section VII — Special Protection Data	
Respiratory Protection:	None normally required
Ventilation:	None normally required
Protective Gloves:	None normally required
Other Protective Clothing or Equipment:	None normally required
Section VIII — Storage and Handling Data	
Precautions to be taken in handling and usage:	Store in original container; keep tightly closed. Do not reuse container for other purposes. KEEP OUT OF REACH OF CHILDREN.
Other precautions:	Read and observe all precautions on product label.

Product # 2

TABLE 1.14

Section VIII — Personal Protection	
Respiratory protection:	None required if in well-ventilated area.
Clothing:	Wear gloves, coveralls, long-sleeved shirt, and head covering to avoid skin contact. Contaminated equipment or clothing should be cleaned after each use or disposed of.
Eye protection:	Wear face shield, goggles, or safety glasses.
Ventilation:	If ventilation is not enough to maintain PEL, exhaust area.

General Cleanup

Household cleaning products are among the most toxic substances we encounter on a daily basis. It is ironic that our efforts to clean up often produce further contamination by spreading noxious fumes throughout the house. Moreover, these products end up down the drain, where they pollute air, soil, and water.

Most commercial cleaning products are made from synthetic chemicals derived from crude oil. Labeling laws and the Trade Secrets Act make it difficult to know exactly what is in any particular product. The product may contain highly toxic substances, but consumers have no way of knowing. Some of the harmful ingredients found in commercial cleaning products include phenol, toluene, naphthalene, pentachlorophenol, xylene, trichloroethylene, formaldehyde, benzene, perchlorethylene, other petroleum distillates, chlorinated substances, ethanol, fluorescent brighteners, artificial dyes, detergents, aerosol propellants, and artificial fragrances.

Commercial Cleaning Products

Professional strength formulas, which are even more dangerous than household cleaning products, are often used when residential construction cleanup is contracted out to janitorial service providers.

Green Seal is an independent nonprofit organization that has created environmental

CASE STUDY 1.2

Toxic Fumes from Cleaning Products

L. G. is a 53-year-old woman who was in reasonably good health until two years after she began working for a hotel as a housekeeper. At that time she consulted Dr. Elliott complaining of rashes, headaches, joint pain, and fatigue. After extensive questioning, Dr. Elliott concluded that the source of her symptoms was probably at her place of employment. Through a process of elimination, it became apparent that she had become sensitized to the pine-scented product she used to disinfect bathrooms. Although this woman was unable to convince her employer to switch to less toxic cleaning products, her symptoms improved when she was transferred to a different job within the same building.

Discussion

Certain strong-smelling cleaning products and disinfectants contain phenol, which is known to sensitize the immune system in some people, as happened to this unfortunate woman. When checking for phenol as an ingredient in a product, a generally safe rule of thumb is to look for any ingredient including phenol in its name or ending in "ol."

and health standards for industrial and institutional cleaners. Based on information provided by the manufacturers, Green Seal has recommended cleaners that meet the following criteria:[8]

- are not toxic to human or aquatic life
- are readily biodegradable
- contain VOC levels under 10 percent by weight when diluted for use
- are not made of petrochemical compounds or petroleum
- do not contain chlorine bleach
- are free of phosphates and derivatives
- do not contain phenolic compounds or glycol ethers
- are free of arsenic, cadmium, chromium, lead, mercury, nickel, and selenium
- have acceptable pH levels
- work optimally at room temperature

The following industrial/institutional strength cleaners are among those that are recommended by Green Seal[9] and that we have found to be reasonably available for use by contractors:

- **Earth Friendly Products**: A complete line of floor care, all-purpose, and specialty cleaners
- **ECO 2000**: A multipurpose cleaner and degreaser derived from naturally occurring, renewable, rapidly biodegradable resources (can be used from a 1:5 dilution as a degreaser and stripper all the way down to a 1:64 dilution as a window cleaner)
- **Enviro Care**: Cleaning products for all washable surfaces
- **Formula G-510**: A multi purpose concentrated colloidal cleaner/degreaser
- **Green Unikleen**: An industrial strength degreaser/cleaner
- **The Natural**: A complete line of naturally derived, fragrance-free cleaning products, with an all-purpose cleaner, a degreaser, and a bathtub and tile cleaner meeting Green Seal requirements

Household Cleaning Products

For normal household cleaning, several effective alternatives to harsh chemical cleaning compounds are available. The following brand-name cleaning products do not contain harsh chemicals:

- **AFM SafeChoice Glass Cleaner**: Virtually odorless glass, mirror, and hard surface cleaner
- **AFM SafeChoice Safety Clean**: Industrial strength cleaner/degreaser and disinfectant
- **AFM SafeChoice Super Clean**: All-purpose cleaner/degreaser
- **AFM SafeChoice X158**: Low-odor, antifungal, antibacterial treatment
- **Auro Awalan Line Cleaning and Care Products**: Full line of natural plant-based cleaning and care products
- **Auro Cleaning and Care Products**: Full line of natural plant-based cleaning and care products
- **Begley's Best**: Cradle to Cradle certified biodegradable all-purpose cleaner
- **BioShield**: A complete line of biodegradable, soap-based household cleaners containing natural and mostly organic ingredients

Maintaining a Healthy Home

BY ATHENA THOMPSON

So the much anticipated day finally arrives. After all these years of dreaming and endless months of planning, your new, healthy home is ready to move into. Now, most people would think that's the end of the story. Mission accomplished! Crack out the champagne! But it's actually a very important new beginning and one that is sadly overlooked by many people. You see, your home is essentially a living organism, and in order for it to remain as healthy and vibrant as when you first move in, you will need a long-term commitment to both occupy and maintain your home in a healthy manner.

Most people assume they already know how to do this. After all, they can arrange the furnishings; decorate or coordinate color schemes; clean their home and even make it smell nice; use the various appliances; and go to the nearest home improvement store if they need to fix something. Surely all this effort makes a home healthy? Unfortunately, most of the time it does not.

One of the most important factors that define whether a home is healthy or not is indoor air quality. If your new home has been built with health in mind, the indoor air quality will be free of the usual toxic chemical soup found in conventionally built new homes. However, it is possible to ruin a healthy home's indoor air quality (even within minutes of moving in) if you aren't aware of a few key facts.

Usually the first thing people do when they move into a new home is bring everything with them from their previous home, whether they need it or not. Let's take a look at how some of the most common items can ruin your healthy home's indoor air quality:

1. Old sofas and chairs made of polyurethane foam: The foam breaks down over time, releasing fine particulate matter into the air. This "dust" can contain chemicals such as toxic fire retardants and antimicrobials.
2. Furniture and household items impregnated with toxic cleaning products and synthetic fra-

- **Bio-Wash**: Environmentally friendly household cleaners
- **Bon Ami Polishing Cleanser**: Nonchlorine all-purpose scouring powder
- **Enviro Care**: Environmentally preferred green cleaning products, some Green Seal certified
- **Green**: Personal care cleaner; contains fragrance
- **KD Gold**: All-purpose biodegradable natural soap
- **Mystical**: Odorless cleaner and deodorizer
- **Naturally Yours**: A complete line of "eco-nomological" household and personal cleaning products
- **Spectracidal Disinfectant Agent**: An EPA approved nontoxic germicide
- **Trewax Nature's Orange**: Scientific Certification Systems certified biodegradable cleaner/degreaser; contains citrus oils
- **Trewax Neutral Cleaner**: Scientific Certification Systems certified biodegradable all-purpose cleaner for no-wax floors, marble, terrazzo, pavers, etc. (not for unfinished wood floors)
- **Wow!**: Scientific Certification Systems certified biodegradable stainless steel cleaner

grance: These items will outgas chemicals into the air around them, often indefinitely.

3. Fragranced laundry products: These products may be loaded with petrochemicals and are frequently a major source of unhealthy indoor air quality. Not only do these products outgas in your laundry but as soon as you start laundering your clothes, towels, and bedding your whole house may also become polluted. I know many people love the smell of their dryer sheets, but just remember those are synthetic chemicals you are smelling, not real fragrance. Many of these chemicals have never been tested for their effects on human health.
4. Cleaning products: Like laundry products, many of these contain synthetic fragrances as well as a host of other toxic chemicals that will outgas into the air and leave an invisible chemical coating on all the surfaces with which they come in contact.
5. Pillows, duvets, and blankets: These are often full of dust mites and their feces, another indoor polluter and common allergen.
6. Old paints, adhesives, stains and finishes, garden and home pesticide products, car maintenance products, and a whole array of miscellaneous products people tend to store in the dark recesses of their cupboards and their garage: These products will frequently outgas even with their lids or caps in place and may pose a serious poisoning risk around small children and pets.

Moving into a new home often requires buying a few new things too. Everything from mattresses to curtains to furniture made of particleboard now contains staggering amounts of chemicals, many known to cause everything from cancer to reproductive harm. All these products will outgas vigorously when new and ruin your home's indoor air quality.

and protectant with no petroleum distillates

Common Household Products That Clean

The following common household products may also be used for cleaning:

- **Baking soda** cleans, deodorizes, scours, and softens water. It is noncorrosive and slightly abrasive and is effective for light cleaning.
- **Borax** cleans, deodorizes, disinfects, and softens water. It is also effective for light cleaning, for soiled laundry in the washing machine, and for preventing mold growth.
- **Hydrogen peroxide** (H_2O_2) is effective in removing mold stains from nonporous surfaces. Purchase a 10 percent food-grade solution. (The solution most commonly sold off the shelf is only 3 percent.) Use protective gloves to apply. A 10 percent solution will bleach many types of surfaces. A 35 percent food-grade H_2O_2 is available through many health food stores. The container must be refrigerated and kept clean. The 35 percent solution will burn skin and must be carefully diluted before it can be safely used.
- **Soap** (as opposed to detergents) biodegrades safely and completely. It is an effective and gentle cleaner with many uses. For hands, dishes, laundry, and light cleaning,

---

As you can see, this combination of old and new household items can quickly ruin all your efforts to create a healthy home. The good news is that much of this damage can be prevented. Here's some advice:

1. Replace old, worn furniture with new items made of natural materials, such as natural latex foam instead of polyurethane foam, and fabrics without flame retardants and other chemical treatments. If this isn't within your budget, at least give your furniture a good vacuuming outdoors and if possible let it sit outside in fresh air and sunshine for a few hours. Wipe furniture down with either a damp microfiber cloth or a mild solution of acceptable soap and water to remove old cleaning product residues. Vinegar may also help remove certain alkaline residues such as soap films. It shouldn't be mixed with the soap but should be used separately. Replace particleboard furniture with solid wood items free of toxic finishes and adhesives and whenever possible choose certified wood.
2. Replace laundry products with healthier, nonfragranced ones. If you want your laundry to smell good, the best remedy is to hang it outside in the sunshine for a while. Many laundry products simply are not needed.
3. Replace cleaning products with nontoxic ones or make your own from common kitchen ingredients such as baking soda or vinegar. (Don't mix these two together since they are a mild alkali and an acid that will neutralize each other's cleaning effectiveness.)
4. Microfiber cloths often eliminate the need for any cleaning product at all.
5. If you need a vacuum cleaner, make sure it's a HEPA model. Conventional vacuum cleaners miss and recirculate about 70 percent of fine dust particles.

use the pure bar or soap flakes without perfume additives.

- **TSP** (trisodium phosphate) can be used according to the manufacturer's instructions for grease removal. TSP is available in hardware stores. Surfaces cleaned with TSP should be neutralized with baking soda prior to the application of finishes. Fluids containing TSP should not be disposed of in septic systems or sewer systems because of their high phosphate content.
- **Vodka** is effective for dissolving alcohol-soluble finishes. Use a high-proof (high alcohol content) product.
- **Washing soda** (sodium carbonate) cuts grease, removes stains, disinfects, and softens water. It is effective for washing heavily soiled laundry and for general cleaning.
- **White vinegar** cuts grease and removes lime deposits. A safe and useful all-purpose cleaning solution can be made from distilled white vinegar and plain water in a 50:50 ratio. For window cleaning, add five tablespoons of white vinegar to two cups of water. The solution should be placed in a glass spray bottle. Glass is preferred because plastics are known to release hormone-disrupting chemicals into bottle contents. Vinegar has been used to clean and control mold growth, but the thin film of residue left on the surface may supply nutrients for new growth.

6. Avoid fragranced air fresheners of all kinds.
7. As your budget allows, replace bedding with naturally dust mite resistant organic wool pillows, duvets, and blankets. Mattresses made of true natural latex are also dust mite resistant. Organic cotton pillowcases, sheets, and duvet covers are well worth the investment when you can afford them.
8. Develop the habit of reading labels. Don't bring any product into your home that contains the words "warning," "danger," or "poison." If in doubt, err on the side of caution and find a safer option.

Over time, situations may arise that need special attention. If you plan to decorate, remodel, or make repairs, you will need to plan ahead to be sure to make the healthiest choices. In case of any unexpected problems, be sure to get them resolved immediately. For example, if you have a burst pipe, dry the area out quickly, hiring qualified professionals, so there is no time for mold to grow.

Understanding how to live in and maintain your home for optimum health is as important as building your home correctly in the first place. With these basic ideas, you can protect the health of your whole family, including pets, and avoid the ever-increasing list of problems associated with living and sleeping in an unhealthy home. May you never know what you have prevented!

Athena Thompson is a certified Building Biology Practitioner. A natural health specialist for over 20 years, she focuses on environmental health, specializing in children's health issues. She is the author of the popular book *Homes That Heal (and those that don't): How Your Home May be Harming Your Family's Health* and cofounder of **Humabuilt** — Healthy Building Solutions.

Contract Close-Out

Once construction is complete and before a home is handed over from the contractor to the owner, various tests should be run on the building. This testing provides the opportunity for tuning and adjusting various systems and either assures that the building is operating as intended or detects errors and omissions in the building system so that the contractor or appropriate subcontractor can correct them prior to occupation. This also provides an opportunity for the contractor to do a walk-through with the owner to explain how the systems work and how the owner needs to maintain and monitor them.

Throughout this book we suggest various tests that the owner may wish to include as part of the contract, to be conducted either by the contractor and his subcontractors or by a third party. Some of these are:

- testing for air leakage in the HVAC system
- pressure balancing of HVAC or start-up and balancing of radiant floor heating
- cycling all appliances
- testing for magnetic fields
- testing air and water quality
- blower door tests to determine if there is sufficient air tightness in the finished building

We also suggest that the owner obtain various documents from the contractor including:

- photo documentation of the building process showing location of utility trenches, electrical wiring, plumbing piping, blocking in the walls, and any other pertinent information that has been covered up in the finished home
- an owner's manual containing equipment, material, and labor warranties, schedules for required maintenance, contact numbers for major subcontractors, and certificates of inspection and occupancy
- "as-built" drawings, which are marked-up copies of the original drawings, and specifications indicating any changes that have been made in the course of construction and locating any pertinent information that was not on the original documents (refer to the section on occupant education in the Overview chapter)

Further Reading

Ashford, Nicholas and Claudia Miller. *Chemical Exposures: Low Levels and High Stakes.* 2nd ed., John Wiley and Sons, 1998. A scientific discussion of the mechanisms underlying chemical sensitivities.

Bower, Lynn Marie. *The Healthy Household.* Healthy House Institute, 1995. Contains a useful section on household cleansers.

Dadd, Debra Lynn. *Nontoxic, Natural and Earthwise.* J.P. Tarcher, 1990. Has a good selection of alternatives to toxic cleaning products.

Lab Safety Supply, Inc. *Preparing, Understanding, and Using Material Safety Data Sheets.* This booklet can be obtained from Lab Safety Supply, Inc. at 800-356-0783.

McDonough, William and Michael Braungart. *Cradle to Cradle: Remaking the Way We Make Things.* North Point Press, 2002. Described on their website as "a manifesto calling for the transformation of human industry through ecologically intelligent design."

Wilson, Cynthia. *Chemical Exposure and Human Health.* McFarland, 1993. A reference to 314 chemicals, with a guide to symptoms. We use this handy guide to supplement information from the MSDS.

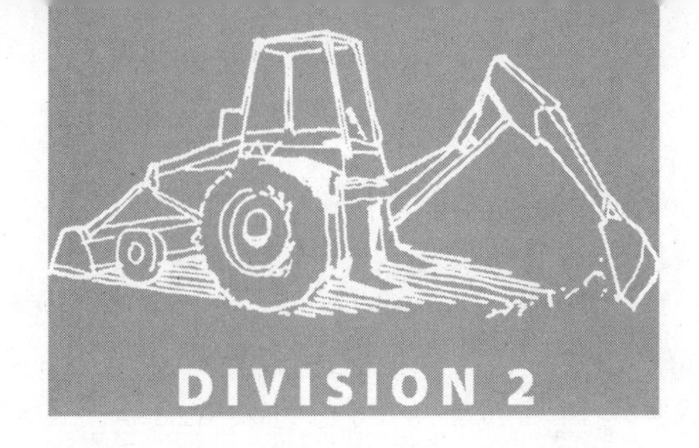

Site Work

Introduction

This Division contains information on site selection and on site maintenance and restoration during the construction process.

Site Selection

Long before construction begins, you will choose the appropriate site. When the ancient Romans selected a site for housing, they paid careful attention to the health-giving qualities of the land. To test a potential homesite, cattle were confined to graze in the area for a specific period of time, after which they were slaughtered and the innards examined. If the animals had unhealthy livers, the site was abandoned.

Unfortunately, the health consequences from the natural conditions of almost any site today pale in comparison to the potential hazards created by humans. Keep the following guidelines in mind when choosing a site:

- Choose a location where the air is relatively unpolluted.
- Evaluate levels of light and noise pollution.
- Determine the direction that prevailing winds blow and how they change seasonally. Consider what is upwind from you.
- Avoid industrial areas, power plants, agricultural lands with heavy pesticide use, and other major pollution producers.
- Avoid proximity to high-voltage power lines, microwave relay stations, and cellular phone and broadcast towers. In general, distances of one-tenth mile from high-voltage power lines and one-half mile from microwave cellular and broadcast towers are adequate. Many public utilities will provide free site measurements for background electromagnetic field levels. Ensure that measurements are taken at a time when power lines in the area are operating at peak load, or have the field calculated based on peak load projections. Utility companies should provide this information in writing.

- Avoid sites adjacent to parking lots and traffic corridors.
- Crest locations generally have better air quality and more air movement than valley sites.
- If you are considering a site in a populated area, analyze the present use and future development of your neighborhood. How are nearby empty lots zoned? Do the neighbors use pesticides? Is there smoke from woodstoves and fireplaces in the winter?
- Investigate water quality in the area.

Professional Assistance in Site Selection

You may require assistance in selecting your site, especially when remedies to suspected

Earth Energies: Choosing the Right Site

J. DAVID MCAULEY

Choosing a site that avoids hazardous pollutants and then building with healthy materials are vital for creating a healthy home. The naturally occurring Earth energies, known as geopathic stress, are another important factor to consider. These energies result from polar magnetism, underground domes, veins and streams of water, radon gas emissions, electromagnetic waves, and seismic activity. Their effects can be seen in rock faults, fissures and geological stresses, power spots, vortices, mineral and ore deposits, and underground caves.

Their health effects can range from subtle to severe, with some being well accepted and others less recognized and sometimes controversial. California prohibits new construction over earthquake faults, and the US Environmental Protection Agency recommends that all homes be checked for radon gas emissions. Switzerland and Germany have mandated testing for geopathic stress before hospitals, schools, and multifamily dwellings are constructed.

Increasingly, the human body is also subjected to the effects of artificially produced electromagnetic forces. These result from mining, building foundations, excavations, underground transportation, sewers, water pipes, communication systems, electrical generation, and transmission infrastructure as well as microwaves, satellites, radar, cell phones, and wireless technologies.

In the 1940s, German researchers Ernest Hartmann and Manfred Curry identified a tightly woven network of magnetically charged, naturally occurring energy lines crisscrossing the Earth and penetrating buildings. When geopathic stress is combined with human-caused stress conditions over a prolonged period of time, our health can be profoundly affected.

Our five senses pick up an infinitesimal part of the spectrum of information about these stresses. In the past, known locations with high levels of naturally occurring harmful Earth forces were avoided. Indigenous people were aware of places where subtle energies supported the abundant growth of plants and trees and the health of animals. We are all familiar with special places that make us feel comfortable, warm, or inspired. Similarly, when we walk into other spaces we become disturbed, cold, or restless. Over time, the places where we live and work will have an impact on our health.

Our understanding of these subtle health effects is growing. According to the Dulwich Health Clinic in London, geopathic stress is present in

problems may be costly. Industrial toxins in the soil, poor percolation for installing a septic system, and unstable soils are examples of conditions that might be causes for concern. We recommend that you make your offer to purchase contingent on inspections by professional consultants. In this way you can prevent being obligated to purchase a contaminated or otherwise unacceptable site. The following sections describe some of the more common consultant specialties.

Phase I Environmental Inspector

If you are considering a property with a past of industrial or agricultural use or underground fuel tanks, or if old buildings are suspected of containing lead or asbestos, then a Phase I environmental audit should be conducted to

people with most types of serious and long-term illnesses. "Geopathic stress does not cause any specific type of illness but lowers your immune system and your ability to fight off viruses and bacteria."[a]

In 1989, Otto Bergsmann found measurable changes in levels of serotonin, melatonin, calcium, and zinc when a person was subjected to noxious Earth energy emissions.[b] Hans Nieper concluded that the incidence of cancer was higher over geopathic zones: "Geopathic zones increase the risk of gene lability," or genetic errors. He strongly advised those suffering from these ill effects to remove themselves from the site of geopathogenic exposure.[c]

Kathe Bachler has linked children's poor school performance to geopathogenic "interference zones."[d] After investigating noxious geopathic lines and chronic fatigue syndrome in 14,000 cases, Alf Riggs concluded that geopathic stress is a major factor in 72 percent of cases of the syndrome and that measurable improvement occurred when a patient's bed was moved to a neutral location. There was even more improvement when a wooden bed was substituted for a metal bed and mattress springs.[e]

Other physical indicators have included:

- sleep disorders (strong resistance to going to bed, insomnia, nightmares, sleepwalking, sweating, cold/shivers, waking feeling tired/unrested, waking feeling nauseous)
- an aversion to lying in certain spots in one's bed
- experiencing a feeling of falling out of bed
- depression, stress, rapid heart rate, or cramps

Some physicians suggest that, if symptoms do not respond to normally successful treatments, Earth energies may exist in their patient's home.

Conventional electronic scientific instruments can be used to indicate zones of geopathic stress by measuring parameters such as conductivity of the ground and air, DC magnetic fields, changes to air ionization, ground temperature, above-normal soil or air humidity, and seismic activity. These sophisticated instruments are expensive and not generally usable by the public.

Plant life and animal behavior can indicate areas of geopathic stress. Cats, bees, and ants are drawn to these areas. Cattle, horses, sheep, pigs, swallows, chickens, and dogs avoid them. In traditional cultures, animals were herded onto building

identify the risks. Remember that up-front costs are minor compared to hazardous waste cleanup costs, which may far exceed property value.

Geotechnical Consultant

If you are concerned about the geological structure of the site, you should consult with a geotechnical engineer, who will be able to troubleshoot problems such as high water tables, unstable soils, expansive soils, earthquake faults, and sink holes. Engineering solutions can be devised for many of these problems so that the costs of development can be determined before you purchase the land.

Septic Engineer

In many locations where municipal sewers are not available, an engineered septic system plan is required before a building permit will be issued. The septic engineer, who is often a geotechnical engineer as well, will study the

---

sites and their behavior was observed to ensure avoidance of geopathic stress. Oak, ash, elm, and willow trees thrive in areas of high geopathic stress whereas fruit trees do not. Trees can also be observed to see if they lean, twist, or grow knurls.

Lightning has been reported to strike where underground water veins cross and geopathic stress appears to be more prevalent in areas of exposed fractured igneous or sedimentary rock and less common in areas with a thick overburden of gravel or soil. Clay soils seem to accentuate the stress. Even observation of buildings can be useful since cracks, moisture, mold, crumbling plaster, discoloration and damaged materials in existing construction, and patterns of alignment or deterioration of stone, masonry, concrete, or pavement correspond to areas of geopathic stress and can indicate its presence.

For centuries, dowsers or diviners have located water veins, energy grids, and points of elevated energy (power spots). Levels of skill and techniques for assessing, locating, and correcting these forces vary considerably, but results are reported to be consistent among experienced practitioners.

Geopathic stress can be reduced or reversed, but the most important corrective measure is avoidance. Architects and designers should take land energies into account and avoid them when siting buildings. In its top 25 principles, Building Biology considers geobiology in the process of selecting building sites and materials. It recommends avoiding certain materials such as steel structural frames, metal furniture, electrical wiring, and ductwork, which conduct and transmit Earth energies throughout a building.

Various correction techniques and devices have been proposed. Individual research and testing by experienced practitioners is recommended to ensure that any corrective measures are effective and do not have any unhealthy consequences.

Choosing building sites with a balanced quality can positively influence our health. It is not a good idea to spend extended time in negatively stressed areas or to inhabit places of high energetic activity. Pay attention to how you feel on a potential building site. Applying information about Earth energies known from ancient universal practices will have a profound effect on our health and well-being in our homes and workplaces.

Further information:

land formation and perform percolation tests to determine how the sewage waste projected for your development can best be handled. In areas with limited percolation, steep slopes, or high water tables, the installation of a proper septic system could be costly or even impossible. If such conditions exist, it is best to be informed prior to purchasing the land.

Water Quality Specialist

If a site lacks water, it is important to determine the cost of obtaining it. If the site is served by the local municipality, the water company may be able to give you an estimate. If the site is rocky, you may need to excavate trenches by blasting the surrounding rock. If you must drill a well, the neighbors or the local well driller can inform you of the depth of surrounding wells and give you information about water quality. If the site already contains a well, ensure that the submersible pump was manufactured after 1979, or that it is safe. If the

The American Society of Dowsers Inc., dowsers.org
BioGeometry, biogeometry.com and vesica.org
The British Society of Dowsers, geomancy.org
The Canadian Society of Dowsers, canadiandowsers.org
The Canadian Society of Questers, questers.ca
International Institute for Bau-Biology & Ecology, buildingbiology.net
Pyramid School of Feng Shui, Nancilee Wydra, fengshuibydesignonline.com

a. Information provided by Dulwich Health and available at dulwichhealth.co.uk.
b. Alf Riggs. "Harmful Effects from Earth Radiation & Electrical Fields" [online]. [Cited December 19, 2007.] whale.to/v/riggs1.html
c. Hans Nieper. "Modern Medical Cancer Therapy Following the Decline of Toxic Chemotherapy." *Townsend Letter for Doctors & Patients*. November 1996, pp. 88-89. *Dr. Nieper's Revolution in Technology, Medicine and Society.* MIT Verlag, 1985, pp. 206, 222. Lecture notes from a medical seminar in Los Angeles, July 4, 1986, pp. 13–15, 22, 28, available from Brewer Science Library, mwt.net/~drbrewer/other.htm. See also Hans A. Nieper et al. *The Curious Man: The Life and Works of Dr. Hans Nieper.* Avery, 1998.
d. Kathe Bachler. "Noxious Earth Energies and Their Influence on Human Beings" [online]. [Cited December 19, 2007.] whale.to/v/bachler.html. See also Kathe Bachler. *Discoveries of a Dowser.* 5th ed., Veritas, 1984 and Kathe Bachler. *Earth Radiation.* Wordmasters, 1989.
e. Alf Riggs. "Myalgic Encephalomyelitis" [online]. [Cited December 19, 2007.] alfredriggs.com

J. David McAuley has practiced architecture in Canada for 29 years using Building Biology, feng shui, and Earth energy dowsing. He is currently studying BioGeometry. David designs buildings to support health in balance with the environment, including sacred spaces, healing retreat centers, and socially conscious spaces for those in need. He can be contacted at 519-823-2441 or jdm-arch.com.

oils in older pumps contain PCBs, they represent a serious health threat should a rupture occur. Whatever the source of potable water, it should be tested by a professional and filtered or purified as required. Water quality will be discussed further in Division 11.

Site Clearing

Although it is more convenient for a contractor to build on a site without obstacles such as trees, native vegetation, and boulders, some but not all contractors will go to great lengths to preserve as much natural vegetation and as many other landscape features as possible. Do not assume that the preservation of your site will be a priority of the same magnitude for a contractor as it will be for you. To clarify your desires and the contractual obligations of the contractor in this regard, you can formalize site preservation intentions by stating them as part of your contract.

Here is an example of site specifications created for the purpose of preserving the natural features of the site and preventing pest infestations as a result of the clearing process.

It is the owner's intention to preserve the natural vegetation and land features of the site to the greatest extent possible.

- **The owner and architect shall approve the site layout prior to the digging of the footings.**
- **Topsoil and large boulders shall be stockpiled for future use.**
- **All trees designated for removal from the building site are to be marked for review by the owner or architect.**
- **All tree stumps and dead foliage shall be fully removed from around and under the building site and disposed of offsite so they do not attract termites and other pests.**
- **The owner and architect shall determine which trees are to be transplanted or maintained during construction.**
- **The construction area and access to it shall be as small as is reasonable to facilitate construction of the home. This area is to be clearly demarcated and roped off to prevent any destruction of natural terrain outside the area by construction vehicles.**

Grading

Many mold problems originate with poor drainage around the building perimeter, which can cause water to puddle against the building and sometimes to seep inside. Although less prevalent in dry climates, mold is still a serious health threat, especially in flat-roof construction where canales or scuppers are used for roof drainage and erosion around the discharge is common. An adequate roof overhang will be the first line of defense in keeping water away from the building envelope. Good site grading will be the second line of defense and a perimeter drainage system in combination with stem wall dampproofing as described in Division 7 will constitute the third component of a comprehensive rainwater management plan. The following specification for surface water runoff management is recommended:

- **Water shall have positive drainage away from the building at all points along its perimeter. Ground shall slope away at a minimum of 5 percent and soil used to grade around the building shall be of an impervious nature with high clay content.**

- **All canales, scuppers, and downspouts shall have splash blocks and an adequate drainage path away from the building.**

Soil Treatment

Sometimes the soils under brick walkways, under interior brick pavers, surrounding the structure, or under the structure itself are treated with insecticides or herbicides. This practice should be avoided. Many people have become sensitive to very low levels of pesticide exposure. Children are especially vulnerable. Some harmful agents will remain potent long after the building is gone. Where soil treatment is mandated or otherwise unavoidable, we recommend the use of boric acid, diatomaceous soil, or other least toxic measures. (Refer to the section on integrated pest management in Division 10.) You may wish to specify the following:

- **Do not treat soil with manufactured chemical treatments.**
- **Treat sand surfaces under floors and brick or stone walkways with diatomaceous soil. Inhaling dust from diatomaceous soil is hazardous and proper precaution should be used during application.**
- **Use barrier cloth under exterior walkways to prevent weed overgrowth.**

Pavement

Petroleum tar, which is the main component of asphalt or "blacktop" paving, is carcinogenic and should be avoided. Not only does it emit harmful vapors during installation but it also will volatilize when heated by the sun. More healthful options include concrete slab, concrete or brick pavers, and paving stone or gravel over a well-drained and compacted base.

The following products are innovative ways to stabilize a road base without the use of asphalt or concrete paving:

- **NaturalPAVE XL Resin Pavement**: A combination of nontoxic, environmentally friendly organic and inorganic resin materials that creates a high- strength pavement.
- **Perma-Zyme**: A biodegradable and environmentally safe road stabilization enzyme product that works by lowering the surface tension of water, promoting penetration and dispersal of moisture. This causes hydrated clay particles to fill voids in soil so that it forms a tight, dense, and permanent stratum.
- **Stabilizer**: A colorless, odorless psyllium-based concentrated powdered soil additive for dirt or crushed stone surfaces. Stabilizer binds and flocks aggregate screenings to provide a firm natural surface for pathways, trails, and driveways.

Where asphalt paving already exists or is the only paving option available **AFM DynoSeal Driveway/Asphalt Sealer** may be used. It is a low-odor elastomeric sealer and top coating for asphalt surfaces that helps to reduce the outgassing and odors generated by new asphalt.

Further Reading

International Institute for Bau-Biologie & Ecology. Home study courses, online study, and seminars. PO Box 387, Clearwater, FL 33757, 727-461-4371, buildingbiology.net.

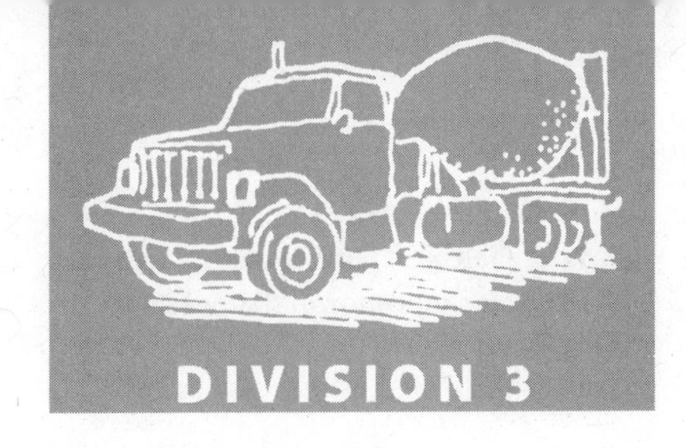

Concrete

Introduction

Concrete is widely used in residential construction for footings, stem walls, and exposed basement flooring, as a subfloor for slab-on-grade construction, and as a finished floor material. Concrete consists of cement (usually Portland cement), water, and sand and other aggregates.

Once cured, concrete becomes an inert product and is not usually associated with toxic exposure, although there may be some more subtle health effects. (Refer to the essay by George Swanson to learn more about these effects and about products that can be substituted for Portland cement.) Certain common construction practices can make concrete harmful to human health and should be avoided. These practices are discussed in the following sections.

Components of Concrete

Cement

Cement is the "glue" that holds the various components of concrete together and comprises approximately 18 percent of the concrete by volume. Concrete is high in embodied energy because of the tremendous heat required to make cement. Cements are often advertised as "green" because they substitute a waste product for Portland cement. The replacement of Portland cement with fly ash has become a common practice. However, fly ash can be a byproduct of the incineration of toxic or hazardous waste. We therefore believe that cement products containing fly ash should be used only if it can be determined that it is derived from a nonhazardous source.

Although it is difficult to build a home today without the use of some concrete, there are many strategies, discussed throughout the book, that we can employ to reduce our use of Portland cement.

Water

Clean, potable water should be specified for mixing concrete:

- **Water shall be of potable quality, free of taste, color, and odor, and should not foam or fizzle.**

Aggregate

The aggregate component accounts for 60 to 80 percent of concrete volume. The size and characteristics of the aggregate will affect the quantities of cement and water required and the compressive strength, weight, and surface character of the finished concrete. Aggregate materials range in size from fine sand to crushed rock pieces. Sometimes recycled materials are used as aggregate and these may be a source of contamination. Recycled industrial waste products may contain hydrocarbons and sulfur. If the source is an industrial process with residual heavy metals or toxic compounds, it can result in a product with toxic properties.

Magnesium-Based Cements

GEORGE SWANSON

Before the widespread use of Portland cement, magnesium oxide-based cements were among the world's most popular cement products. By the late 19th century, the use of Portland cement had spread around the world. Although Portland cement has now essentially cornered the market, it has some inherent drawbacks when compared to the magnesium oxide-based cements used by our ancestors. Portland cement manufacturers are currently allocating enormous R&D funding to overcoming deficiencies that impact the environment, human health, and the strength, durability, and usability of Portland cement. Billions of dollars are being spent in an effort to make Portland cement do what magnesium phosphate- and magnesium oxychloride-based cements do naturally.

No one ever purposely set out to make a problematic cement; quite the opposite. When Joseph Aspdin invented his water-activated Portland cement in his Leeds, England, kitchen in 1824, it seemed to be a viable and exciting advance in addressing the needs of the Industrial Revolution, which was hungry for construction materials. His new product was convenient to use and the raw materials to make it were in abundant supply.

Portland cement is created by heating raw materials to 2,700 degrees Fahrenheit to create clinkers. It is common knowledge that the worldwide production of Portland cement, which is increasing at a rate of 5 percent annually, currently creates as much as 12 percent of the greenhouse gas emissions responsible for global warming.

Some of the most harmful effects of concrete made with Portland cement come when it is "enhanced" with plastics. The concrete never cures, or does so extremely slowly, which may enhance the strength of the concrete but not the health of a building's occupants. Furthermore, concrete treated with these plastics outgasses and is toxic, particularly when it is mixed with mold. The high temperatures used in the production of Portland cement make it extremely thirsty for water (hydrophilic), causing a number of problems including the promotion of mold growth.

In many buildings today, 50 to 90 percent by weight of a solid concrete envelope is involved in holding up its own "dead weight." In the future, the

Other recycled materials such as crushed brick are highly absorbent and may have been exposed to atmospheric pollutants prior to being used in concrete. Aggregate that is free of toxins and acquired odors should be specified as follows:

- **Only clean, natural mineral aggregates are acceptable. The following are unacceptable aggregates: crushed brick, crushed sandstone, crushed concrete slag, fly ash (unless it is possible to verify that it contains no heavy metals or toxic substances), cinder, and volcanic material (other than pumice). The contractor shall verify the aggregate content with the concrete supplier prior to pouring.**

Admixtures

Many different types of admixtures may be added to the concrete mix to modify various

use of ultra-high-strength magnesium oxide cements could reduce the use of structural cement materials significantly, thereby increasing the percentage of more insulative, nonstructural infill elements and creating far more energy-efficient envelopes.

Magnesium cements have consistently proven to be superior to Portland cement in strength, versatility, and environmental integrity. Yet until recently magnesium cements had virtually fallen into disuse over the past 175 years. A brief history of magnesium cements will explain why these ancient building materials are of such great historic importance and, more importantly, why they may now hold the key to the future of worldwide sustainable building practices. This cement alternative (often called ceramic cement) provides unique advantages over Portland cement.

Blends of magnesium oxide were used in ancient times in Germany, France, Mexico and Latin America, Switzerland, India, China, and New Zealand, among other countries. The Great Wall of China and many of the stupas in India, still standing today, were made with magnesium-based cements. Ancient European artisans used a timber frame with magnesium oxide infill in constructing homes. No gaps are visible in the 800-year-old walls that remain in use.

Magnesium deposits exist in abundance in every corner of the Earth and cover roughly 8 percent of its surface. Depending on where they are mined, magnesium oxide cements require only 20 to 40 percent of the energy used to produce Portland cement.

Magnesium-based cements have exceptional health-promoting properties for the occupants of homes in which they are used as a building material. For example, research at Argonne National Laboratories has documented that occupants of homes made with traditional cow dung and magnesium oxide located right next to the Chernobyl nuclear power plant had less radiation sickness from the nuclear accident than any other group. Occupants of modern stud frame and concrete homes, even miles away, succumbed at higher rates to radiation sickness.

These natural cements bind exceptionally well to all things cellulose (such as plant fibers

properties. For example, air entrainment admixtures disperse air bubbles throughout the concrete to improve resistance to freezing and thawing. Water reducing admixtures decrease the amount of water required. Retarders and accelerators modify the setting time of concrete. Super plasticizers allow for lower water to cement ratios. They frequently contain sulfonated melamine, formaldehyde condensates, sulfonated naphthalene, and other potentially harmful ingredients.

Water reducing agents and air entrainment admixtures are frequently added to concrete mixtures even when not specifically requested. The exact ingredients of an admixture are usually proprietary. Although admixtures generally make up a very small portion of the concrete and do not pose a significant problem to any but the most sensitive individuals, they can be completely eliminated if concrete work is scheduled for warm weather and if the concrete supplier is aware of this requirement. Even with admixtures, concrete must never be poured on frozen soil or when there is a risk

and wood chips) and are often referred to as living cements. Although the cost of magnesium oxide cement is currently considerably higher than that of Portland cement, a wide variety of indigenous rock, plant and wood fibers, and other cellulose granules can be added to it as aggregate, extending the basic cement material by up to 95 percent and thereby reducing its cost. This is in sharp contrast to Portland cement, which repels cellulose.

Magnesium-based cements commonly achieve compressive strengths of 9,000 to 45,000 pounds per square inch and tension strength of over 800 pounds per square inch, many times stronger than conventional concrete. Combined with clays and cellulose, magnesium oxide forms cements that "breathe" water vapors, a significant plus. The clay in magnesium oxide balances and enhances the movement of moisture. The material never rots because it always expels moisture.

Magnesium-based cements are completely nonconductive of electricity, as well as heat and cold, and have been used for flooring for radar stations and hospital operating rooms.

Until the early 1930s almost all terrazzo floors were made with magnesium phosphate or magnesium oxychloride. These materials were used extensively throughout the United States until Portland cement offered what appeared at the time to be a less costly, more user-friendly alternative. The successful manufacture, marketing, and proliferation of Portland cement occurred at a time when energy was cheap and public awareness of environmental health concerns was virtually nonexistent.

Recently magnesium-based products have become available from several sources:

Argonne National Laboratory (anl.gov) and others have now licensed firms to market magnesium-based cements under the name Ceramicrete. These companies have patents on their products. US Gypsum, the original American maker of Portland cement, is also introducing magnesium oxide as a nontoxic accelerant and additive. Aquacast is one magnesium oxide product being marketed by US Gypsum.

Grancrete, a spray-on structural cement, has been developed by scientists at Argonne National Laboratory and Casa Grande LLC as one of

that frost may penetrate under the slab while it cures. If you wish to avoid additives, you must specify this. The following is a sample specification:

- **No admixtures shall be used in the concrete. It is the contractor's responsibility to comply with the necessary climatic parameters so that required strengths and finishes are obtained without additives. Verify with the supplier that all concrete is free of admixtures, including air entrainment and water reducing agents, accelerants, and retardants. Air entrainment is acceptable for garage slabs.**

Slab Reinforcement

Metal throughout a structure can contribute to electropollution (see Division 16). Placing a mesh of welded wire fabric within a concrete slab to help prevent cracking is common, but this practice can distribute unwanted voltage throughout the home. Several types of

the modern applications of a magnesium oxide-based cement. According to a paper by Argonne (anl.gov, search for "Grancrete"), Grancrete is "a tough new ceramic material that is almost twice as strong as concrete [and] may be the key to providing high-quality, low-cost housing throughout developing nations."

The Bindan Company in Chicago (bindancorp.com) makes twelve different products with magnesium oxide. Their magnesium oxide/phosphate cements and concretes are some of the strongest ever tested.

A useful application of magnesium oxide is four- by eight-foot panels imported from China and known commercially as Strong-Enviro Board, Dragonboard, and MagBoard. These panels are commonly available in many standard US thicknesses from ⅛ to ¾ inch and can fully take the place of plywood, OSB, and drywall in virtually all construction applications. The fiber-reinforced sheets typically meet all UL, ASTM, and ICC requirements as replacements for conventional interior and exterior sheeting materials. They have a two- to four-hour fire rating, depending on the thickness, are 100 percent nontoxic, and produce no toxic gases if they burn. More information can be obtained from the manufacturers' websites, strongenviroboard.com, dragonboard.com, and mag-board.com.

George Swanson holds a Bachelor of Science degree in industrial design from Western Washington University (1975) and is a graduate of the International Institute of Bau-Biologie & Ecology (1992). His firm, Swanson Associates, specializes in the design of healthy and ecological structures using a variety of alternative wall systems. He is currently involved in product development in China and in the importing, distributing, and application of magnesium oxide-based building materials. See geoswan.com.

approved nonmetallic reinforcing fibers are now readily available to do the same job with very little or no increase in cost. Check with local code officials to determine acceptability in your jurisdiction. If wire mesh reinforcing is being excluded, you should add the following specification:

- **Slab reinforcing shall be ½" fiberglass or polypropylene fibers as manufactured by Fibermesh 650 or Novomesh or equal.**

Stem Wall Reinforcement

Steel bars are placed in footings and stem walls to reinforce the concrete. In situations where the ground is higher than the floor level, such as in a basement or behind a retaining wall, steel reinforcing is also present, often at horizontal and vertical intervals of 12 inches or less.

If an owner wishes to eliminate large amounts of conductive metal from structures, it is possible to use fiberglass reinforcing bars. These rebars were originally designed for bridge construction because they do not rust, corrode, or dissolve from galvanic action. Because fiberglass rebar cannot be bent onsite and must be preordered, you should plan well in advance if you wish to use this product. It can be ordered through **Tillco** or **V-rod**. If you plan to use fiberglass rebar, ask your local code enforcement officials prior to purchase whether they will accept a particular product. We have used fiberglass rebar successfully in a few homes but have found it to be expensive and inconvenient. You also can reduce electric fields by grounding metal rebar, but the presence of the metal can still provide a potential pathway for stray magnetic fields.

Form Release Agents

Concrete formwork is usually coated with release agents so that it can be easily removed and reused once concrete has cured. Although many inert products may be used for this purpose, diesel fuel and other equally noxious substances are commonly used because they are least expensive and readily available. These practices should not be allowed in a healthy house and we suggest the following be specified:

- **The use of petroleum-based form oil as a release agent is prohibited. The following are acceptable for use as form release agents:**
  - **Non-rancid vegetable oil or an acceptable paint specified in Division 9**
  - **Bioform: 100 percent biodegradable form release agent, environmentally safe, VOC compliant, does not freeze**
  - **Crete-Lease: Very low-odor, non-toxic, nonflammable, biodegradable spray-on concrete form release agent**
  - **ELM Concrete Form Release WS: Very low-odor, nontoxic, biodegradable spray-on concrete form release agent**
  - **SOYsolv: Very low-odor, water-based, nontoxic, nonflammable, biodegradable spray-on concrete form release agent**

Concrete Curing

After pouring, concrete can cure and gain strength only if it remains nearly saturated with water for a minimum of 28 days. The curing process stops if the relative humidity of the concrete drops below 80 percent. Improperly cured concrete will develop structural weaknesses and cracks that can become pathways for unwanted moisture and soil gases to creep into the building. Rushing the drying process may also weaken the surface so that concrete dust continually sloughs from the surface into the home. Pouring slabs in cold weather is also risky since cold temperatures impede the curing process. The use of propane heaters may cause the concrete surface to become weak and crack as combustion gases enter the material and interfere with its chemical composition.

Improperly cured concrete will have high alkalinity levels that can cause certain substrates and finishing materials to breakdown or rot. Testing pH can help determine whether a concrete surface has been properly cured and whether problems will develop with certain finish applications. This simple test is described in the materials testing section of Division 13.

Concrete Finishes

An exposed concrete slab can be an attractive finished flooring surface. Usually when a slab will be used as a finished floor it must be troweled to a smoother finish than a slab slated for use as a subfloor. Smooth-surfaced concrete requires the expertise of an experienced tradesperson. When it is first poured, the concrete will have more water than it needs to complete the setting reaction. Some of this extra water will come to the surface. If the concrete is finished before the extra water has fully migrated upward, it will become trapped in the upper layer of the concrete, resulting in a weakened surface that will release concrete dust into the indoor environment. The window of opportunity for properly smoothing the surface is short. If too much time has elapsed, the surface will have set and will remain rough.

For exposed finished slabs, control joint locations must be carefully planned for their esthetics, and often more joints are added to minimize random cracking. Color is often added, either mixed into the wet concrete or applied after the concrete sets. Because the slab is usually poured near the beginning of the construction, it must be kept covered during the course of construction to ensure that it is not damaged or stained. All of these factors will add to the price of the concrete work, but the process will still be cost-effective when the price of covering the concrete with another material is considered.

Both the coloring agents and the surface treatment must be selected carefully to achieve a healthy finish. One process uses muriatic acid to stain floors. Although the finished floor will not outgas, muriatic acid is a highly toxic chemical that requires protective equipment for the installers, and the wash-off is considered hazardous waste that must be properly disposed of.

More benign methods for staining or coloring exposed slabs may be specified:

- Do not use aniline-based coloring agents.
- Use only high-quality mineral pigments such as **Chromix Admixture** and **Lithochrome Color Hardener** or **Davis Colors**. Verify with the manufacturer that the selected color is free of chromium and other heavy metals.
- **PureColor** is a two-stage stain formulation of pure mineral ions and oxygen catalyst for concrete surfaces. Colors can be custom mixed.
- A solution of **iron sulfate** (fertilizer) reacts with the concrete, producing yellow,

orange, red, and brown stain hues depending on the chemical composition of the concrete.

Acceptable sealers are listed in the next section.

Slab and Stem Wall Treatment and Detailing

Concrete can act as a wick for ground moisture, thereby promoting water damage and fungal growth in other materials through moisture transfer. A layer of coarse gravel under the slab with no fines smaller than half an inch will break capillary action. A layer of continuous, unpunctured polyethylene directly under the slab will help prevent water vapor and soil gases such as radon from finding their way through cracks in the slab. A fully cured slab can also be sealed to further prevent moisture and soil gases from entering the building and to create a more finished floor surface. Some sealers are solvent based and should be avoided. The following sealers are more benign:

- **AFM Safecoat CemBond Masonry Paint**: Water-resistant coating for cement, concrete block, and masonry
- **AFM Safecoat DecKote**: Waterborne coating for use on concrete, magnesite, walkways, breezeways, and patios
- **AFM Safecoat MexeSeal, AFM Safecoat Penetrating Waterstop**: Water-based sealers and finish coats
- **AFM Safecoat Watershield**: Water repelling sealer for masonry and painted surfaces
- **AgriStain for Concrete**: Sealer and stain for concrete, plaster, and porous tiles
- **Vocomp-25**: A solvent-reduced, water-based sealer
- **Weather-Bos Masonry Boss Formula 9**: A water reducible sealer for all above-grade concrete and masonry surfaces; helps reduce dusting, powdering, efflorescence, spalling, cracking, and freeze-thaw damage
- **Xypex**: A nontoxic (according to manufacturer), zero-VOC chemical treatment for the creation of moisture resistance and the protection of concrete; creates a non-soluble crystalline structure that permanently plugs the pores and capillary tracts of concrete. Xypex concentrate **DS-1** and **DS-2** are dry-shake formulations designed for horizontal surfaces.

Further Reading

Timusk, John. *Slabs on Grade*. National Building Envelope Council, Building Science Treatise, Construction Canada 92–07.

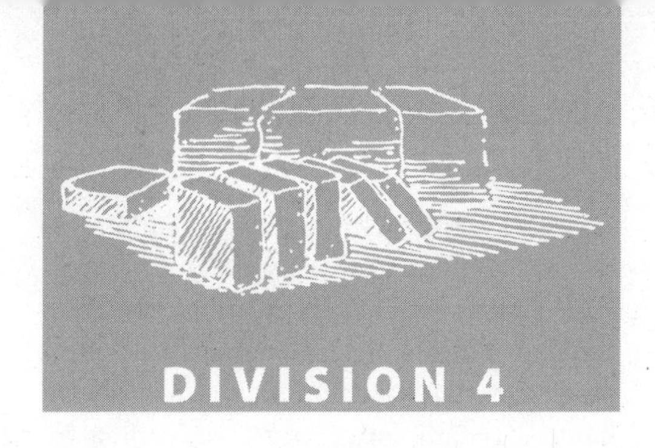

Earth Masonry and Other Alternatives to Frame Construction

Introduction

Most code-approved building materials in North America are manufactured using industrialized processes that create components of uniform size and form, with predictable performance characteristics such as fire resistance, permeability ratings, insulation values, and structural properties. Since the process of testing such materials for code approval is extremely expensive, only large manufacturers who intend to produce, package, and sell a product for wide distribution can afford to test. This product-oriented approval process is not geared toward the analysis and acceptance of nonproprietary unprocessed natural building materials and it has all but closed the door on 9,000 years of preindustrial building technology.

There is at least one exception to this trend that perhaps serves as a model in this country for future code approval of other natural building materials. Wood is a naturally occurring, minimally processed building material that has universal code acceptance even though it is flammable and subject to shrinkage, comes with inconsistent structural properties, and will rapidly deteriorate through rot and insect infestation if left unprotected. In spite of its embarrassingly preindustrial nature, it remains the dominant building material in residential construction, and building codes have succeeded in creating safe guidelines for its classification and use.

Why consider alternative natural materials such as earth and straw as an option for healthy housing? These historically derived methods of construction differ from standard cavity wall construction in that manufactured petrochemical-based barriers are not installed to retard the flow of vapor through the walls. Instead, vapor is allowed to flow naturally. The massive walls employ hygroscopic natural materials to increase the capacity of the wall to handle the transfer of moisture from the interior and the exterior surroundings and to release vapor back into the surroundings as climatic conditions change. Because temperature change occurs very slowly in the flow-through process, and because dried clay-based materials have the ability to absorb and desorb large amounts of moisture without deteriorating,[1] accumulation from condensation is insignificant. When a home is properly constructed using these mass wall techniques it will be an extremely comfortable environment with superior temperature and humidity stability. Furthermore, because the solid walls provide insulation and can be finished with a covering of plaster or furred-out wood applied directly to them, the need for synthetic exterior sheathing, batt insulation, gypsum board, joint fillers, and paint is eliminated. Many volatile organic compound contamination sources are thereby eliminated as well.

In the philosophy of Building Biology, a

The Breathing Wall Concept: Misconceptions

KATHARINA GUSTAVS

The breathing wall concept goes back to Max von Pettenkofer (1818–1901), one of the most accomplished hygienists of his time and the pioneering founder of the occupational and environmental hygiene sciences as we know them today. He was instrumental in stopping the cholera epidemics in Munich, one of the largest cities in Germany, during the second half of the 19th century. By initiating the construction of a central water supply and sewage treatment system, he greatly improved public health and achieved celebrity status.

In his dedicated search for better living conditions, von Pettenkofer introduced carbon dioxide measurement as an important indicator of overall indoor air quality. His measurements of air exchange rates in a room with brick walls, a masonry heater, and sealed windows led him to hypothesize that the brick walls must let air pass through. Even with the keyhole and other cracks sealed, the air exchange rate dropped only about a quarter compared to the rate prior to sealing.[a]

He seems to have forgotten to consider the effect the masonry heater would have on the ventilation rate. Thus he proceeded to demonstrate that when air is pumped through a brick cylinder, sealed on the outside except for both ends, a candle flame at the other end could be extinguished. In his eagerness to prove his hypothesis, he overlooked the fact that the maximum natural air pressure across a wall of about 30 pascals is many times lower than the pressure required in his candle-extinguishing experiment (between 700 and 10,000 pascals).

Von Pettenkofer's celebrity status may have been one of the reasons his hypothesis of natural ventilation through walls was not scientifically debunked until the 1920s.[b] Though he never used the term "breathing wall," this concept took on a life of its own that continues to this day. The Institute of Building Biology and Ecology Neubeuern in Germany recommends avoiding the use of the term because it does not reflect the reality of the complex processes occurring in a wall and usually leads to misconceptions.[c]

In Building Biology, a natural home is considered to be a living organism in the sense that it should be — as much as possible — self-sufficient, energy-efficient, and built from materials that are part of the natural cycle and do not contribute to toxic waste. The roof and wall systems are often re-

wall made of unprocessed materials through which the flow of vapor is unhindered is called a breathing wall. The concept is central to the Building Biology goal of creating a healthy dwelling. (The term "breathing wall" is really a misnomer because the walls of course are not the primary ventilation source for the building. The term "vapor-permeable wall" would perhaps be more accurate.) Another Building Biology concept is that of the building envelope being our third skin (clothing being our second skin). This analogy is a more useful one in describing how a breathing wall works. Our skin is the organ of contact with the outer environment and regulates the balance of moisture and temperature of the body in relation to the environment. Skin must remain permeable to facilitate a healthy interaction between the natural environment and the human organism. So too, according to Building Biology,

ferred to as our third skin, implying that, just like human skin, the building envelope is in constant contact with the environment and plays a crucial role in maintaining a healthy inner climate despite unfavorable weather conditions outside. Let us have a closer look at what does or does not permeate a wall with regard to air and moisture.

A constant supply of oxygen-rich air and the reduction of carbon dioxide are essential to a healthy indoor climate, but it is a misconception that walls can "breathe" air, especially massive walls built from earth, masonry, or solid wood, despite their varying degrees of porosity. The air pressure difference between outdoor and indoor air is never high enough to promote an air exchange through such a massive wall. If air does get through a wall, it is not through the wall itself but through poorly sealed joints and cracks. This, however, is the least desirable way to supply fresh air because it promotes high heat loss in winter, makes for very unpleasant drafts, and invites moisture problems.

To ensure the Building Biology recommended rate of about one complete change of air per hour, either mechanical ventilation with a heat recovery system or cross-ventilation through open windows several times a day is necessary. Massive wall systems are especially well suited for natural ventilation methods because their extraordinary heat storage capacity keeps heat loss at a minimum during brief opening of the windows in winter.

It is interesting to note here that human skin does not breathe air either. All oxygen for our inner organs is supplied by the air inhaled through the nose and mouth, which in keeping with the analogy of the third skin would be comparable to the windows and doors in a house. Though the outermost layer of our skin (up to 0.4 millimeters) can extract oxygen from the ambient air, the oxygen does not cross into the body.[d]

It is true that wall structures without vapor barriers allow for the free flow of moisture or water vapor. Moisture always moves from a warmer area to a colder one, from a higher vapor pressure concentration to a lower concentration. As a result, water vapor tends to flow from the inside out in the north and from the outside in down south. In mixed and moderate climate zones, it has a tendency to flow from the inside out during the winter and from the outside in during the summer.

must our third skin, the walls of our dwellings, remain permeable in order to achieve an optimal environment for health.

There is an intimate connection between the health of an individual and the health of the environment. All building processes involve the extraction of raw materials from nature and the disruption of the natural ecosystem. The alternative materials and methods described below use these materials in a minimally processed state with far less environmental impact than the highly refined and processed materials prevalent in conventional construction. When one considers that 40 percent of the material resources entering the global economy are related to the building industry,[2] it becomes clear that the building material choices we make have a global impact on the health of the ecosystem, the ultimate determinant of our own health.

In recent years, with renewed interest in environmental concerns and energy

Massive wall systems made from earth, clay, or solid wood also have a high capillary activity that is capable of wicking away liquid water. Though any wall system should be designed to prevent vapor condensation from occurring, the wicking capacity of natural building materials provides additional insurance that liquid water will not get trapped in the wall. This, of course, works only as long as all wall finishes are also highly permeable to water vapor.

The actual amount of water vapor an exterior wall can shuttle to the outside of a building is rather low. For example, in winter, when outside temperatures are low in northern and moderate climates, only about 1 to 2 percent of the indoor moisture can make it through a brick wall.[e] Again, it is obvious that the majority of the moisture that is usually generated inside a home needs to be removed through active ventilation, using windows and/or mechanical ventilation systems.

Building and finishing materials with a high moisture buffer or hygric capacity improve indoor air quality tremendously because they help mitigate temporary humidity highs. Nearly all natural building materials are highly hygroscopic, especially wood, earth, lime, and cellulose. Lime plaster (13 grams per square meter) or clay plaster (30 grams per square meter) can absorb large amounts of water vapor. But as soon as you finish a lime plaster with a standard latex paint, water vapor absorption drops (to below 9 grams per square meter).[f] Therefore it is important to choose surface treatments that are highly permeable to water vapor, such as lime wash, silicate, or casein paint. Note that this moisture buffering effect relies on only the first 1 to 1.5 centimeters of the interior wall surface. Thus almost any wall structure can benefit from the moisture buffering effect of adding a material such as a clay plaster.

It is unclear why the breathing wall concept persists when it is riddled with misconceptions. What is clear, however, is that any building envelope has to meet two major challenges: first, not to let any water in and second, if water does get in, to let it out again. In contrast to the widespread use of polyethylene vapor barriers, which often makes no sense from a building science point of view, Building Biology favors the so-called flow-through design, which allows water vapor to pass through the wall assembly's components without

efficiency, several alternative methods of building have enjoyed a limited renaissance among environmentally concerned homeowners, designers, and builders. Since the last edition of this book in 2001, the negative impact of human activity on the global environment has become increasingly evident, and in our efforts to lessen this impact the green building movement has experienced exponential growth. The Bau-Biologie or Building Biology study course states that "there is almost always a direct correlation between the biological compatibility and ecological performance of a given building material." This statement is exemplified in the proper use of natural, minimally processed, and locally found and crafted building materials.

Methods of Earth Construction

Earth is widely available at little or no cost. It is nonflammable, is infinitely recyclable, is

condensing. Even if water does condense, there is always an exit pathway for it. Natural building materials such as earth, cob, and masonry are especially well suited for this task. To create a fully functional wall based on the flow-through design, any healthy home project must take into account all the climate-specific details of its location.

a. Max von Pettenkofer. *Über den Luftwechsel in Wohngebäuden*. Literarisch-Artistische Anstalt der J. G. Cotta'schen Buchhandlung, 1858.
b. Erwin Raisch. "Die Luftdurchlässigkeit von Baustoffen und Baukonstruktionsteilen." *Gesundheitsingenieur*. Issue 30 (1928).
c. Winfried Schneider. "40 Jahre Baubiologie – Klischees, Innovationen, Trends." *Wohnung und Gesundheit*. Vol.120 (2006), pp. 12–14. See also baubiologie.de/site/zeitschrift/artikel/120/12.php.
d. M. Stücker et al. "The Cutaneous Uptake of Oxygen Contributes Significantly to the Oxygen Supply of Human Dermis and Epidermis." *Journal of Physiology*. Vol. 538 (2002), pp. 985–994.
e. W.Schneider and A. Schneider. *Baubiologische Baustofflehre + Bauphysik*. Course Module 7 of IBN Building Biology Correspondence Course 1998, p. 67.
f. Moisture uptake of building materials within three hours while ambient air humidity increased from 40 to 80 percent. W. Schneider and A. Schneider. *Baubiologische Baustofflehre + Bauphysik*. Course Module 7 of IBN Building Biology Correspondence Course 1998, p. 37.

Katharina Gustavs, BBEC, CT, is a Building Biology environmental consultant living on Vancouver Island, British Columbia, who specializes in electromagnetic field testing and healthy lifestyle programs for environmentally sensitive individuals. As a professional translator, she is also translating and researching the original Building Biology Correspondence Course from Germany for the International Institute for Bau-Biologie & Ecology in Florida. Contact her at gustavs@buildingbiology.ca.

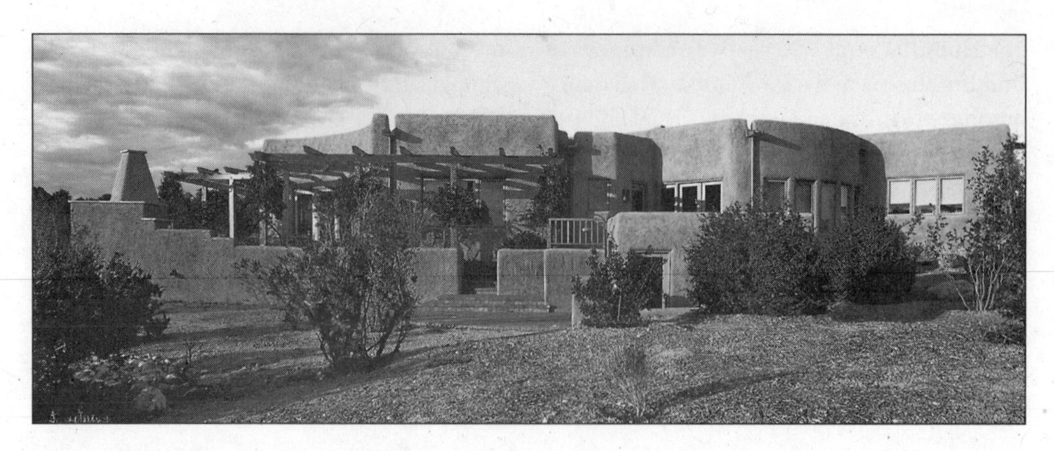

Adobe home, Santa Fe. Architect Baker-Laporte &Assoc. Builder: Prull & Assoc.
Photo: Robert Laporte.

not subject to insect infestation, is a natural preservative, has excellent thermal mass storage capacity,[3] has the ability to handle large amounts of water vapor diffusion and stabilize humidity without mechanical augmentation, and, unlike postindustrial manufactured building materials, has a proven record of longevity with intact examples dating back more than 7,000 years.

Earth is the predominant preindustrial building material. Earth construction, in all of its various forms, has not been codified on a national level in this country, and in spite of the fact that it is the wall-building material for more than a third of the world's homes its use is considered by most building departments to be experimental. In Germany, simple standardized tests for measuring various structural properties of mud have been developed and codified. The work done there could pave the way for wider acceptance here if more performance-based criteria for code compliance are permitted in the future. For the most part, approval is currently at the discretion of the local building authority.

Earth Block Construction

Earth block construction is used in every hot, dry subtropical climate throughout the world. Examples have been found in Turkestan dating back to 6,000 BC. The historical core of Shibam in Yemen, consisting of eight-story buildings, is constructed entirely of adobe. These magnificent buildings have scarcely been altered since the time of their last rebuilding in the mid-16th century.

Earth blocks are primarily used in modern construction in three forms. Adobes are mixed wet, poured into formwork, and then sun dried. Pressed blocks are made from moist soil that is compacted by a mechanical or hand press. Green bricks are extruded in a brick-making plant and used unfired.

In the US Southwest, adobe is a traditional building material that has remained in continuous use and is the material of choice for some of the most exclusive residences being built today. It has been jokingly called the building material for "the idle rich" or "the idle poor" because stacking the heavy blocks is labor intensive.

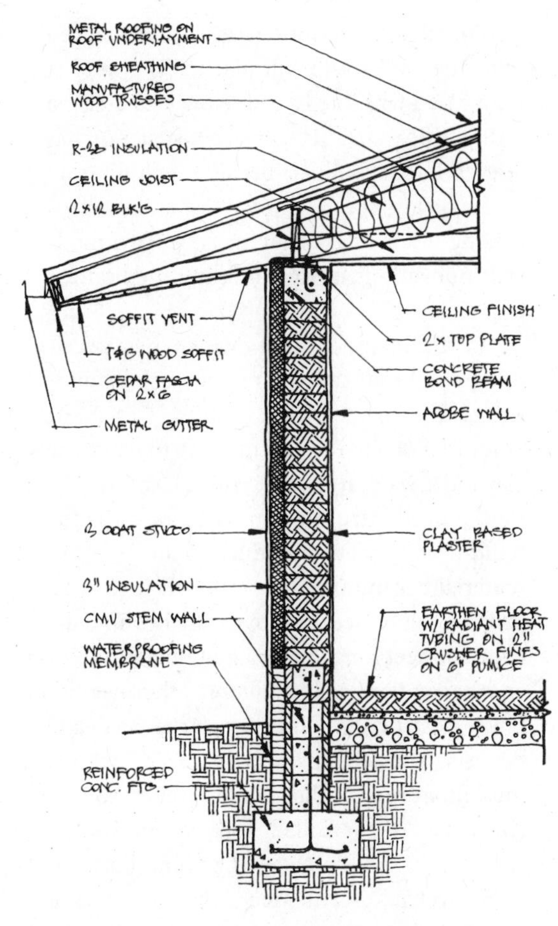

Section through adobe wall.

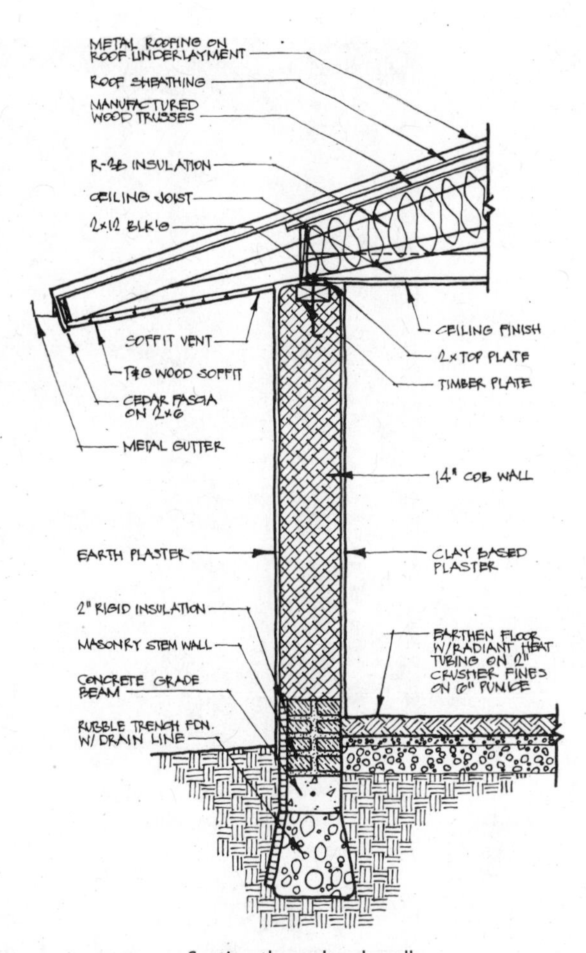

Section through cob wall.

Because the R-value[4] of earth blocks is fairly low, walls require additional insulation to meet energy requirements in all but the warmest parts of North America. A higher R-value is usually obtained by adding foam insulation to the exterior of the building, which affects the "breathability" of the wall and creates a dubious marriage between natural and synthetic materials. Although most earth block is currently used in desert climates and for exterior wall construction, its excellent mass and acoustic properties make it a superb product for interior mass walls in any climate where it is available or can be produced.

Adobe blocks are frequently "stabilized," mainly to make them more water resistant and to prevent breakage during transport. The most common stabilizer is asphalt, a carcinogenic material that should be avoided in the healthy home. Unstabilized adobes can be purchased from some adobe yards and can be special-ordered. Compressed earth blocks can

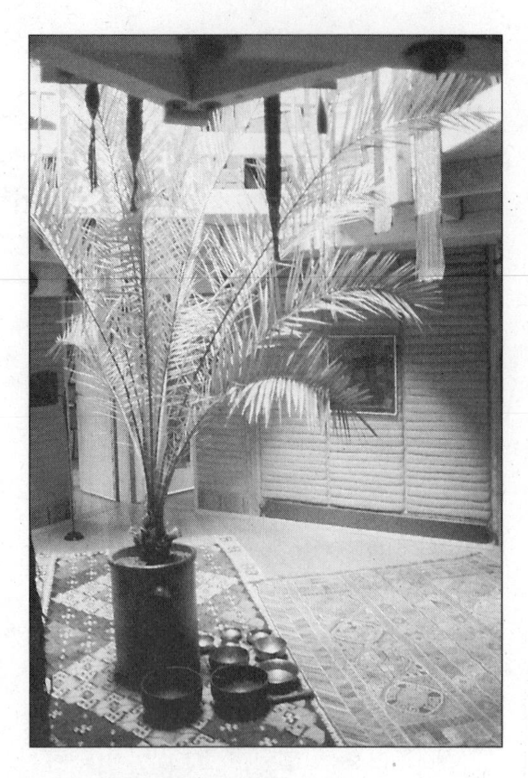

Home of Professor Gernot Minke showing the "stranglehm" wall components.
Photo: Robert Laporte.

be made onsite with an adobe press, thereby eliminating the need to protect blocks during transportation. However, earth blocks that are not stabilized must be protected from ground water damage. This can be accomplished by holding the first course of blocks off the floor by installing a layer of concrete block first.

New Mexico has developed its own comprehensive code for load-bearing adobe construction, which has served as a model for parts of Colorado and Arizona.

Cob and Other Wet Clay Techniques

Throughout history, several methods for mud construction have evolved using wet mud fashioned into various shapes and stacked onto the wall while still plastic. The mud is then fused with the layers below it to create a monolithic wall. This type of construction has lent itself to laybuilders because it requires no formwork or special equipment and no processing other than onsite mixing. Two modern innovations in this building method are of note.

In Germany, Gernot Minke has developed a method called stranglehm for building with extruded clay profiles. Casein or whey is added to the clay mixture to make the clay more water resistant. Minke has created a mechanized extrusion apparatus for use at the building site that can produce about six feet of material per minute. The uniformly extruded profiles, which are three by six inches and just over two feet long, are stacked one on top of another and pressed to adhere to the layer below. Construction joints are placed vertically between the ribbons and "caulked" with a mud mixture after the ribbons are dry so that shrinkage is controlled and air infiltration can be blocked. Being used as infill between wooden structural members, the system is not load bearing. Insulation must be added to the exterior in colder climates.

In North America, the Cob Cottage Company has been responsible for the revival of cob, or wet mud, construction. Founders Ianto Evans, Linda Smiley, and Michael Smith have developed a stronger mix using a more controlled formulation process than their predecessors did. The Oregon Cob method that they have developed is characterized by small, free-flowing, sculpturally shaped homes with arched windows and doors and a strong solar orientation. Their designs emphasize maximum space utilization through curvilinear

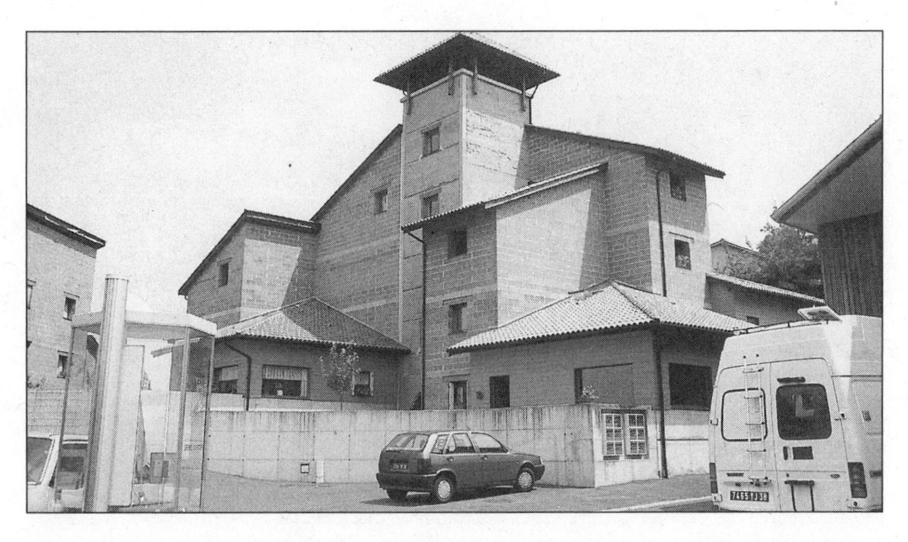

5-storey rammed earth and compressed earth block in Multiple Housing complex in Lyon, France by Craterre. Photo: Robert Laporte.

formations and built-in benches and platforms. In England, this traditional form of building has been revived by Katy Bryce and Adam Weismann of Cob in Cornwall Ltd.

Cob construction uses moistened earth containing suitable clay and sand content that is mixed with straw and formed into stiff loaves of a size that can be moved, person to person, from the mix site to the building site. The loaves are then piled onto a wall and blended with the previous layers. The result is a monolithic, load-bearing mud wall.

Cob has R-values comparable to adobe construction and is best suited to warmer climates where less insulation is required and high thermal mass is effective. Cob is also valuable for adding thermal mass in the interior of buildings, especially for heat storage in passive solar designs. Anecdotal evidence has indicated that it exhibits better seismic performance than adobe because the walls are monolithic.[5]

Rammed Earth

Historically, rammed earth construction has been found not only in hot, arid climates but also throughout the cold, wet regions of Europe. Thousands of rammed earth structures, some dating back 400 years, can be found in the Rhone River valley.

Earth with the proper moisture, sand, gravel, and clay content is rammed into formwork in six- to eight-inch layers. When formwork is full it can be immediately removed and reused for the next sector of wall. Because of the low moisture content, the walls, if properly constructed, will not shrink or crack. No curing time is required and construction can continue without any delay in sequencing.

The finished walls are thick, precise, and beautiful. Different colors of earth can be used to create decorative effects. Rammed earth walls are usually left exposed without any further finishing. Unlike adobe or stone masonry, where the joints are pathways for

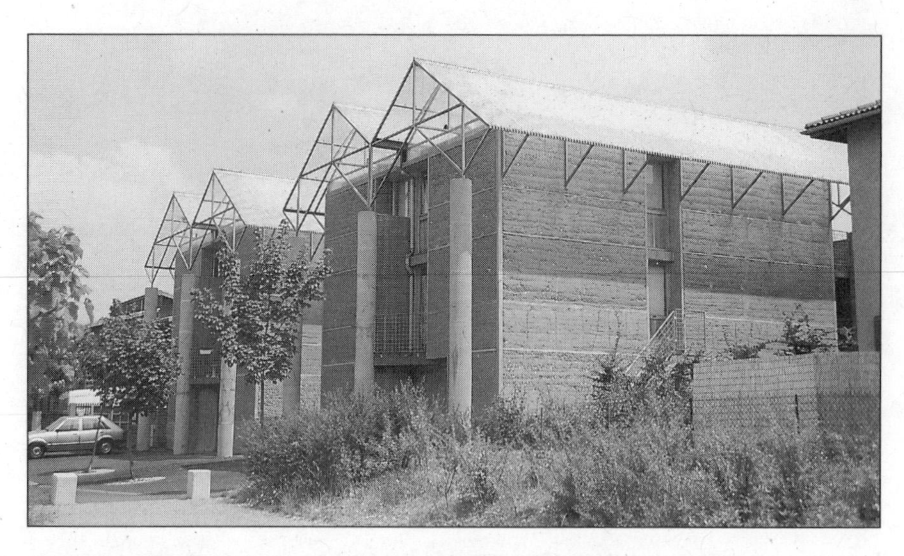

Rammed Earth or "pise" multi-storey housing complex by Craterre in Lyon, France. Photo: Robert Laporte.

erosion caused by the expansion of water, the monolithic surface of rammed earth has proven to hold up extremely well to freeze and thaw cycles. With modern comfort and energy demands, this technique is most suitable in warmer climates. However, innovations, such as placing a two-inch board of rigid insulation at the center of the wall, have been used to adapt this method for cold climate use.

Of all the earth building techniques described in this chapter, rammed earth technology has advanced the most through the use of modernized machinery. It has been calculated that historic homes of rammed earth took as many as 30 worker-hours per cubic meter of wall construction, whereas highly mechanized techniques can take as few as two worker-hours per cubic meter of wall.[6] Adaptation to mechanization, improvements in formwork, high compressive strength, and short curing time make this type of earth construction suitable for large projects. Highly refined, multistory buildings have been created using this technique, including the five-star Kooralbyn Hotel and Resort in Australia.

With more test data being accumulated in both the US and Europe on the structural properties of rammed earth, it is becoming easier for professional engineers to create reliable structural designs and predict how the material will act under extreme conditions. In earthquake zones, some concrete has been added to the mix, and steel reinforcement has been used in much the same way as in concrete structures, allowing permits to be granted throughout earthquake-prone California, where David Easton, a pioneer and innovator in the rammed earth revival, lives and works.

Light Clay-Straw Construction

For construction in colder climates, where higher insulation values are required than can be provided by mud alone, several methods

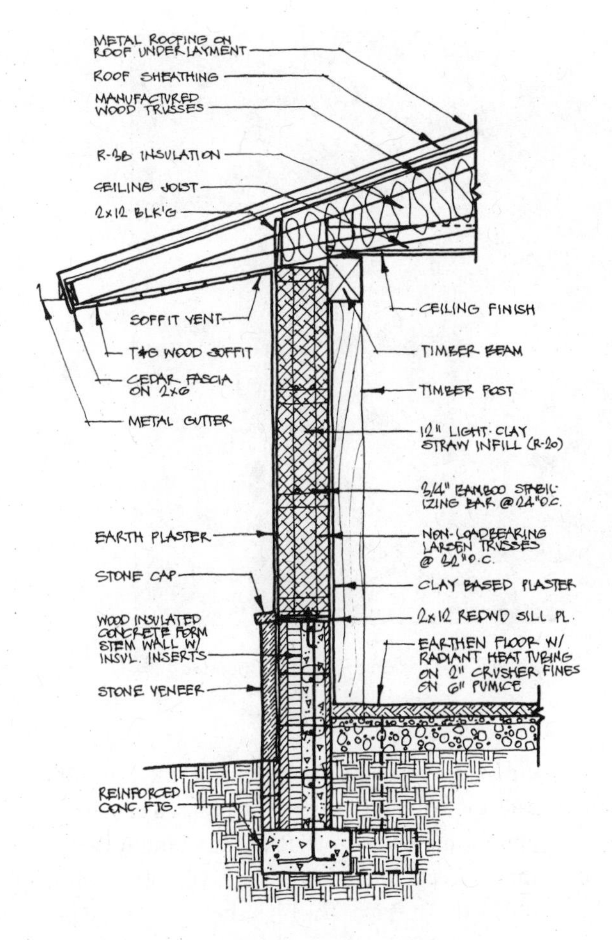

Section through light clay straw wall.

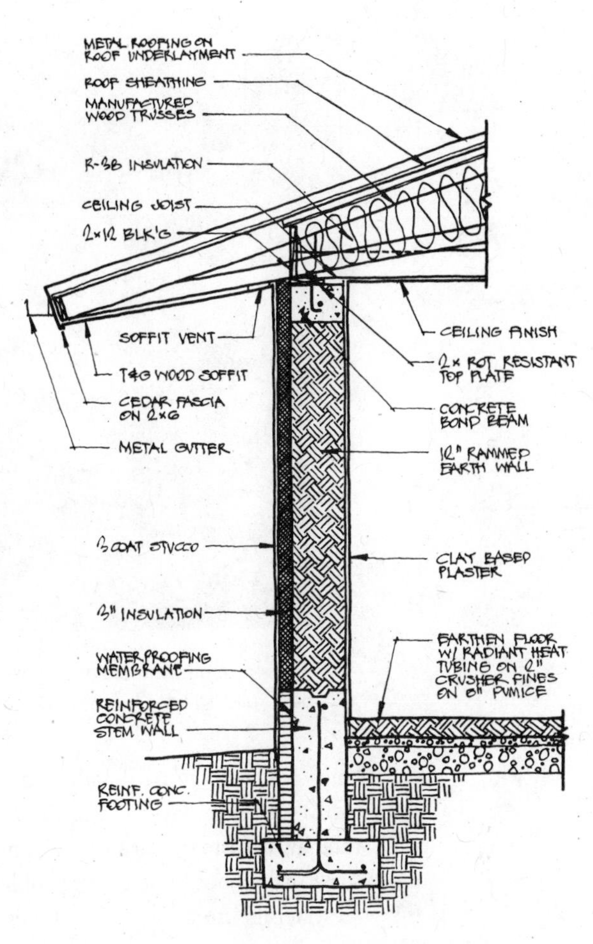

Section through rammed earth wall.

that combine earth with lightweight natural aggregates have evolved. These include mixing mud with pumice, volcanic rock, straw, wood chips, expanded clay, or vermiculite. In the US, clay-straw construction has become the most well-known of these methods because of the work of Robert Laporte of the Econest Building Company, who has taught workshops and built clay-straw structures throughout North America. The Laporte technique uses a lightweight mixture of clay and straw as an "outsulating" wall around a timber-frame structure. Clay-straw can also be used as an infill material between deep structural members.

Straw is mixed with a clay slurry so that each strand is coated. The wet material is then compacted into a 12-inch-wide formwork, which is removed the same day. The result is a precise wall that has enough texture to accept plaster without any further wall preparation

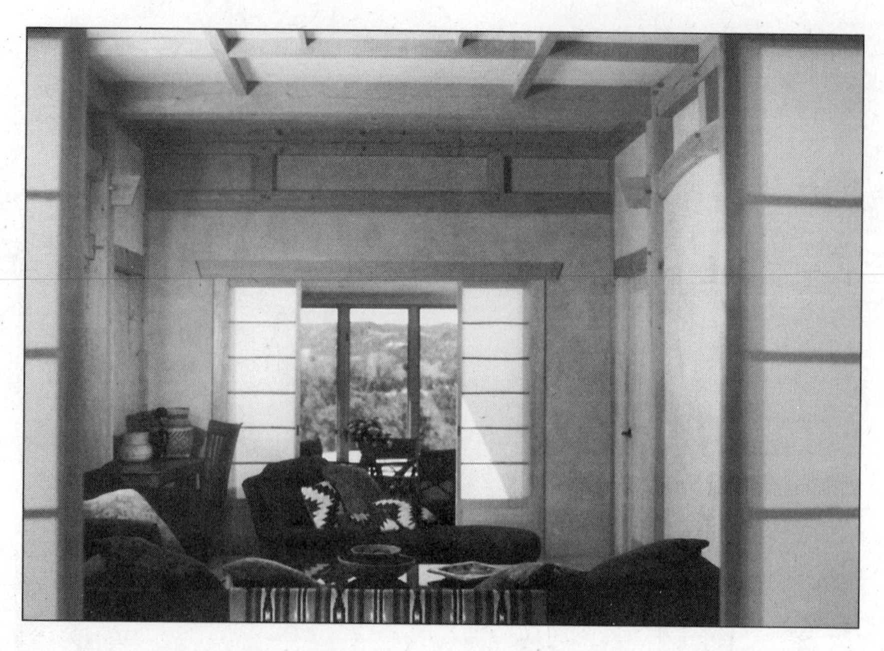

The timber frame structure and light-clay walls of the Baker-Laporte Residence. Builder: Econest Building Co.; Photo: Lisl Dennis.

or lathing. The walls must be allowed to dry thoroughly. Because clay has the capacity to wick water away from the straw that it encases, mold growth has not posed any problem in this wall system if initial full curing takes place in a timely manner. A completed wall that accidentally becomes wet will dry out without developing mold, but the walls must be finished with materials that will allow for sufficient vapor diffusion. Earth and lime plasters, or wood siding with a vented air space and an air barrier of earth plaster on the clay-straw (for wetter climates with driving rain), are ideal for this purpose.

A clay-straw wall weighs approximately 50 pounds per cubic foot. The density can be varied to provide more mass on the south side of a building and more insulation on the north side, with weights of 60 and 40 pounds per cubic foot respectively. The average R-value of a 12-inch-thick clay-straw wall has a range of approximately R-19 to R-24,[7] making it thermally acceptable in all but the coldest regions of North America. The high thermal mass also makes it an excellent material for use in hot, dry regions. In areas with rainfall of more than 30 inches a year, an exterior sheathing of wood with a vented air space between the wood and clay-straw is advised.

Clay-straw is less suitable for locations that do not have a predictable dry season of at least three months duration for proper curing to occur. A similar technique combining clay and cedar wood chips has been used successfully in wetter climates. These buildings can be dried from the inside out during the winter with a wood heat source. Many examples, including some that are several hundred years old, can be found in Germany, which has an extremely damp climate. The older examples of mud and straw wall construction found in Europe are denser and have a higher clay content than our modern formulas, which are designed to have higher insulation values. As with all natural systems, a good above-grade stem wall or plinth and large roof overhang will help protect the walls and increase longevity.

Because clay-straw is non-load-bearing, permitting has been readily granted in many localities. However, if you are interested in building with clay-straw, check with your local building department to determine whether approval will be forthcoming. New Mexico has passed official guidelines for clay-straw construction, and this information, which is available on the Econest website at econest.com, may be helpful for obtaining approval from code officials elsewhere.

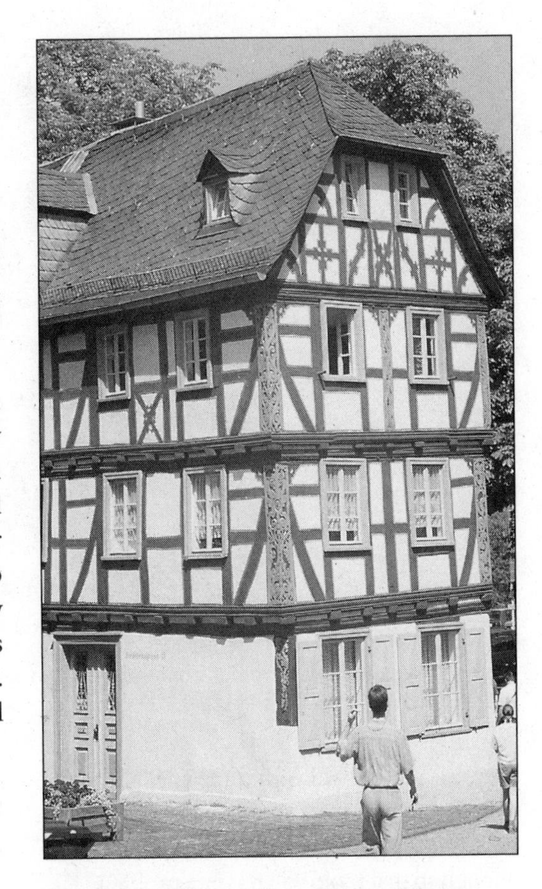

One of many 800 year old structures in Germany. Composed of timber frame and earthen and straw wall materials it stands as a testimonial to the beauty and longevity of natural building materials. Photo: Robert Laporte.

Other Alternative Building Systems

Straw Bale

Although straw has been an important component of natural building for centuries, straw bale is a relatively new form of alternative construction that appears to be an innovation of the early settlers of the Nebraska plains, where unsuitable soils and a scarcity of wood made necessity the mother of invention. The high insulative value of straw bale (between R-33 and R-57, depending on the type of bale and the testing facility) and the aesthetics of the thick walls have quickly made it a popular alternative building material.

Because much of the straw grown in the United States is heavily sprayed with pesticides, we recommend looking for straw that has been organically grown. *The Last Straw*, listed in the bibliography at the end of this chapter, has published a list of organic straw sources.

Because cellulose is a perfect food for mold, bales of straw often contain mold. This means that it is very important with straw bale building to incorporate rigorous water and moisture management strategies into the design. If the walls are allowed to breathe — that is, if

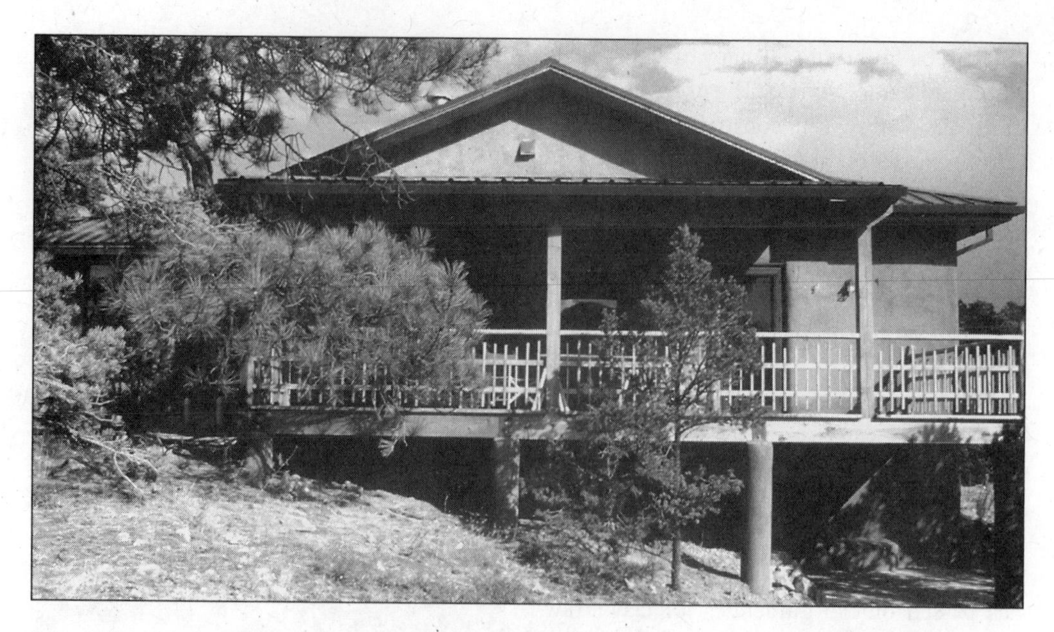

Straw bale residence in Santa Fe, New Mexico. Metal roof, wide roof overhangs and rain gutter system protect the stucco finishes from the occasional high desert rains. Architect: Baker-Laporte and Associates; Builder: Prull and Associates; Photo: Julie Dean.

they are not covered with impermeable membranes that will trap any moisture in the wall — in theory the bales will always remain dry enough so that mold will not be a problem. Using earth-based instead of cement-based plasters on interior walls will help keep water away from the bales and allow them to dry out more readily when they do get wet. On the exterior of the building, earth-based plasters that are augmented to prevent water penetration may prove more desirable from a moisture movement standpoint than cement-based plasters, which are less flexible, tend to crack more, and allow less vapor diffusion. Should water become trapped in the wall through roof failure, plumbing leaks, poor drainage, or other building systems failures, mold can become a problem.

Many techniques have evolved for straw bale construction. Building permit approval is greatly simplified when structures are non-load-bearing and most straw bale construction relies on a variety of structural systems, including exposed and buried post and beam, steel posts, and poured or masonry concrete piers. Load-bearing straw bale examples have been built in Colorado, Arizona, and Canada. Several jurisdictions have adopted straw bale codes, including New Mexico and California; Pima County and Guadalupe, Arizona; Austin, Texas; Boulder and Cortez, Colorado; and McCook, Nebraska. Nevada has a legislative mandate to ensure that local jurisdictions develop building codes allowing straw bale construction. While some jurisdictions permit load-bearing straw bale construction, others permit straw bale only as a non-load-bearing wall system.

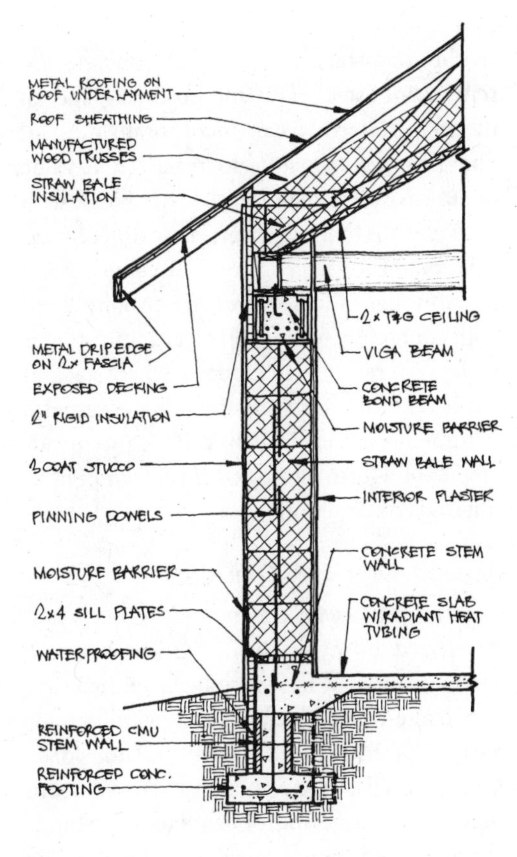

Section through straw bale wall.

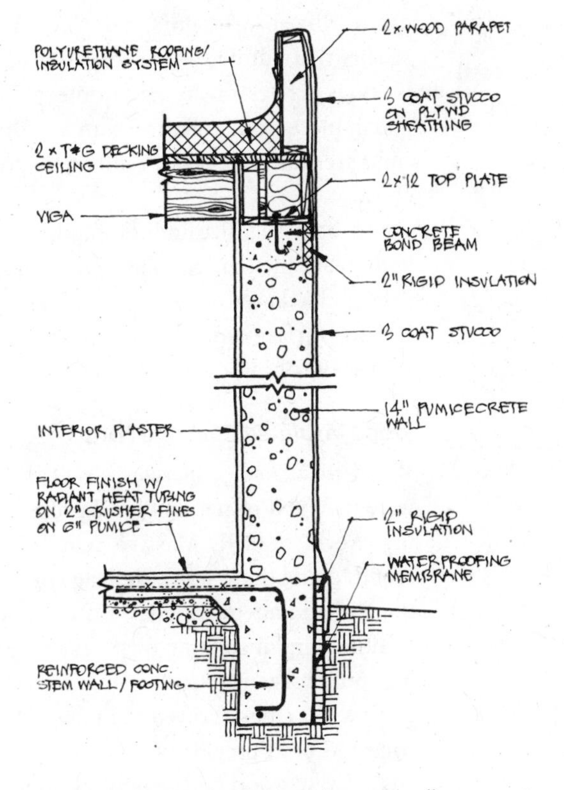

Section through pumicecrete wall.

Pumice-Crete

In this method, 14- to 24-inch-thick walls are created by mixing pumice, a very porous volcanic rock, with a light, soupy concrete. The mixture is poured into formwork. The resulting walls have both thermal mass and a high insulation value, and are ready to accept plaster without further preparation. When used with a concrete bond beam at the top, the walls are load bearing. In Europe, pumice and other naturally occurring lightweight volcanic aggregates have been used with mud in place of the concrete. However, these walls are not used in a load-bearing situation.

Because of the simplicity of this system and the absence of organic matter in the wall construction, pumice-crete is very suitable for persons with chemical sensitivity, who are often also highly sensitive to wood terpenes, mold, and pesticides that may be found in small quantities in other building materials. Since the wall uses cement, the rules for concrete formwork and cement composition, outlined in Division 3, must be followed.

Pumice can be radioactive. Samples should be tested with a Geiger counter to be sure they are free of radioactive material. (Refer to the section on radiation in Division 13 for testing methods.) Because pumice is highly porous, it can readily absorb odors and it is prudent to specify that pumice be free of acquired odors when it arrives onsite and protected onsite and in place from pollution sources. Once the walls are plastered, this should no longer be of concern.

To help stabilize indoor humidity levels and create further thermal mass storage capacity, clay-based plasters can be applied to interior surfaces and will adhere well without the use of lathing.

Wood Insulated Concrete Forms

Wood insulated concrete forms (WICFs) were invented of necessity in Europe following World War II. Massive rebuilding was required and there was a shortage of conventional building materials. Waste wood was plentiful, and insulating forms made by mixing mineralized (clay impregnated) wood chips with cement proved to be a good way to conserve both precious fuel and scarce concrete. These wood and cement masonry units had many excellent building properties. They were lightweight and noncombustible, had a high strength-to-weight ratio, and were dimensionally stable, insulative, and resistant to freeze-thaw, rot, insects, and fungus growth. The resulting structures were more durable, energy efficient, and economical than structures built by prewar methods. In continuous use since the 1940s under various brand names, WICFs are still a preferred method of construction throughout Europe.

In North America, WICFs are available through **Durisol, Faswall,** and **Healthy Buildings Made Easy**. They come as interlocking hollow blocks similar to cinder or masonry unit blocks. They are dry-stacked (without mortar) and filled with concrete and reinforcing steel. Durisol produces special thermal units that can incorporate mineral fiber insulation inserts to reach an R-value of 28. Faswall is a shorter, heavier block with thicker walls that can incorporate different insulation inserts to produce an R-value of 26.

Although all the cores are usually filled with concrete, a more ecological application is to use concrete only in the cores where steel rebar is required and to fill the other cores with natural insulation or earth. WICFs are considered to be a form of vapor diffusible or breathing wall construction.

Aerated Autoclaved Concrete

Aerated autoclaved concrete (AAC) was first developed by a Swedish engineer between 1920 and 1932. It has since been refined into a concrete-based block material with high insulation used for both load- and non-load-bearing walls. AAC is manufactured from quartz sand, lime and/or cement as the binding agent, aluminum powder, and water. The aluminum powder reacts with calcium hydroxide and water to form tiny hydrogen gas bubbles. At the end of the foaming process the hydrogen escapes into the atmosphere and reacts with air to form water, and air replaces the hydrogen in the formed bubbles. The finished block does not contain aluminum. The final block form is autoclaved under heat and pressure to reach full strength.

AAC block construction uses standard masonry skills and is installed in a manner similar to regular cinder block, using a thinset instead of a cement mortar. Where reinforcing is required by code, special units with bored cylindrical holes can be vertically stacked and filled with rebar and cement grout, thus

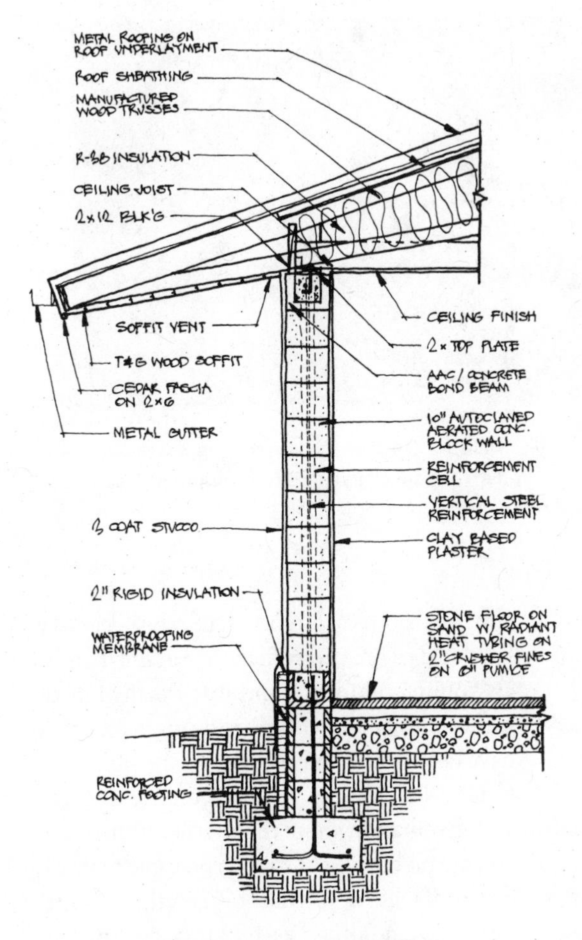

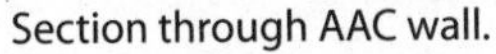
Section through AAC wall.

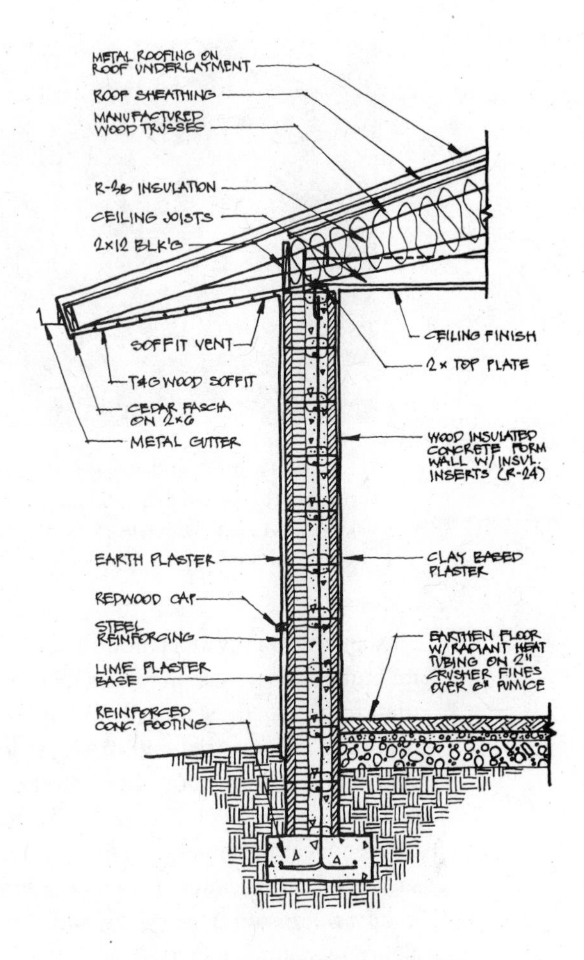

Section through wood insulated concrete form wall.

minimizing the use of cement. No blocking is required, and shelving and other attachments can be screwed directly into the walls. The blocks can be sawn, cut and shaped with woodworking tools. The solid, lightweight walls combine thermal mass and high insulation values. They have outstanding seismic, acoustic, and fire performance. The walls can be plastered inside and out and are inert and stable, with no toxic outgassing. This system has worked well for people with chemical sensitivities, but sensitive individuals should pretest the thinset mortars for acceptability. In North America, aerated autoclaved concrete is manufactured by **Aercon**, **Contec**, **Humabuilt HumaBlock,** and **TruStone.**

Conclusion

A variety of natural materials can be used to create heirloom quality buildings that are ecologically sound, promote health, and have

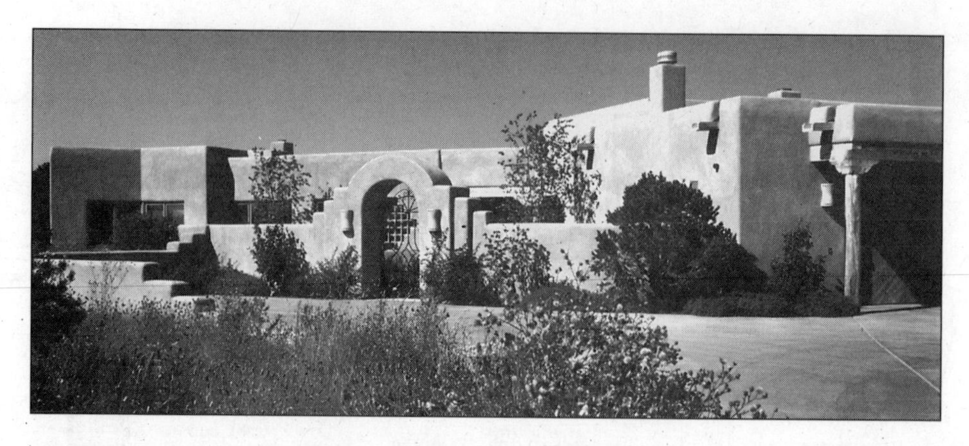

This "Santa Fe Style" residence features pumice-crete walls, hard trowelled plaster interior wall finishes, sustainably harvested maple flooring, central air filtration and specialty finishes throughout. Architect: Baker-Laporte and Associates; Builder: Prull and Associates.
Photo: Lisl Dennis.

outstanding energy efficiency. In short, natural building materials may be superior in all these respects to the standard building systems prevalent in industrial countries. An owner choosing to use a natural alternative building system is a pioneer who may be well rewarded for an adventuresome spirit. Regional factors such as drainage, rainfall, temperature, humidity, freeze and thaw cycles, and the availability of natural materials will make some natural building systems more suitable for certain locations than others.

When planning to build with alternative materials, make careful inquiry to determine the status of these materials with local building authorities to ensure that the alternative you choose will be permitted in your jurisdiction. Each of the model building codes used in the United States has a provision for alternative methods and materials. Building officials of the jurisdiction in which a project is located have the authority to approve any building they deem adequately meets the intentions and provisions of the code. It may be necessary to educate a building official about the materials you intend to use, and it is worthwhile to gather information about code approvals that have been granted elsewhere for the same materials. If a building official is unable to make a determination about the alternative material you are presenting, it may be possible to move forward with approvals by creating a legal document holding the building department harmless. **DCAT** is a nonprofit organization dedicated to addressing the challenge of institutional barriers to sustainable building and development found in building codes.

Earlier in the 20th century it was incumbent upon industrial manufacturers to prove to code officials that their products performed as well as their preindustrial counterparts. The powerful forces of industry, with their financial capability to test manufactured products, have now completely reversed the situation to the point where nonproprietary materials and methods of construction are viewed as inferior.

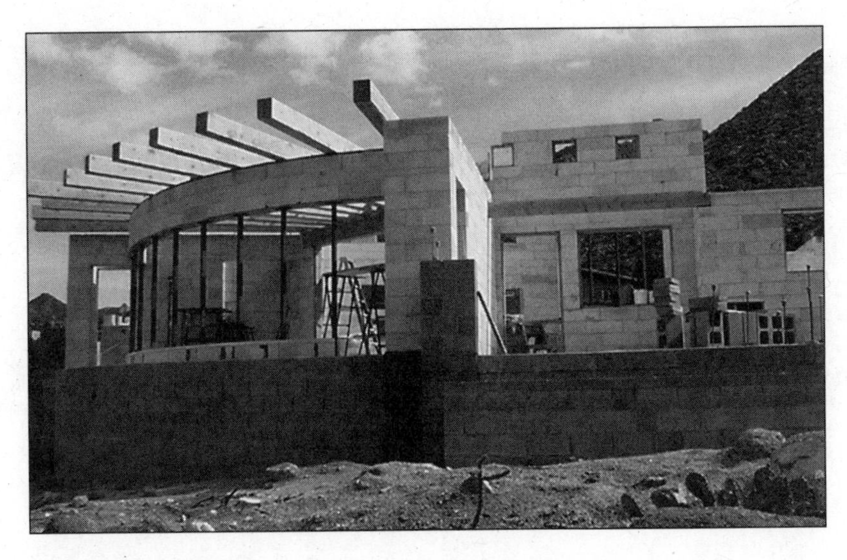

AAC home under construction. Photo: Paula Baker Laporte.

Ironically, this is so in spite of the thousands of years of research and development that have gone into the refinement of natural building techniques. In order to gain more widespread acceptance into mainstream building venues in this country, each example of natural building must be well-conceived, well-documented, and based on a sound knowledge of the laws of nature. In fact, a thorough understanding of building science is even more important for designers and builders using these alternative systems because of the high degree of experimentation involved in adapting ancient techniques to modern comfort and performance demands.

We would like to emphasize that the use of natural construction materials does not automatically create a healthy home. The material used in the building's walls is only one of many components that go into creating a home environment. However, when the alternative systems described in this chapter are used in conjunction with the other principles of healthy building outlined in this book, it is possible to produce buildings of exceptional vitality.

Further Reading

Baker-Laporte, Paula and Robert Laporte. *EcoNest: Creating Sustainable Sanctuaries of Clay, Straw and Timber*. Gibbs Smith, Publisher, 2005.

Chiras, Daniel D. *The Natural House*. Chelsea Green Publishing Company, 2000.

Cob Cottage Company. *Earth Building and Cob Revival: A Reader.* 3rd ed., Cob Cottage Company, 1996.

Easton, David. *The Rammed Earth House*. Chelsea Green Publishing Company, 1996.

Elizabeth, Lynne and Cassandra Adams, eds. *Alternative Construction: Contemporary Natural Building Methods*. John Wiley and Sons, 2000.

Evans, Ianto et al. *The Hand Sculpted House*. Chelsea Green Publshing Company, 2002.

Kennedy, Joseph et al., eds. *The Art of Natural Building*. New Society Publishers, 2002.

King, Bruce. *Buildings of Earth and Straw.* Solar Living Center, 1996.

The Last Straw: The International Quarterly Journal of Straw Bale and Natural Building. See thelast straw.org.

MacDonald, S.O. and Matts Myhrman. *Build It With Bales: A Step-by-Step Guide to Straw-Bale Construction.* Treasure Chest Books, 1997.

McHenry, Paul G. *Adobe: Build It Yourself.* University of Arizona Press, 1985.

Minke, Gernot. *Earth Construction Handbook: The Building Material Earth in Modern Architecture.* WIT Press, 2000.

Roodman, David Malin and Nicholas K. Lenssen. *A Building Revolution: How Ecology and Health Concerns Are Transforming Construction.* Worldwatch Paper 124, 1995.

Steen, Athena Swentzell et al. *The Straw Bale House.* Chelsea Green Publishing Company, 1994.

Steen, Bill et al. *Built by Hand.* Gibbs Smith, Publisher, 2003.

Wanek, Catherine. *The New Straw Bale Home.* Gibbs Smith, Publisher, 2003.

Weismann, Adam and Katy Bryce. *Building with Cob: A Step-by-Step Guide.* Green Books, 2006.

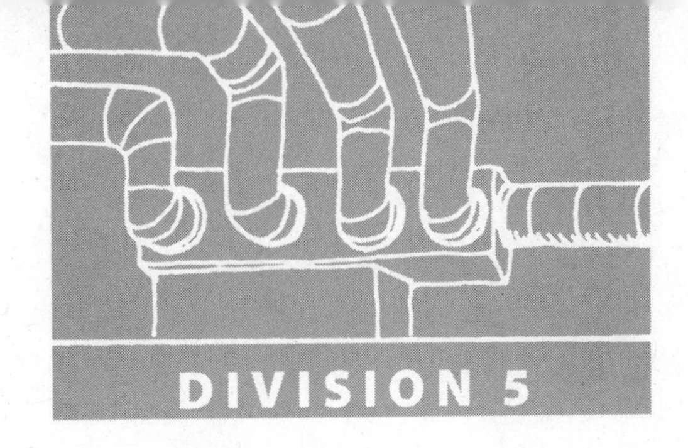

Metals

Oil Residue on Metals

Expanded metal lath and other metal goods are often shipped to sites coated in rancid oil residues left over from the manufacturing process. Such residues will be odorous for a prolonged period of time unless the metal is cleaned. When these oils are left in metal ductwork, hot air blown through the ductwork distributes these odors throughout the house. To avoid this unwanted pollution source, consider adding the following to your specifications:

- **Remove oil residue from all coated metal products using a high-pressure hose and one of the acceptable cleaning products listed in these specifications.**

Some builders have found that the high-pressure hoses at self-service car washes are effective for removing oil residues.

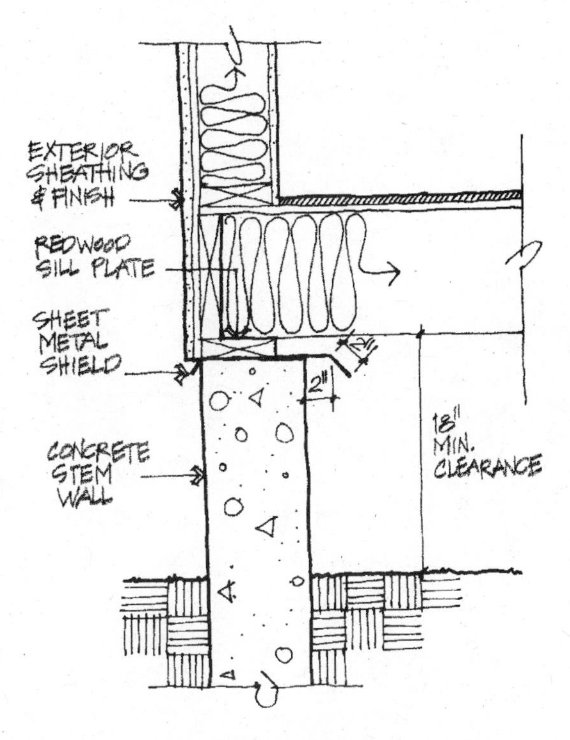

Termite Shield Detail.

Metals and Conductivity

The role that metals play in the electroclimate of a building, along with proper grounding considerations, will be discussed in Division 16.

Metal Termite Shielding

Where floors are joisted, the proper application of metal termite shielding, as illustrated, will create a physical barrier that is effective against subterranean termites.

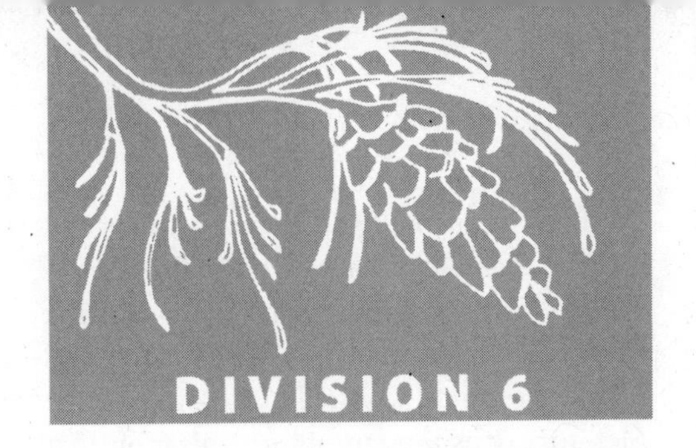

Wood and Plastics

Use of Sustainably Harvested Wood

The history of lumber harvest in the United States is long and complicated. On one hand, the relentless removal of the aboriginal forests built great cities and industries and made way for the agricultural abundance necessary for building a nation. On the other hand, the destruction of the aboriginal forests in all regions of the country was for the most part wanton, complete, and without regard for ecological, biological, and human costs.

As a nation we have moved beyond the idea of limitless resources. Wood can be used in an ecologically conscious manner through sustainable harvesting and replanting, along with a commitment to building methods that produce structures with greater longevity than the growth periods of the trees from which they are built. A sustainably harvested forest is one in which the forestry practices are continuously monitored and improved to ensure the present and future quality of both the wood resource and the forest itself. This approach includes consideration of the economic and social impacts on the communities involved and the protection of regional biological diversity.

Sustainably harvested wood can often be obtained for the same price as lumber harvested by environmentally damaging methods such as clear-cutting. By specifying the use of sustainably harvested woods for a building project, you are helping to raise awareness and increase market demand. Specifying sustainably harvested wood can be done by describing the standards the wood must meet in order to be classified as sustainable, or more simply by listing local suppliers of wood that has been reputably certified. In residential construction, where the builder may not have a sizable research and purchasing department, the second method is more effective.

The **Forest Stewardship Council** (FSC) is a leading international organization that sets standards for sustainability and accredits third-party, independent certifiers. In the

US there are currently nine organizations that are FSC accredited. These include the **SmartWood Certification Program** and **Scientific Certifications Systems** (SCS). The **Certified Forest Products Council** has now become **Metafore**. It is a nonprofit organization that provides information on sources for purchasing FSC certified wood, with state-by-state listings and more than 4,500 certified locations on its website. It also provides sample specification language tailored for use in the Construction Specifications Institute (CSI) Master Format.

Home Depot, the world's largest buyer of forestry products, adopted the FSC principles in 2001 and Lowe's, the world's second largest buyer, soon followed suit. Both now offer FSC products in a relatively wide range.

Health Concerns with Wood Frame Construction

Wood has historically been used as a component of a breathing wall system, whether it be the half-timber, wattle-and-daub constructions of medieval Europe or the log cabins of our ancestors in North America. (See Division 4 for an explanation of the breathing wall concept.) Wood is an advantageous material in a healthy home because it has the property of hygroscopicity. This means it has the ability to absorb and release moisture, thus helping to balance humidity levels and the electroclimate. However, for many chemically sensitive individuals the natural terpenes found in wood, especially soft or aromatic woods such as pine or cedar, are intolerable. Certain woods may need to be eliminated from, or sealed when used in, a home for a chemically sensitive person.

In standard home construction, the air space between the wood studs may be filled with insulation laden with chemicals. The exterior sheathing often contains formaldehyde-based glue or asphalt backing. The gypsum board applied to the inside face of the studs may be finished with harmful joint compounds. If the home was built before 2004, the studs sit on a sill plate that is most likely pressure treated with a pesticide to prevent rot and insect infestation. When standard construction is the only option, we recommend that the most benign wall construction materials available be used and that a barrier be installed between the wall construction and the living space. Refer to Division 7 for air barrier product and installation information.

In some instances, creating a barrier for the purpose of blocking fumes can cause other problems when moisture from condensation becomes trapped inside the wall. Applying the gypsum board in an airtight manner will help block fumes but will not in itself block the normal movement of water vapor. See Division 9 for more specific details on creating a barrier using gypsum board.

Construction lumber is at risk of contamination by pesticides when farmed, when milled, during transportation, and in storage. For those who have severe sensitivities to pesticides, it is important to locate a source for uncontaminated wood. Wood that is sustainably harvested can be traced from source to sawmill to distributor and its pesticide history can be determined. Certified producers and processors are encouraged to use least-toxic pest management. Some regional certification organizations have mandated a ban of pesticides for sustainably harvested wood in their jurisdictions. Certain imported woods may be

CASE STUDY 6.1

Pesticide-Treated Lumber

Although Germany has been a leader in the Bau-Biologie and healthy housing movement, it was only two decades ago that the general public there became aware of multiple chemical sensitivity disorder. This awareness followed the experiences of thousands of people who were exposed to lumber treated with both the preservative pentachlorophenol and the pesticide lindane. Hundreds of people developed chronic neurological complaints, chronic fatigue, and an unusually heightened sensitivity to chemicals that were previously tolerated. Lindane has subsequently been banned in Germany as a wood treatment.

dipped in pesticides that are now banned in the US. In some cases, uncontaminated lumber can be picked up directly from a local mill, where the sawyer will be closer to the source of the lumber and will know whether pesticides are used where the wood was grown.

Wood Selection and Storage

Kiln-dried framing lumber is drier than air-dried lumber. It is therefore more true to size and less susceptible to shrinkage and mold infestation. Certified, sustainably harvested, kiln-dried framing lumber is now becoming widely available. Framing lumber of this type is currently slightly more expensive than standard lumber, which is often logged using unsustainable practices.

Wood may occasionally be delivered to the site containing mold. It can also become moldy while stacked onsite if it is unprotected. To avoid these problems, you should include the following instructions in your specifications:

- **Framing lumber shall be kiln dried.**
- **Only wood that is free of mold and mildew is acceptable.**
- **Fir, spruce, and hemlock are preferred over pine where available at no additional cost to the owner.**
- **Wood stored onsite shall be protected from moisture damage by elevating it off the ground and covering it with a tarp during precipitation.**
- **Wood that becomes wet must be quickly dried by cross-stacking to promote aeration. It should have less than 16 percent moisture content, as tested by a moisture meter, and must be free of all signs of mold in order to be acceptable. (See Division 13 for moisture meter testing.)**

Wood Treatment

Wood surfaces and edges exposed to the weather will usually be surface treated to make them more weather resistant. Wood that is not naturally rot resistant and that will come in contact with moisture must be treated for rot and mold resistance. Creosote and pentachlorophenol are two commonly used wood preservatives that are quite toxic. Creosote is a dark-colored, oily tar that will outgas harmful vapors long after it has been applied.

Pentachlorophenol has been shown to cause liver damage in adults and fetal death and has been banned in some European countries. These substances should be prohibited for use in a healthy home. The wood treatment products discussed below do not contain these harmful ingredients.

Wood Treatment to Prevent Insect and Mold Infestation

- **BioShield**: Wood preservative oils
- **Bora-Care**: Low toxicity, borate-based, penetrating preservative containing glycol, used for protection against powder post beetles and subterranean termites
- **Livos Donnos Wood Pitch Impregnation**: Penetrating preservative for wood that is in contact with moisture
- **PureColor**: Two-stage stain formulation of pure mineral ions and oxygen catalyst for wood; no solvents, oils, VOCs, odors, acids, or bleaches; has antimicrobial and antifungal properties
- **Shellguard** and **Armor-Guard**: Borate-based wood preservatives for protection against wood-boring insects
- **Timber Pro UV**: Natural, plant-based, oil-based, waterborne breathable stain that seals and protects and is available in five standard and 40 custom colors with optional low-toxicity fungicide/algaecide (1 percent solution) providing mildew and algae resistance
- **Timbor**: Low toxicity, borate-based wood preservative that protects against drywood termites and wood decay fungi
- **Weather-Bos' The Boss**: Four different formulas for protection of exterior wood surfaces

Wood Treatment to Provide Weather and UV Protection

Many wood treatment products for exterior use are solvent-based and highly volatile. They can continue to outgas for several days or even weeks. Although exterior applications will have far less impact on indoor air quality than products used inside the home, they will still affect the applicator and sensitive people who are in the vicinity. This problem can be completely avoided thanks to the wide range of more benign products now available. Some of these lower-impact products are:

- **9400 W Impregnant**: Solvent-free, water-repellent, ultraviolet protective coating for interior/exterior wood; also effective in minimizing mold and mildew growth
- **AFM Safecoat Durostain**: Seven different earth pigment, semi-transparent wood stains for interior and exterior use
- **BioShield**: Wood preservative oils
- **Hydrocote Polyshield**: Interior and exterior polyurethane wood protection
- **LifeTime Wood Treatment**: Protects, stains, and beautifies wood products
- **Livos Donnos Wood Pitch Impregnation**: Penetrating preservative for wood in contact with moisture
- **Livos Dubno Primer Oil**: Undercoat for exterior wood
- **OS Wood Protector**: Preserves against water damage, mold, mildew, and fungus
- **PureColor**: Two-stage stain formulation of pure mineral ions and oxygen catalyst for wood; no solvents, oils, VOCs, odors, acids, or bleaches
- **Timber Pro UV**: Natural, plant-based, oil-based, waterborne breathable stain that seals and protects; available in five

standard and 40 custom colors with optional low-toxicity fungicide/algaecide (1 percent solution) providing mildew and algae resistance

- **Weatherall UV Guard**: Exterior acrylic wood finish that penetrates and seals, forming a protective shield against UV, rot, and decay; comes in clear and semi-transparent finishes
- **Weather-Bos' The Boss**: Four different formulas for protection of exterior wood surfaces
- **Weather Pro**: A water-based, water-repellent wood stain

Wood Maintenance

Common products for stripping, cleaning, and brightening wood often contain harsh solvents. The following product is safer:

- **Dekswood**: Cleaner and brightener for exterior wood.

Wood Adhesives

Wood adhesives commonly contain harmful solvents. However, solvent-free solutions are readily available and may be specified. The following adhesives are healthier choices for various wood related applications.

- 100% pure silicone caulk: Can be used as a subfloor adhesive; specify aquarium-grade caulk without additives
- **Chapco 244**: Acrylic urethane latex wood floor adhesive
- **DAP/Dow Corning**: 100% silicone sealant
- **DriTac 7500**: Solvent-free, zero-VOC wood flooring adhesive
- **Elmer's Carpenter's Glue**: Low-odor, nontoxic, water-based glue for porous materials
- **GE Silicone II**: 100% silicone sealant for a variety of indoor and outdoor applications
- **Roo Glue**: Waterborne, environmentally safe adhesive for cabinetry, flooring, and most other construction materials
- **Taylor Meta-Tec 2086 Tuff Lok-Link**: GreenGuard certified solvent-free, low-odor polymer-based wood flooring adhesive
- **Timberline 2051 Wood Flooring Adhesive**: For laminated plank and parquet flooring
- **Titebond Solvent Free Construction Adhesive**: For plywood, paneling, and hardboard
- **Titebond Solvent Free Subfloor Adhesive**: For subfloors

Rough Carpentry

Sill Plates

Sill plates or mudsills are decay- and insect-resistant wood members used in frame construction wherever wood comes into contact with concrete or soil. For many centuries before toxic petrochemicals came to be used, builders had devised natural means for avoiding rot and insect infestation. They commonly charred the portions of wood that were to be placed in the ground or else used naturally resistant woods. From about 1974 to 2003, the standard building practice was to use lumber pressure treated with chromated copper arsenate (CCA) or ammoniacal copper arsenate (ACA). CCA and ACA contain arsenic salts and chromium compounds that can leach out onsite and be absorbed through the skin or ingested by mouth. They are extremely toxic to

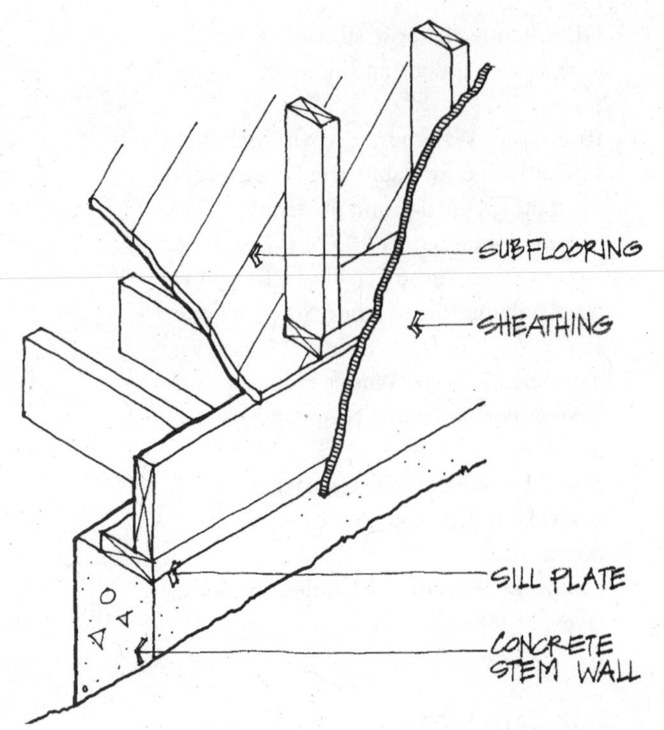

Wood frame construction showing sillplates.

both humans and the environment. The use of these chemicals for sill plates is now banned but they still will be found in most existing frame homes. CCA imparts a green tinge to the wood. You have probably seen this toxic wood used in children's playground equipment.

It is important that no recycled sill plates containing CCA or ACA find their way into new construction, and you may wish to add the following to your specifications:.

- **No wood treated with chromated copper arsenate (CCA) or ammoniacal copper arsenate (ACA) may be used on this job. The following wood treatment products may be used:**
  - **ACQ Preserve: Wood treatment containing alkaline copper quaternary (ACQ)**
  - **Nature Wood: A waterborne wood preservative containing ACQ**
  - **TimberSIL: A nontoxic, arsenic-free wood treatment process that uses sodium silicate technology (SST)**
- **The heartwood of untreated farmed cedar or redwood is acceptable for use as sill plates where approved by local code officials.**
- **Where the sill plate is at least 18 inches above grade, a metal termite shield may be used instead of a treated sill plate if acceptable to local code officials.**

Framing

Wall Framing

Where wood 2x wall framing is used, follow the guidelines for wood selection and storage in this Division.

Roof and Floor Framing

Solid beams, round logs, or 2x joisting are commonly used for shorter roof spans. Manufactured trusses, typically made of composite wood products and assembled into profiles engineered for strength, are commonly used for longer spans. They have several advantages over solid lumber. They are less expensive, use wood resources more efficiently, have greater span capabilities, provide a deep pocket for roof insulation, and can be fabricated with a built-in slope for flat roof application.

Truss joists, commonly called TJIs, are manufactured beams containing either plywood or dimensional lumber for top and

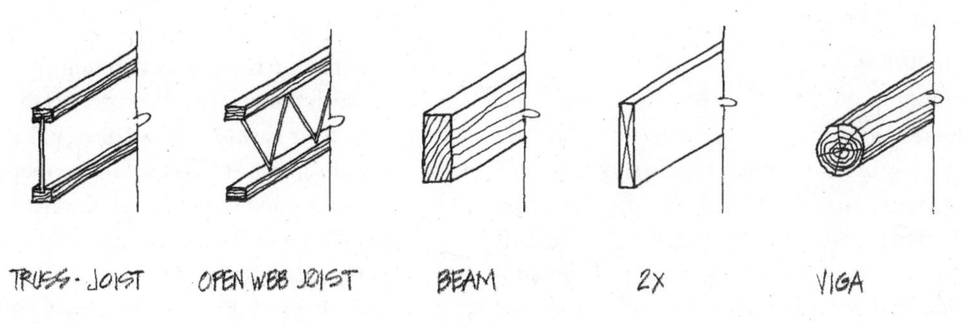

Ceiling framing components.

bottom chords, and either plywood or pressboard for the webs. Because they are a very cost-effective way to frame large spans, truss joists are widely used in residential construction. The members are subjected to heat during manufacturing, which helps cure them, reducing the quantity of VOCs they emit into a new home. A small amount of formaldehyde remains. In new home construction, the cumulative effect of several low emissions can add up to unacceptable levels. Where an airtight gypsum board assembly or air barrier is applied between the structure and the living space, these fumes will be fairly insignificant. If there is still concern, however, the TJIs can be sealed. **BIN Primer Sealer** is particularly good for this purpose because the white color allows you to visually inspect the job and make sure everything has been well coated. Another option is to use open-web roof trusses with dimensional lumber for the top and bottom chords and webs, thereby avoiding the use of pressboard entirely.

Special Procedures for Interior Garage Walls

Ideally, to prevent harmful automobile fumes from entering the home the garage should not share walls with it. If this is not possible, a series of extra procedures should be followed:

- **Follow procedures for airtight gypsum board installation (as outlined in Division 9) between garage and home.**
- **Apply Type X gypboard to garage walls per code.**
- **Use a solid core, weatherstripped door between home and garage.**
- **Thoroughly seal the door sill with one of the sealants listed in Division 7.**
- **Make all electrical penetrations in the wall airtight. (See section on gasketed electrical boxes in Division 16.)**
- **Seal and tape any plumbing penetrations between garage and home with aluminum tape.**
- **Provide automatic mechanical exhaust ventilation in the garage as outlined in Division 15.**

In addition to these built-in barriers, the homeowner can greatly reduce the risk of these fumes entering the home by opening the garage door before starting the car and turning off the motor as soon as the garage is entered, or by using an electric or hybrid car that does not burn fuel while idling or at slow speed.

Sheathing

Subflooring

Interior-grade plywood and particleboard are typically used for subflooring in standard construction. Urea-formaldehyde glues are used to bond the wood during manufacturing. This is a concentrated, volatile form of formaldehyde that contributes significantly to indoor air pollution. In addition, the subflooring may then be attached to the framing underneath with solvent-based glues that will also contribute to the pollution level.

Solid wood, as well as the cementitious subfloor sheeting more commonly used in commercial building, can be considerably more expensive, but exterior-grade plywood can substitute for interior-grade plywood for only a small increase in cost. While exterior-grade plywood contains less-volatile phenol-based formaldehyde glues, it will still release significant amounts of formaldehyde into the air when new. Airing out the wood by cross-stacking it onsite is better than installing it immediately after delivery. Sealing the wood after it has been aired out will provide the most protection against toxic fumes and this extra step may be taken for chemically sensitive individuals. We suggest the following specifications for healthier subfloor installation:

- **The use of subflooring materials such as interior-grade plywood, pressboard, or oriented strand board (OSB) containing urea-formaldehyde glues is prohibited.**
- **Subfloor adhesive must be solvent free. (Refer to the section on wood adhesives.)**
- **The following may be used for subflooring in place of products containing urea-formaldehyde binders:**
  - **structural cementitous sheeting**
  - **1x finish floor boards laid parallel to walls over 1x subfloor laid diagonally to walls may be a good solution when a finished wood floor is desired; verify for proper span conditions with the architect or engineer**
  - **exterior-grade plywood that has been aired out; may be sealed with BIN Primer Sealer or another acceptable sealer on all six sides for extra protection for chemically sensitive individuals**

Exterior Sheathing

Exterior sheathing in wood frame construction is attached to the outside of the frame and makes up the surface to which the exterior finish is applied. Before manufactured sheet goods such as plywood were available, 1x or 2x material was nailed to the studs for this purpose. In standard wood frame construction today, exterior-grade plywood or OSB (oriented strand board, also known as waferboard) is typically used as exterior sheathing for the entire building or at corners where shear strength is required. These materials contain varying degrees of formaldehyde and isocyanates and do not have the longevity of solid wood products.

Many problems with the use of OSB in roof and wall sheathing have recently been identified. In fact, one prominent manufacturer was the subject of a class action suit. When the board gets wet it is vulnerable to fungal invasion and rapidly deteriorates. Asphalt-impregnated fiberboard or asphalt-sheathed insulating board is commonly used as infill between the corner shear panels. Since asphalt is a known carcinogen, we believe that any exposure level is too high when other alternatives exist.

When an air barrier or airtight drywall assembly is used on the interior face of a wall, sheathing material will not have as great an impact on the indoor air quality as the materials exposed to the interior. Moreover, the sheathing will have had several weeks in place to air out before it is covered up. In a permeable or breathing wall system, where vapor barriers are eliminated with the intent of allowing vapor movement through the wall, the type of exterior sheathing must be more carefully considered in terms of both permeability and harmful chemical content. The following may be included in your specifications to reduce the pollution generated by exterior sheathing:

The following products are unacceptable for exterior sheathing:

- **products containing asphalt**
- **odorous foam insulation boards**
- **pressure-treated plywood**

The following products and methods are acceptable for exterior sheathing:

- **1x recycled lumber laid diagonally with diagonal metal or wood bracing as structurally required (a more labor-intensive and expensive solution, most suitable for breathing wall frame applications)**
- **CDX-grade plywood that has been aired out (purchase as far in advance of installation as possible and stack to allow air flow on all sides of each sheet while protecting it from moisture damage)**
- **non-odorous foam boards such as bead board**
- **AdvanTech: very low emissions, durable composite wood sheathing for walls, floors and roof**

Roof Sheathing

Roof sheathing is placed on top of roof framing members and under the roofing. As with exterior sheathing, exterior-grade plywood or OSB is most commonly used for this purpose. Unlike wall sheathing, roof sheathing will be exposed to high temperatures and will therefore be subject to more intense outgassing. Roof sheathing usually has less time to air out in place since it is roofed over as soon as possible to avoid water damage from precipitation. We therefore recommend that plywood, if used, be stickered and aired on site. We do not recommend OSB because it can develop mold and deteriorate more rapidly if it happens to get wet. When roofing members are exposed to the interior, as is often the case when beams or vigas are used, solid wood or tongue-and-groove planking is commonly used.

For sloped roofing, when structural conditions permit, purlins or skip sheathing may be acceptable in place of solid sheathing. Purlins are wooden members spaced to receive metal roof panels, while skip sheathing consists of solid wooden members spaced more closely together for shingle and tile roof applications. Both purlins and skip sheathing eliminate the need for sheet goods and allow ample air movement to ventilate the roof space. However, they do not provide the shear strength that plywood provides and their use must also be weighed from an engineering standpoint.

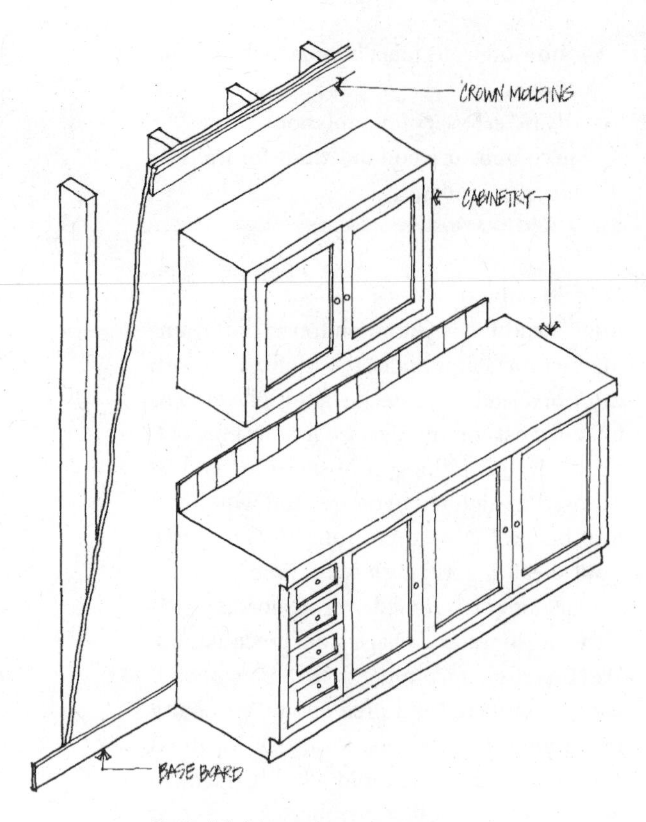

Typical finish carpentry components.

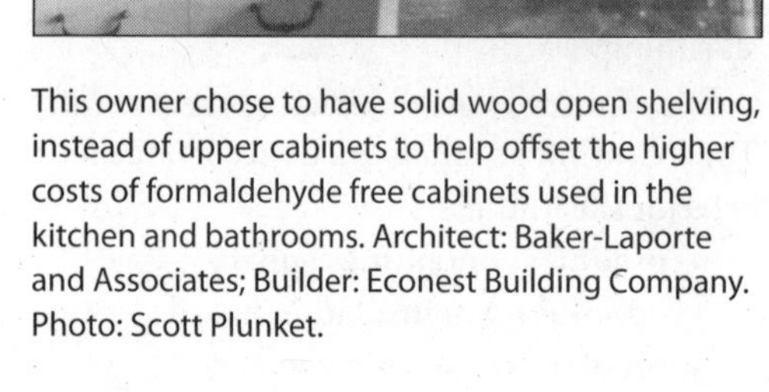

This owner chose to have solid wood open shelving, instead of upper cabinets to help offset the higher costs of formaldehyde free cabinets used in the kitchen and bathrooms. Architect: Baker-Laporte and Associates; Builder: Econest Building Company. Photo: Scott Plunket.

Where a continuous air barrier is installed between the framing members and the living space, the choice of sheathing material is less crucial.

Consider the following guidelines for inclusion in your specifications:

- **The use of solid wood boards, tongue-and-groove board, solid wood skip sheathing, or purlins is preferred where structurally acceptable.**
- **CDX-grade plywood, when used for roof sheathing, should be purchased as far in advance as possible to allow time to air out. Provide protection against moisture damage.**
- **Provide a continuous air barrier on the inside face of the ceiling assembly as outlined in Division 7.**

Finish Carpentry

Many manufactured composite board products designed for interior use contain urea-formaldehyde binders. They outgas formaldehyde for many months and contribute significantly to the indoor pollution level. In standard construction, these interior-grade composites are used in many finish applications including cabinetry, molding, shelving, and trim. They should not be used in a healthy home. The following may be specified:

- **No sheetgoods or trim pieces containing urea-formaldehyde shall be used.**
- **Exposed interior finish wood shall be comprised of solid wood and finished with a low-VOC finish as specified in Division 9.**
- **Where sheet goods are used, choose one of the low-emission boards listed in the section on cabinets, or exterior-grade plywood that has been aired out, thoroughly sealed on all edges and surfaces with an acceptable vapor barrier sealant, and finished with one of the paints specified in Division 9.**
- **Trim pieces shall be milled of solid wood or made of formaldehyde-free composites such as Medite II or equal.**

Medium Density Fiberboards

Medium density fiberboard (MDF) is sheetgood material used for interior nonstructural applications such as cabinetry boxes and shelving. Traditionally, MDF has been bound with urea-formaldehyde-based glues, making their use unacceptable in a healthy house. The following products are formaldehyde-free and may be available laminated with plastics or hardwood veneers:

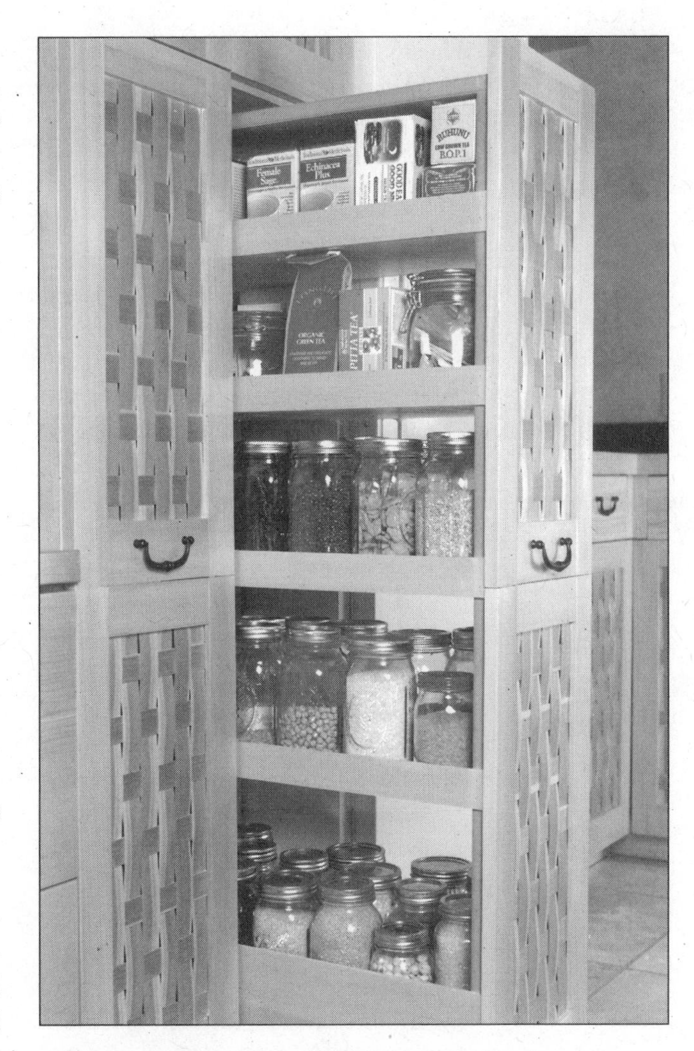

Efficient kitchen storage can obviate the need for some upper cabinets thus helping to offset the higher costs of formaldehyde free cabinetry. Photo: Lisle Dennis.

- **Arreis**: Scientific Certification System certified medium density fiberboard with no formaldehyde added in the manufacturing process
- **Glacier Clear**: Scientific Certification System certified medium density fiberboard with no formaldehyde added in the manufacturing process
- **Medex** or **Medite II**: Scientific Certification System certified medium density fiberboard manufactured without formaldehyde

- **Wheatboard** or **Wheatstraw**: Medium density fiberboard made from straw fiber and containing no incremental formaldehyde emissions

Cabinets

Although the drawers and doors on cabinetry are often made of solid wood, the boxes or cases are usually composed of particleboard, interior-grade plywood, or melamine, which has a particleboard core that is exposed where holes have been drilled for adjustable shelving. Cabinets are most often finished with solvent-based finishes that may outgas high levels of VOCs for several months.

Because standard cabinetry contributes significantly to poor indoor air quality, it is not acceptable in the healthy house. You will pay more for healthier cabinets, but in terms of indoor air quality, this is money well spent. If your budget is tight, we suggest you explore strategies that will reduce the amount of cabinetry necessary. For example, you may choose to consolidate some of your kitchen storage in a pantry area, or to use attractive solid wood open shelving for dishes or cookware as a less expensive alternative replacing some of the upper cabinets.

Finishes on wood cabinet doors and drawers are commonly solvent-based applications that will take many months to fully cure. Some of the lacquer finishes, although odorous when first applied, will completely cure before they are brought to the jobsite and will not require refinishing for many years. If these are applied in quality controlled, well-ventilated shops, they may be worth considering. Ask for a recently applied, dated sample to help make your determination. Low-VOC, water-based finishes that are more suitable for jobsite or factory application are listed in Division 9.

As cabinetmakers are becoming more familiar with the need for healthier cabinetry, and as low-VOC finishes and materials become available, the price gap between standard and healthy cabinets is decreasing. The following companies manufacture formaldehyde free or low emissions cabinetry:

- **Cervitor**: Distributors of metal cabinetry with a baked-on enamel finish that may be used with metal or solid wood doors and drawers
- **Core Home**: Cabinets manufactured to European E1 emissions standards with FSC certified products
- **Humabuilt Wheat Core Cabinets**: Pressed wheatboard boxes, premium-grade woods and veneers assembled with ultra-low-VOC adhesives and finishes, free of synthetic formaldehyde
- **Neff Cabinets**: Manufactured cabinets with a 98% reduction in formaldehyde content
- **Neil Kelly Cabinets**: Cabinetry system designed to meet the needs of the chemically sensitive, with cores of wheatboard or Medite II with wood veneers, and a wide variety of door and case veneers. Door and drawer fronts available with certified woods, prefinished with AFM clear sealers or paints.

For all options, specify the use of a solvent-free carpenter's glue in the fabrication process.

The following products are formaldehyde-free sheetgoods that can be used for making cabinet boxes:

- **Environ Biocomposites**: Line of formaldehyde-free, agri-based sustainable panel

CASE STUDY 6.2

The Radioactive Countertop

John Banta was called to the home of a woman who was employed as a cook by the television industry. Her task was to create samples of the same recipe in various stages of preparation, from raw ingredients to oven-ready mixtures to finished product. The prepared foods were then delivered to the television studio so a celebrity on a culinary arts program could demonstrate the recipe.

During the investigation, John discovered that his client was being exposed to an unexpected occupational hazard. The orange-colored tile used for her counter was glazed with uranium oxide, a highly radioactive substance that was making the numbers on the Geiger counter spin too fast to count. For over 30 years this woman had worked at a radioactive counter, slicing, dicing, mixing, and arranging her creations.

When she learned of the radioactivity, the client revealed to John that she had recently had a precancerous lesion removed from her intestines. Her surgical scar was located at the level where the counter pressed against her while she cooked. The client was advised to have her countertop replaced. Her physician concurred.

products for interior finishes and cabinetry (see Resource List for products)

- **Medex** or **Medite II**: A medium density fiberboard manufactured without formaldehyde
- **Multi-core**: A low-emissions plywood with a variety of hardwood veneers
- **PureKor**: Specify their formaldehyde-free board
- **Roseburg SkyBlend Particleboard**: Scientific Certification Systems certified, low emissions, certified recycled content, no urea-formaldehyde added during manufacturing process
- **Temstock-Free**: No added urea-formaldehyde particleboard underlayment and industrial-grade particleboard
- **Terramica**: Scientific Certification Systems certified no added urea-formaldehyde particleboard underlayment and industrial-grade particleboard
- **Tru-Spec**: Line of urea-formaldehyde-free, millwork-quality wood strand engineered wood products for interior wood finishes and cabinetry, GreenGuard certified

Alternatives to Hardwood

Because hardwoods take a long time to grow and are therefore not as sustainable as faster growing alternatives, you might consider the following healthy alternatives to hardwood for your finsh carpentry and cabinetry:

- **Allowood**: Hardwood lumber substitute manufactured from faster growing softwoods and agri-based materials
- **Environ Biocomposites**: Line of formaldehyde-free, agri-based sustainable panel products for interior finishes and cabinetry
- **Bamboo**: Refer to Division 9 for bamboo sources

Countertops

The ideal countertop material for a healthy home would have a solid, nonporous surface that is stain- and scratch-proof. It could be attached by mechanical means directly to the cabinet boxes, thus avoiding the need for underlayment and adhesives. It would be beautiful, inexpensive, and manufactured in a variety of colors. Unfortunately, all of these characteristics are not found in combination in a single countertop option. Chart 6.1 reviews the most common countertop materials and outlines specification concerns for each.

Chart 6.1: Countertop Comparisons

Type	Relative cost	Advantages	Disadvantages	Comments	Specify
High pressure laminates (e.g., Formica, Wilsonart)	Lowest initial investment	• Wide variety of colors, patterns, textures, and sheens • Low cost • Seamless surface	• Glued to particleboard with toxic glues • Particleboard outgasses formaldehyde • Not stain- or acid-resistant • Will scratch • Cannot be resurfaced • Short life; deteriorates quickly if the particleboard gets wet	• Not a good choice for a healthy home	• Fasten to cabinetry with mechanical fasteners • Seal all exposed edges and surfaces of particleboard with foil or one of the vapor barrier sealants listed in Division 9
Solid-surface materials (e.g., Corian, Avonite, Swanstone, acrylic or plastic colored with resin)	Expensive	• Nonporous • Sanitary; integral sinks and rolled backsplashes are easy to clean • No substrate needed for most • Scratches and stains are easily sanded • Attractive marble- and granite-like surfaces • Can be mechanically fastened	• Can be more expensive than granite or marble	• Select a type that does not require substrate	• Fasten to cabinetry with mechanical fasteners

Chart 6.1: Countertop Comparisons (cont'd.)

Type	Relative cost	Advantages	Disadvantages	Comments	Specify
Tile	Can be moderate	• Hard, scratch-resistant surfaces • Large variety of sizes, colors, and textures to choose from	• Grout joints are subject to staining and mold and bacterial growth • Glazes may contain heavy metals or be radioactive • Tiles can crack or chip under heavy impact	• Choose large tiles to reduce the number of grout joints • Choose presealed tiles • Choose commercially rated tiles • Choose tiles requiring the narrowest grout joints • Choosing porcelains with integral color will disguise chips	• Follow recommendations in the tile section of Division 9 for underlayment, tile setting, and grout sealing
Butcher block	Moderate	• Warm, inviting aesthetics • Natural material • Can be refinished by sanding • Does not require underlayment • Can be mechanically fastened	• Porous surface stains easily and can harbor mold growth	• Seams might have been glued with formaldehyde-based adhesives	• Finish with odorless, nontoxic oil such as walnut oil • Fasten to cabinetry with mechanical fasteners • Use adhesives that are solvent- and formaldehyde-free
Solid sheet granite	Expensive	• Wide selection of very beautiful stones • Hard, scratchproof, stain-resistant surface that will last forever • Solid, seamless surface • Can be mechanically fastened or glued with silicone • May not require substrate	• May be cost prohibitive • Surface must be finished with impregnating finish	• Oil or butter left on surface will stain it • Must check for radioactivity	• Examine MSDS of surface impregnating finish for toxicity • Fasten mechanically or with 100% pure silicone caulk (aquarium/food grade)
Engineered stone quartz — 93% quartz, 7% resin (e.g., Silestone, CaesarStone, Cambria, Zodiaq)	Expensive	• Does not require sealing • Stain-, scratch-, and heat-resistant • Hygienic • Can be mechanically fastened	• Heavy • Requires professional installation	• Good choice for durability and hygienic properties and because it does not require use of impregnating finish	• Fasten mechanically

Chart 6.1: Countertop Comparisons (cont'd.)

Type	Relative cost	Advantages	Disadvantages	Comments	Specify
Granite tile	Moderate	• Can resemble granite but is less expensive than slab • Very thin grout joints can be sealed with transparent silicone • Mar- and scratch-resistant	• Requires epoxy-type glues to set • Requires underlayment	• Oil or butter left on surface will stain it • Must check for radioactivity	• Examine MSDS of surface impregnating finish for toxicity • Refer to section on underlayment for tile in Division 9
Stainless steel	Expensive	• Nonporous, nonstaining • Easily cleaned continuous surface	• Thinner gauges require underlayment • Noisy • Must be special-ordered	• Conducts electricity • Proper ground fault interrupters are essential to prevent potential electrocution	• Use formaldehyde-free underlayment and mechanical fastening
Solid slate	Comparable to granite	• Nonporous, nonstaining	• Softer than granite and can chip	• Can be mechanically fastened • Does not require finish	

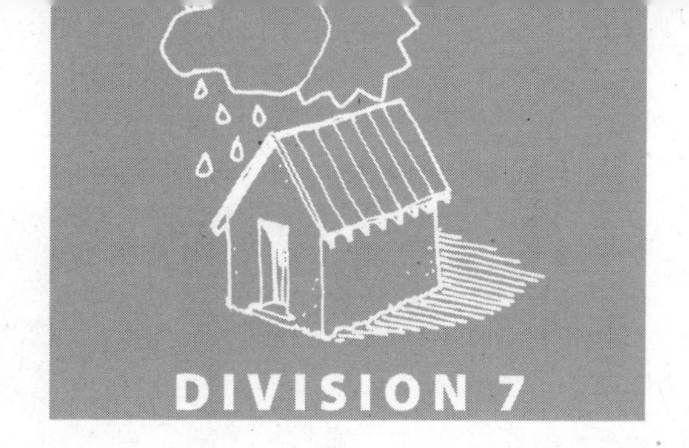

Thermal and Moisture Control

Foundation Water Management

Dampproofing is used to form a water-resistant barrier on the outside of stem walls where they come into contact with the earth. This treatment is especially important wherever there is a crawl space or basement below grade. Along with proper grading and perimeter drainage, dampproofing is used as protection against the migration of moisture through the wall. Water migration can result in a damp environment under or inside the home, which can lead to structural deterioration of the building. This is a frequent and serious cause of mold infestation throughout the country.

Dampproofing of stem walls is only one component of the creation of an effective water barrier. Proper drainage backfilling and final grading are also essential in order to drain unwanted water away from the wall and relieve hydrostatic pressure that, if present, will drive water through any imperfection in the dampproof barrier and the stem wall. Conscientious and thorough workmanship are of the utmost importance. The following sample specifications describe the proper installation of perimeter drainage.

Installation of Perimeter Drainage

A drain system shall be installed around the perimeter of the foundation footing. The drainage system shall consist of the following:

- **Positive drainage shall be away from the building along the entire perimeter, with a slope of no less than 5 percent and a top layer of impervious soils.**
- **Dampproofing of all exterior wall surfaces that are below grade or in contact with soil shall be carefully applied according to the manufacturer's directions to form a watertight barrier. (See below for a list of acceptable products.) Care shall be taken during backfilling and other construction to prevent damage to the dampproofed surface.**

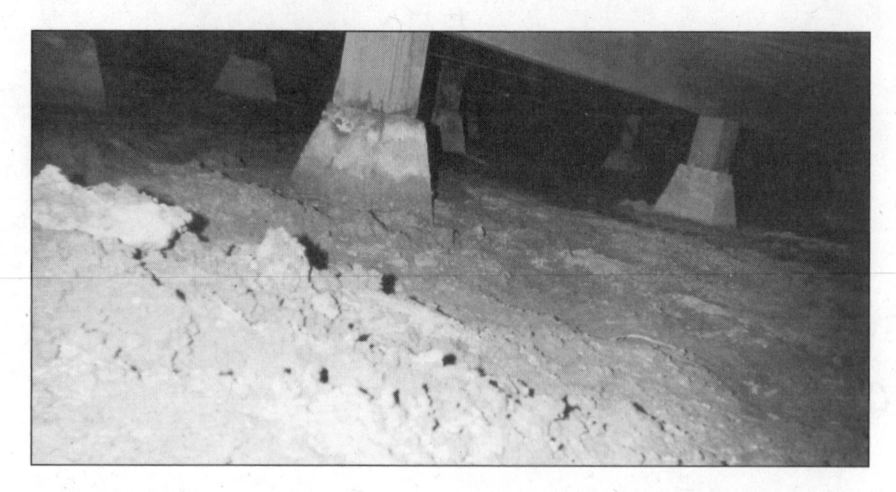

The Problem: Saturated crawl spaces created perfect conditions for mold growth. Recommendation: Crawl spaces should be dry. Perimeter drainage and detailing should keep water out of the crawl space and a barrier placed over the soil can prevent soil moisture from creating moldy conditions.
Photo: Restoration Consultants.

- A free-draining backfill of ¾-inch minimum crushed stone or gravel that is free of smaller particles shall be used to line and fill the excavation for all below-grade walls.
- An engineered drainage system may be substituted for a free-draining backfill. These systems frequently incorporate perimeter insulation with the drainage. The engineered drainage system must be installed in strict compliance with manufacturers' specifications.
- A french drain shall be installed so that all perforated pipes are located below the level of the bottom surface of the footing. French drain perforated pipes shall be installed with the holes down to allow water to rise into the pipe. If holes are present in more than one side of the pipe, at least one set of holes shall face downward.

  French drains shall be sloped downward a minimum ¼ inch per foot of run and be connected to daylight. If a french drain cannot be connected to daylight, it may have to be connected to an underground engineered collection pool, a sump pump, or a storm sewer system. The architect or engineer should then provide drawings that explain the exact requirements. This situation is not ideal because sump pumps can fail and storm sewers can back up. If these problems are not quickly corrected, water damage may result. If the storm sewer is connected to the sanitary sewer — a situation that is usually not permitted in new construction — any backup may also result in sewage on the exterior side of underground walls.
- The perforated pipe shall be surrounded and set in a minimum 2-inch depth bed consisting of a minimum ¾-inch size of crushed stone free of smaller particles.

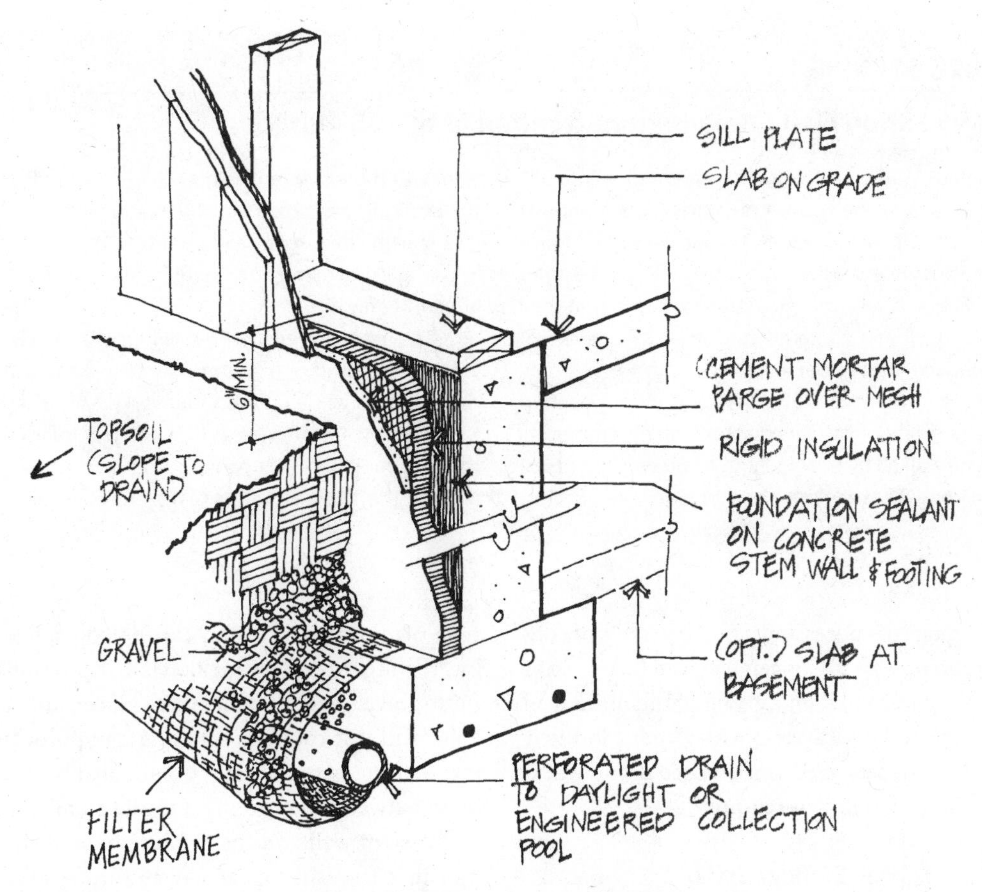

Perimeter drainage and stem wall treatment.

- **The perforated pipe and crushed stone shall be surrounded by a filter membrane to prevent adjacent soil from washing into and clogging the french drain system.**

Dampproofing for Foundation Walls

The use of asphaltic and bituminous tar mixtures for dampproofing is standard practice. These petrochemical-based materials are known carcinogens. There are several other readily available products made for this purpose that are more healthful choices. The following products may be specified for dampproofing foundation walls or other walls adjacent to soil:

Cementitious Dampproofing

- **Thoroseal Foundation Coating**: A cementitious dampproofing for concrete and concrete masonry unit (CMU) surfaces.
- **Xypex**: A nontoxic (according to manufacturer), zero-VOC chemical treatment for dampproofing and protection of poured concrete, it creates a nonsoluable crystalline structure that permanently

CASE STUDY 7.1

How Radon First Came to the Attention of the US Public

Stanley Watras had worked as an engineer for 11 years at a nuclear power plant in Pennsylvania. At the end of each workday, he and other plant employees were checked by a monitor that measured radiation levels. This procedure ensured that they had not been contaminated by unsafe levels of radioactivity while at work.

In December 1984, Watras suddenly began setting off the buzzers on the radiation monitors as he walked by the machine on his way out of the building. The readings showed high levels of contamination over his entire body. For several days this scenario was repeated, with Watras subjected to a lengthy decontamination ordeal. Where was Watras picking up this radioactivity and why was it affecting only him?

The mystery was solved when Watras decided one morning to go through the monitors at the exit door as he entered the workplace. When the alarms went off, Watras immediately realized that the radiation was coming from somewhere outside the nuclear power plant. The local elec-

plugs the pores and capillary tracts of concrete. Xypex Concentrate can be used as a single-coat dampproofing membrane or in a two-coat system with Xypex Modified. Xypex Modified can be used alone where dampproofing is required.

Fluid-Applied Dampproofing

- **AFM Safecoat DynoFlex**: A topcoat for use over DynoSeal
- **AFM Safecoat DynoSeal**: A flexible vaporproof barrier
- **Rub-R-Wall**: Asphalt-free moisture resistant membrane products for various foundation applications

Bentonite Dampproofing

- **Volclay**: A self-healing bentonite-based moisture resistant panel

Creating a Capillary Break

Under some conditions, water will move upward through the soil by capillary action. This type of moisture invasion can be controlled by creating a capillary break. Half-inch minimum gravel, free of smaller fines, placed under a slab will stop capillary action. A dampproofing coating or membrane should also be applied between the footing and the stem wall or the stem wall and the framing to stop any moisture from being carried up through the concrete and entering the framing.

Soil Gas Management

A variety of natural and human-caused soil gases can infiltrate structures and lead to indoor air quality problems. Soil gases can be sucked into basements, crawl spaces, and floor slabs if negative pressurization exists within or under a structure. You can prevent this problem by creating a physical barrier between the soil and the home and by controlling the air pressure conditions under and within the home.

Harmful human-source soil gases include

tric company sent a team of specialists to his house to investigate. The readings on the Geiger counter showed levels 700 times higher than the maximum considered safe for human exposure. Researchers concluded that the culprit was radon, a naturally occurring radioactive gas derived from underground uranium.

Discussion

At that time, very little was known about radon and its health effects. The Watras house was used as a laboratory for radon researchers who wanted to learn how radon gets into a house and how to get it out. Low-grade uranium ore was discovered beneath the basement of the structure, in direct contact with the house. The foundation of the house was removed, along with the soil underneath, to a depth of four feet. Ventilation fans were installed to pull radon-laden air out from under the house. Watras and his family were eventually able to move back into their home.

pesticides, herbicides, and gases from nearby landfills or industrial sites. In new construction, most of these problems can be avoided through careful site selection and through home and yard maintenance that is free of toxic chemicals.

Water vapor and radon gas are two naturally occurring soil gases that may infiltrate a structure and result in health problems. The intrusion of water vapor into the home may cause structural damage and mold problems. These gases are both easily dissipated or blocked from entry by installing appropriate controls during the construction process.

Radon Gas Infiltration

Radon is a clear, odorless gaseous byproduct of the natural breakdown of uranium in soil, rock, and water. While radon gas dissipates in open spaces, it tends to cling to particulate matter and accumulates when enclosed. When inhaled, radioactive particles become lodged in the mucous membranes of the respiratory system. The Surgeon General has stated that radon exposure is second only to tobacco smoke as a cause of lung cancer.

It has been estimated that as many as one in 15 homes in the United States contains elevated radon levels. The EPA recommends mitigation at levels higher than 4.0 picocuries per liter of air. Even at 4.0 picocuries per liter, there is an increased risk of lung cancer. Therefore, reducing radon to between 1.0 and 1.5 picocuries per liter is a prudent target, ensuring a margin of safety.

Radon mitigation is most effective and least costly when incorporated into the construction of the home. If you are building a new home and there is reason to suspect a radon problem, a soil test is advisable. Although the test will not tell you definitively what the radon levels will ultimately be in the finished home, it will help you decide whether to include mitigation measures in your construction plans. For more information about this test, refer to Division 13.

Water Vapor Infiltration

The infiltration of water vapor as a soil gas is a common problem that may be due to several conditions, including high water tables, underground springs, or hardpan soils that cause excess water to remain at the surface. Certain soils hold moisture so that, instead of percolating through the soil, water vapor evaporates and travels upwards. Even with proper perimeter drainage around the building, which will take care of flowing water, this residual water vapor may be sufficient to cause damage.

Soil Gas Mitigation and Prevention

Foundation detailing and design affect the amount of soil gases that will accumulate in a building if they are present in the soil. The basement is the most vulnerable to radon and other soil gas seepage because it has the largest surface area in contact with the soil. Crawl spaces under buildings, especially unvented ones, can concentrate these gases. The gas is easily transferred to the living space if there is not an effective air barrier separating the living space from the soil under the crawl space. A slab-on-grade can form an effective barrier against soil gas, but any cracks, joints, or penetrations in the slab will create routes for soil gas to enter. Where elevated soil gas levels are suspected, clay-based and other types of permeable floor systems that come into direct contact with the ground are not recommended without supplementary controls.

Methods of Soil Gas Mitigation

The EPA conducts radon mitigation training programs for contractors. State offices can provide you with the names of contractors who have been trained and qualified under the EPA's Radon Contractor Proficiency Program. Contractors who understand radon mitigation will have a basis for understanding any type of soil gas mitigation. A good strategy for soil gas mitigation consists of the following three components:

- **Blockage of all potential entry routes**: Concrete slabs and basement walls must be properly reinforced to minimize cracking. (Refer to Division 3 for information on concrete reinforcement.) Cracking in concrete floors is a common occurrence. Cold joints and expansion joints help control where cracking will occur so it can be more easily and reliably sealed. Plumbing penetrations must be sealed with a flexible caulk. (Refer to recommended caulking materials in this chapter.) Special barrier sheeting placed under the slab or over the soil in the crawl space will further block soil gas from entering. Basement walls must be thoroughly parged. Concrete floor slabs and block or poured concrete walls can by coated with **AFM Safecoat DynoSeal** or another low-emissions flexible membrane to further seal cracks and joints.
- **Prevention of negative pressurization of the building envelope**: A home that has lower air pressure than the surrounding outside environment will be negatively pressurized. This creates a vacuum that will suck air and soil gases into the building wherever there happens to be a route of entry, including tiny cracks in the slab, crawl space soil barrier, or basement walls. To prevent negative pressurization, it is important to provide sources for the controlled supply of outside air into the home to replace the air lost through the operation of various appliances such as exhaust fans and clothes dryers. Creating a condition

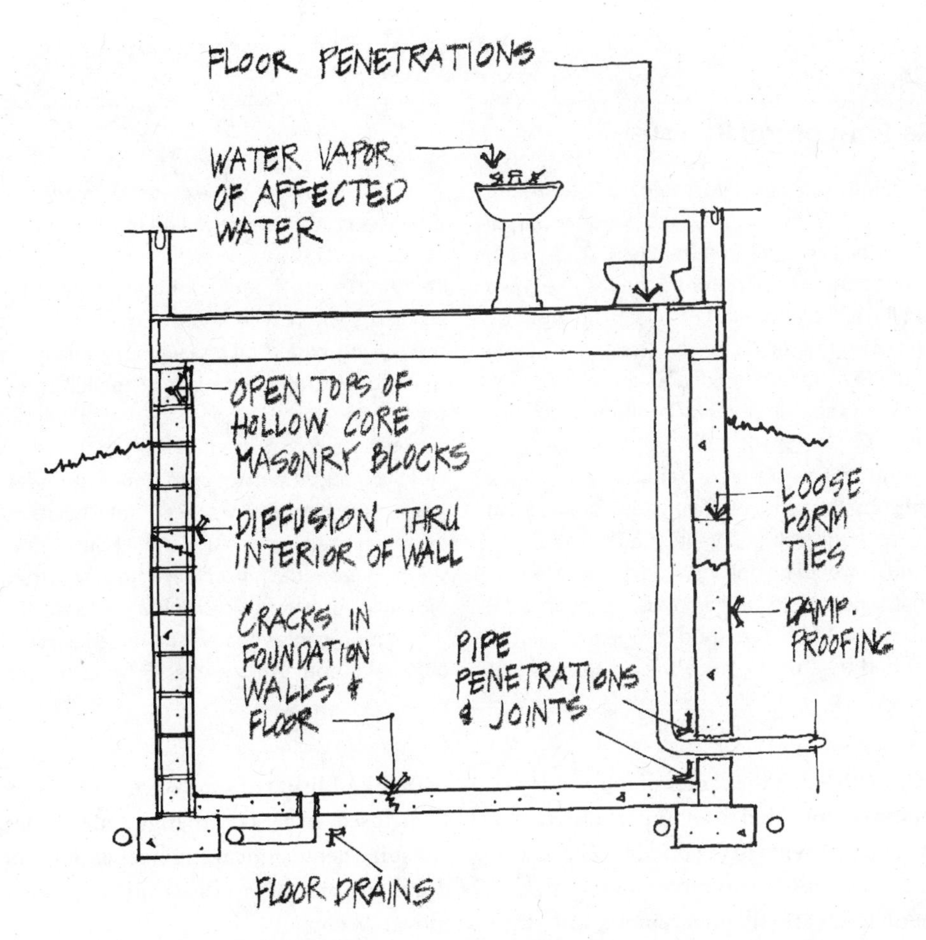

Potential entry points for radon and other soil gases.

where there is a slight positive pressurization can be an effective means of reducing levels of radon and other soil gases. Strategies for providing proper pressurization are discussed in Division 15.

- **Collection of soil gas from under the building envelope and redirection away from the building**: There are several methods for accomplishing this task. **Professional Discount Supply** is a company that specializes in radon mitigation supplies. Many of these same materials are applicable to all soil gas mitigation.

You may want to include the following collection methods in your specifications, along with instructions for proper installation of barriers and sealants:

Method 1: A 4-inch layer of aggregate is placed under the building envelope. A 4-inch-diameter perforated pipe is laid in the

CASE STUDY 7.2

A Radon-Control Retrofit

John Banta was called to evaluate a home for radon. The owner had received a do-it-yourself radon test kit as a gift from relatives. When he finally got around to performing the test, he could not believe the laboratory results. His daughter's room registered 24 picocuries, six times higher than the EPA's recommended action level. John's electronic radon equipment confirmed the test results.

John proposed a radon reduction technique called subslab suction. It involved sucking radon from under the slab and ventilating it to the outside. Holes would be drilled in the downstairs slab so that pipes could be inserted and connected to an exhaust fan, a method frequently used in unfinished basements. Since the owner had just finished installing an expensive marble floor downstairs, he was not willing to accept this proposal.

After some thought, John suggested that the subslab suction technique be modified so that the drilling would take place horizontally under the slab through the outside of the hill on which the first floor rested. A company that drills horizontal wells was contracted for the job. The site was surveyed and the drill set to bore just under the foundation. Six evenly spaced holes were bored horizontally all the way under the house. After the drill was withdrawn from each hole, a perforated pipe was inserted to provide a pathway for gas from radon-contaminated soil to be sucked from under the home. The owner finished the job by

aggregate through the center of the envelope. The pipe is connected to an unperforated riser tube that vents to the outside. The vent tube acts as a passive radon removal outlet. If radon levels are still unacceptable once the building is completed, a fan can be attached to the vent pipe to actively suction out the gas.

Method 2: In place of aggregate and perforated pipe, Soil Gas Collector Matting can be laid on the finished grade prior to pouring concrete. The matting, which is covered in filter fabric, is laid around the inside perimeter of the foundation in a swath about one foot wide, and the concrete is poured directly on top. The matting is connected to a vertical riser vent that extends through the roof. The natural chimney effect will draw the soil gas upward. If deemed necessary, the system can be adapted for active suction with the addition of a fan once the building is enclosed. In areas with high water tables, consult a geotechnical engineer about proper drainage prior to installing any soil gas removal system.

Products for Soil Gas Control

The following low-emission products may be used to block entry of radon from the ground into the living space:

- **AFM Safecoat DynoSeal**: Water-, vapor-, and moisture-proof membrane sealer
- **Cross Tuff**: Specify radon-control grade
- **Tu-Tuf 4**: Crosslinked polyethylene sheeting

Water Management at Doors and Windows

Door and window openings that are improp-

joining all the perforated pipes together with solid pipe. At a short distance from the home he connected an exhaust fan to the pipe to suck radon to the outside, where it dissipated. The pipes were then covered with soil and the area landscaped. The radon in the home was reduced to an acceptable level of approximately one picocurie. If the fan is shut off, however, the radon level will begin to climb. More radon testing was carried out on other buildings located on the property and in the general neighborhood. No other elevated radon levels were found.

Discussion

Radon can exist in isolated spots, depending on underlying geological formations. Some parts of the US are known to have higher radon levels than others. Homes with basements, cellars, or other subterranean structures are the most susceptible to radon accumulation. Yet even homes with slab foundations and ventilated crawl spaces can have elevated levels. The only way to be certain is through radon testing. In John's experience, radon can almost always be reduced to acceptable levels. When building your home, use appropriate techniques to avoid the possibility of radon accumulation if radon is known to be present in your area.

erly detailed are a common source of water intrusion in homes. Often these leaks go undetected until they have caused severe damage when water finds a path directly into the wall cavity without ever revealing damp surfaces visible from within the home.

Until recently, all products for door and window flashing were asphalt-based. The following flexible flashing products do not contain asphalt:

- **Tyvek FlexWrap**: Self-sealing, 70-mil elasticized polyethylene film laminate with a synthetic rubber adhesive for windowsills, round top and custom shaped windows, 3D sill projections, and wall interruptions
- **Tyvek StraightFlash**: Self-sealing, 30-mil polyethylene film laminate with a synthetic rubber adhesive for jambs and heads of rectangular shaped windows
- **VaproFlashing**: Non-self-sealing bonded polypropylene fabric flashing, requiring the use of VaproAdhesive to adhere to most building materials (refer to **VaproShield**)
- **WindowWrap-Butyl**: Self-sealing 20-mil laminated polyethylene film with butyl rubber adhesive for flashing window and door openings and building joints

Thermal Protection

Moisture Problems Associated with Building Insulation

The addition of thermal insulation into wall cavities has had a major impact on moisture control in buildings. As buildings have become tighter and better insulated, the opportunity for water vapor to dry out from wall and roof assemblies has been reduced. Trapped water leads to wall assembly failures.

Buildings in cold winter climates will tend to dry to the outside since moisture flows from the warm interior towards the cold exterior. Under these conditions, water vapor passing through insulated building assemblies will reach a temperature where it will begin to condense. If this condensation occurs before the vapor reaches the exterior of the building, the insulation will become wet. Most insulation acts like a sponge, collecting moisture that is unable to escape. If an adverse moisture condition persists, mold and rot will affect the structure even when inorganic fiberglass insulation has been used.

In hot, humid conditions the situation is reversed but equally problematic. When hot, moist air is allowed to enter the wall from the outside, it may condense in the insulation as it approaches the colder, air-conditioned space.

The insulation alone does not create the problem, but because of its absorbent nature it will often augment the problem. The type of vapor retardant barrier and its position in relation to the insulation are critical in preventing mold and rot from developing. The general principle is to install the vapor retardant barrier so that it prevents the travel of moisture into the insulated cavity without impeding the ability of the moisture to escape. The dilemma is that climatic conditions may vary widely on a daily and seasonal basis, creating mixed conditions. This makes insulation and moisture

Remedying a Mold Problem

DAN STIH

If you think you have a mold problem or if you are sick in your home and suspect mold is to blame, I recommend contacting a reputable professional to do an investigation. The self-test kits found at local hardware stores are not accurate. They may tell you there is a problem when there is not and they are not good at detecting *Stachybotrys*, one of many problematic types of mold. *Stachybotrys* has frequently been referred to as "black mold," but there are many types of mold that are black. You can't judge a mold by its color; there are some types of edible mold that are black and other molds that aren't black but are probably every bit as bad as if not worse than *Stachybotrys*. So getting a competent diagnosis is important.

Several states have licensing requirements for mold inspectors. By itself, having a license does not make one competent. Ever had a bad haircut from a licensed cosmetologist? A bad roof installed by a licensed roofer? One helpful screening tool is checking to see if the inspector has Errors and Omissions (E & O) insurance. Another is asking for references. See if the consultant has been in the business for awhile, if they have complaints on file with the Better Business Bureau, and if they are in good standing with professional or trade organizations. It also makes sense to hire a mold inspector who has experience in other areas of indoor environmental quality, building science, and Building Biology.

A mold inspection should really be called a mold investigation. Unless you see mold there won't be any inspecting, and at least half the time mold is hiding. One way to look for mold is look for damp spots. The inspector should spend time checking the moisture levels of walls and ceilings

control procedures more complicated and requires site- and climate-specific design strategies beyond the scope of this book. Guides that distinguish and explain these design strategies for climate-based moisture control are available through The Energy & Environmental Building Association (EEBA). We highly recommend them. (See Further Reading at the end of this chapter.)

Insulation Products

Fiberglass Insulation

Ninety percent of the homes in the United States are insulated with fiberglass insulation. There has been much debate as to whether or not fiberglass is a human carcinogen, and for a period of time fiberglass insulation was labeled with the warning "probable human carcinogen." Although the material did not change in any way, the labeling was dropped. Whatever the case may be, fiberglass is by no means a healthful substance. Fiberglass insulation can release both particulate matter and gaseous contaminants into the air from formaldehyde binders in the fibers and asphalt in the backing. There are numerous reports linking fiberglass to pulmonary disease in production workers and installers.[1,2] Although healthier alternatives exist, they are generally more expensive and may not be as readily available. However, since the cost of insulation comprises a very small percentage of the overall building cost, even doubling this figure will not constitute a large increase in the cost per

with a moisture meter. If you find a damp spot you will have found a place with the potential for mold growth. The longer it has been wet, the greater the risk that mold has grown. Suspect areas can be tested for mold.

Even if a moisture meter does not detect a damp area, that does not mean there is no mold. Often things get wet, mold grows, things dry out, and mold sticks around waiting for them to get wet again. Just because the building is dry now does not mean the mold is gone. Sometimes when you are looking for mold you just have to start testing the areas that are suspected to have been damp at one time. Since a good percentage of mold problems are due to plumbing leaks, the first places to look are under bathroom and kitchen sinks, inside utility closets, next to hot water heaters, and behind the washing machine.

How do you remove mold? If you are cleaning it from a hard, nonporous surface such as bathtub grout, use a nontoxic detergent and remove the stains with a hydrogen peroxide-based cleaner. Contrary to popular belief, bleach does not kill mold that has grown in your wall cavities or other porous materials. And even if bleach did kill mold, it would not be recommended since dead mold spores are still allergenic. The properties of toxigenic molds are not neutralized by bleach or disinfectants. Mold needs to be removed. If it is removed, there will be nothing left to kill or sanitize.

If mold is present on porous materials or in inaccessible places such as wall cavities, remediation by a qualified professional is strongly recommended. If you are mold sensitive, don't even think about doing it yourself! Effective remediation

square foot of your home. Formaldehyde-free fiberglass insulation is now being produced by major insulation companies and is becoming readily available.

One of the more reasonably priced alternatives to fiberglass is cellulose spray-in or loose-fill insulation. This product has an R-value of ±3.5 per inch. It can contain corrosive or toxic fire retardants, but many brands are available with more benign borate-based treatment that also protects against mold and insect infestation. Recycled newsprint is often used as a major component of cellulose insulation, which may introduce harmful dioxins into the mix. This type of insulation should not be exposed to the ambient air. Some manufacturers provide virgin or cardboard content instead (refer to the list of alternative insulations below). The printing industry has shifted to predominant use of soy-based inks making dioxin exposure less of an issue.

Choosing one of the alternate building systems discussed in Division 4 is another option. In most of these systems, the more massive walls themselves provide the insulation.

Fiberglass Batt Products

The following brands of fiberglass batt contain fewer harmful chemicals or are encased, thus providing safer installations:

- **CertainTeed**: Manufactures undyed, unbacked fiberglass batt insulation.
- **ComfortTherm**: Fiberglass batts that come prewrapped in polyethylene bags. These have limited application, however, since the bags must be cut open and trimmed wherever spacing is irregular.
- **Johns Manville**: A line of formaldehyde-

---

requires specialized equipment, containment, and protective clothing.

To effectively remove mold, porous materials such as wallboard, plaster, insulation, and carpeting need to be cut out and thrown away. Wood may be sanded or wire brushed clean. Even if only a small amount of visible mold is present, there may be hidden mold, When cutting into the walls, using containment and other safety precautions may be necessary. At this level the remediation goes beyond the scope of most homeowners. When selecting a professional mold remediation company, consider one that specializes in mold and water damage restoration. Mold grows only where there is or has been water, so the two go together.

Why not try to prevent mold so you don't have to worry about all this in the first place? Sudden floods from plumbing leaks are responsible for a large number of mold problems. If you have a sudden flood or a plumbing or roof leak, don't merely try to dry things out yourself. If things are not dry within 48 hours you may end up with mold. The first 24 hours are critical. Look in the phone book under Water Damage Restoration. Insurance companies usually pay for sudden and accidental water damage (not floods from outdoor sources), but they frequently don't pay for mold, or they place a low cap on what they will pay. Call your insurance company immediately but don't let a water damage problem become a mold problem by waiting for their approval or for an adjuster to visit your house. Have the emergency water damage taken care of immediately. Once it's dry, you can spend time negotiating with the insurance carrier about the repairs. If mold grows because you did not call

free fiberglass insulation products. Fibers are bonded with a formaldehyde-free thermosetting resin.
- **Knauf Fiber Glass**: Fiberglass insulation products certified by GreenGuard.

Fiberglass Blown-In Blanket System (BIBS)

Loose-fill fiberglass insulation is blown behind netting or sheeting. Noncombustible fiberglass fibers contain no chemicals or binders and are inert. The products average R-4 insulation value per inch. They include **Climate Pro** by Johns Manville and **InsulSafe 4 Premium Blowing Wool** and **Optima** by CertainTeed.

Alternatives to Fiberglass Insulation

The following alternative insulation systems can be cost effective if suppliers and applicators are located in your vicinity:

- **Air Krete**:* A cementitious magnesium oxide insulation that is foamed in place.
- **BioBased 1701**: GreenGuard certified soybean-based polyurethane water-based closed-cell spray-applied foam with an R-value of 5.5 per inch.
- **Celbar**: Cellulose insulation treated with a borate compound for fire resistance, available in loose-fill or spray-in application. The loose-fill can be ordered without recycled newspaper content.
- **Florapan**: Hempwool insulation, although not available in this country, is used in Europe and can be imported.
- **Good Shepherd Wool Insulation**: Wool batt and wool rope (for log buildings) insulation imported from Canada.

a water damage restoration company immediately, your insurance company may even hold you responsible.

Professional drying companies will bring in industrial-strength fans and dehumidifiers that will dry the building quickly. They may drill holes in the walls and in the kick plates of bathroom and kitchen cabinets. The insides of walls are usually the last place to dry out and the first place mold is going to grow. Drilling or cutting holes in the walls is frequently necessary to allow air to circulate into the wall cavities.

What else can you do to prevent mold growth? Mold can't grow without water, so prevent excess moisture in your home. Check for slow plumbing leaks under bath and kitchen sinks and in utility closets. Caulk or grout any cracks in shower tile and cracks or gaps behind and around kitchen sinks. Maintain the roof. Caulk around exterior doors and windows twice a year. Keep water away from the house. If water collects next to the house when it's raining, install gutters and change the landscaping to drain water away. Keep things dry and mold can't grow. It's that simple.

Dan Stih, BSE, CMC, CIEC, is an aerospace engineer, Certified Microbial Consultant, Certified Indoor Environmental Consultant, and Building Biologist. He is the author of *Healthy Living Spaces: Top 10 Hazards Affecting your Health*. Visit healthylivingspaces.com for more information about mold.

CASE STUDY 7.3

Moist Soil in Crawl Space Causes Ceiling Damage

A 15-year-old single-family residence was purchased for year-round occupancy in a popular ski area of Idaho. During the first spring in the home, the family noted water dripping from the ceiling of the kitchen. The dripping continued for a couple of days, and then the condition appeared to resolve itself. The family forgot about the problem until it recurred during the spring of the second year. This time they noted a strong, musty odor developing inside the kitchen cabinets. Once again the dripping soon stopped, but a few days later mold became visible on the kitchen ceiling and inside the upper and lower cabinetry.

Investigation revealed that the soil in the crawlspace under the kitchen was damp. Because the moisture vapor content of the soil under the home was high, moisture was coming into the home as a soil gas. It was traveling through the ceiling, condensing on the cold underside of the kitchen roof, and freezing. During the spring, the ice block melted into the ceiling space above the kitchen, soaking the gypsum board and insulation. The wet insulation acted like a sponge, holding excess moisture long enough to cause mold growth.

The owner was advised to install a vapor retarder on the soil surface of the crawl space. At this point, he admitted with embarrassment that

- **Icynene Insulation System**:* A low-density, sprayed-in-place modified urethane foam insulation that is free of formaldehyde, fibers, CFCs, and HCFCs and according to the manufacturer has no detectable emissions after 30 days. It performs as an air barrier and is vapor-permeable, with an R-value of 3.6 per inch.
- **Ultra Touch**: A formaldehyde-free natural fiber insulation made mostly of recycled content, with thermal and acoustic performance superior to fiberglass batt. No warning labels and no respirator or protective gear necessary for installation. Comes unbacked in 5½-inch R-19 batts or 3½-inch R-13 batts.

(*Wet-applied insulation must be thoroughly dry prior to application of an air barrier in order to avoid trapping excess moisture in the wall cavity.)

Insulation Over Exposed Beam Ceilings

Where structural members of the ceiling are exposed, the air space between the structural members is not available to receive insulation. In flat roof construction, various tapered insulation systems are designed to go over the exposed ceiling decking and create a sufficient slope for proper drainage. The less toxic alternatives tend to be expensive. It may be more cost effective to build cavity area over the existing exposed ceiling and insulate with one of the above-mentioned products.

Insulation Around Doors and Windows

Regardless of the type of construction, the juncture where windows and doors meet the structure is a potential source of unwanted air infiltration and condensation. The industry standard for sealing this gap is to use an expandable urethane foam product.

there had been a layer of plastic on the soil when they had purchased the home. He had noticed damp under the plastic, so he had removed the plastic to allow the soil underneath to dry. Unfortunately, the release of the extra soil gas moisture was sufficient to cause water damage and mold growth. Had the owner left the soil gas barrier in place, he could have prevented the mold problems from developing.

Discussion

Mold infiltration in this home originated with excess moisture in the soil, the cumulative effect of several mistakes and building inadequacies. Better crawl space ventilation would have helped to remove some of the excess moisture. However, because of the extreme cold in Idaho, large amounts of natural ventilation can freeze pipes. Mechanical ventilation would have been a better solution. The roof also lacked sufficient ventilation. Well-built homes have multiple controls. In this case the vapor barrier worked well enough to prevent noticeable moisture problems for 15 years. The removal of the barrier by the owner was the straw that broke the camel's back.

Foam Insulation

The foam may contain toxic chemicals that will outgas in the wet stage but are believed to cure completely after a short time. These foams may also contain hydrochlorofluorocarbons (HCFCs). Because HCFCs play a role in depleting the ozone layer, the United States is phasing out their consumption by first limiting and then ending their production and import in a stepwise fashion, with the eventual phaseout scheduled for 2030.[3]

Because polyurethane foams do an excellent job of sealing and insulating these gaps, their efficacy must be weighed against their environmental impact. A look at any of the product MSDS sheets will reveal several petrochemical-based ingredients that are considered to be toxic. It is possible to lessen the environmental impact by specifying HCFC-free foam. Where the small amount of outgassing from the dried foam is a concern, the foam can be covered, once it has fully cured, with an air barrier material such as aluminum tape. **Polyken Tape 337** is an aluminum tape that has been used successfully by some chemically sensitive individuals for this purpose. Since the tape is moisture impermeable, care must be taken not to trap moisture.

The following widely distributed polyurethane foams do not contain formaldehyde:

- **Great Stuff**
- **Tiger Foam**

Alternatives to Foam Insulation

Recently several natural alternatives to polyurethane foam have become available. Those wishing to avoid synthetic foams may consider the following options:

- **Custom Woolen Mills**: Wool products for home insulation.

- **Eco Wool**: Wool batting products.
- **Florapan**: Hempwool insulation, although not available in this country, is used in Europe for this purpose and can be imported.
- **Log Home Wool**: Sheep wool insulation in batts or rope configuration can be used for sealing around doors and windows.

Air Barriers

Impervious sheeting, applied to the inside face of stud walls behind the finish surface, is often used to block air movement and is mandated by building departments in some localities. In a home built with standard frame construction, such a material is also a means of blocking the fumes generated by undesirable building materials in the wall cavity from entering the living space. The barrier itself must also be free of noxious odors and emissions. (See the list of suitable air barriers below.)

This method is not intended for use in hot, humid climates, especially where air conditioning is used. Because moisture vapor migrates from warm to cold, condensation can occur on the insulation side of the barrier, causing hidden water damage and microbial growth. This type of barrier is often used by chemically sensitive individuals as a temporary measure to block fumes emanating from walls, floors, and ceilings in an existing building. A safer method is to create an air barrier that still allows for the transpiration of moisture through the wall. This can be achieved by applying the gypsum board in an airtight manner. Refer to Division 9, "Creating an Air Barrier with Gypsum Board," for the specifics of this application. When a sheet-type air barrier is to be applied, use only unbacked insulation to avoid creating a double barrier in the wall cavity.

Given the complexities of construction and the number of materials that must be mechanically fastened together, it is almost impossible to avoid punctures in air barrier sheeting. The ultimate success of the barrier will depend on the quality control that is exercised during installation and before all finish surfaces are applied.

Air Barrier Installation

The following instructions can be included in specifications for the proper installation of sheet-type air barriers:

- **An air barrier shall be applied on the inside face of studs, joists, or rafters just prior to the application of the interior facing. After applying the acceptable air barrier (see list below), seal with 100 percent silicone caulk or foil tape. Staple the barrier in pieces that are as large as possible over the insulation and attach them to the window and door jambs with staples and approved caulk to form a complete seal. Caulk all wall openings such as plumbing and electrical boxes. Tape or caulk all seams and joints. Caulk all electrical boxes at the hole where the wire comes through, or purchase gasketed boxes (refer to Division 16 for product information). Note: This type of installation is not recommended in air conditioned climates.**

Air Barrier Products

The following products generate few or no emissions and are suitable for air barriers:

- **Aluma-foil**:* Foil laminated on two sides of kraft paper with nontoxic adhesive.

- **Cross Tuff**: Cross-laminated polyethylene sheeting. If you specify "for a healthy house," the manufacturer will incorporate additional processes.
- **Dennyfoil**:* Virgin kraft paper laminated with foil containing sodium silicate adhesive on both sides.
- **Reflectix**: Foil-faced and -backed over plastic bubbles, especially designed to reflect heat.
- **rFOIL**: Reflective foil insulation product with two layers of plastic bubbles with foil in the middle.
- **Super R** and **Tempshield**: Radiant barriers and reflective insulation.
- **Tu-Tuf 4** or **XF**: High-density, cross-laminated polyethylene sheeting.
- **Tyvek HomeWrap**: Housewrap is generally used for exterior applications and is somewhat vapor permeable while highly resistant to air movement. It can be used to create a suitable air barrier for interior use if it is necessary to block wall, floor, or generated fumes in an existing structure.

(*Not suitable for areas that may get wet.)

Roofing

A well-sloped roof with a sizable overhang is preferable to a flat or low-sloped roof for the following reasons:

The roof overhang plays an important role in protecting the walls and foundation from water damage by directing water away from the building.

Inert roofing materials are readily available and are standard products for sloped-roof construction, while they are an exception in flat or low-sloped residential roof construction.

Sloped roofs shed water quickly, whereas water will puddle and linger on poorly constructed flat roofs.

Flat roofs have a higher failure rate and shorter life expectancy, which may lead to devastating mold problems.

Overhangs can be sized to suit the solar conditions in your region, providing shade in the summer while allowing maximum heat entry in the winter.

Sloped Roofing Materials

Asphalt-based rolled roofing and shingles will outgas when heated by the sun and should be avoided. Clay tile, concrete tile, metal, and slate are all inert, long-lasting slope roof solutions. Wood shingles can be a good roofing material where fire danger is low and humidity is moderate and if rot resistant woods such as cedar are used. Zinc or copper strip applied at the ridge will wash wood shingles with preservatives every time it rains. Availability of roofing materials varies from region to region.

Roofing Underlayments

In many cases, roofers will want to install an asphalt-based felt paper over the roof sheathing. Several non-asphaltic-based underlayments are now available to choose from:

- **RoofShield**: High permeability three-layer spun bond polypropylene underlayment
- **RooftopGuard**: Five-layer polypropylene/polyethylene underlayment
- **StrongSeal Roofing Underlayment**: Contains no asphalt; both nail-down and self-adhering membranes
- **Titanium UDL**: Non-asphaltic, coated synthetic roofing underlayment for sloped roofs

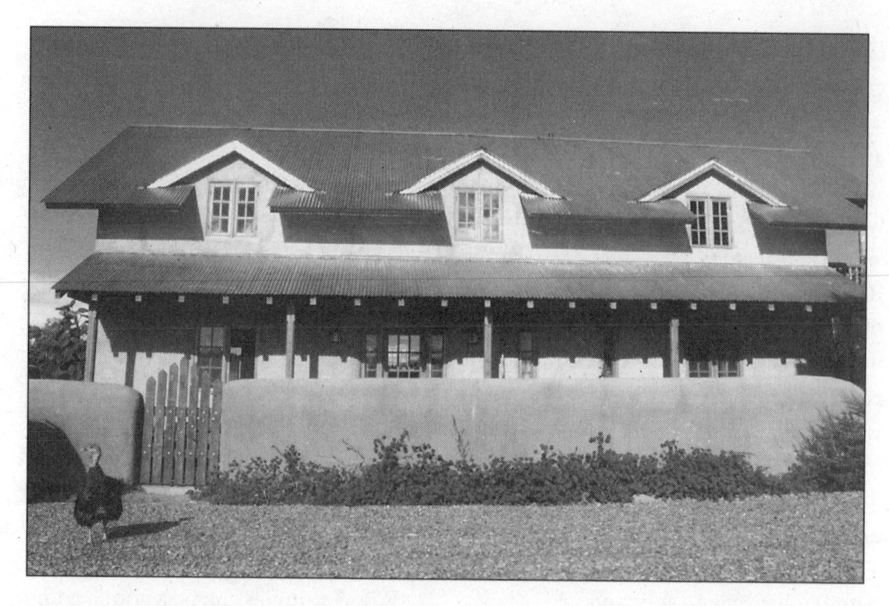

Northern New Mexico style straw bale building with metal roofing. Architect: Baker-Laporte and Associates; Builder: Living Structures.
Photo: Paula Baker-Laporte.

Membrane Roofing

Membranes for flat roofing can be problematic. These roofs are in fact more accurately described as having a very low slope, usually ¼ inch per foot or less. Tile, shingles, and most metal applications that depend on rapid water runoff will not hold up under standing water conditions and are not suitable for low-slope roofs.

Built-up tar and gravel roofing is the most common and least expensive material available for flat roof applications, but we do not recommend it. A tar and gravel roof will emit volatile organic compounds from asphalt, benzene, polycarbon aromatics, toluene, and xylene. It will continually outgas when heated by the sun. Some of these vapors will inevitably find their way into the living space and degrade air quality. Eventually the roof will outgas to the point where it does not adversely affect indoor air quality, but soon thereafter it will require replacement. The average tar and gravel roof is guaranteed for only two to five years and may require replacement in less than 10 years. Since most people are not in a position to move out for several weeks when their roof is repaired or replaced, they will be exposed to high levels of toxic fumes. Chemically sensitive individuals often have difficulty tolerating a tar and gravel roof that is less than one to two years old.

Toxicity is not the only health concern to consider when choosing a product. Many persistent mold infestations begin with an undetected roof leak. No type of roofing installation is foolproof, but the use of high quality roofing materials and skilled installers will reduce the risk of leakage.

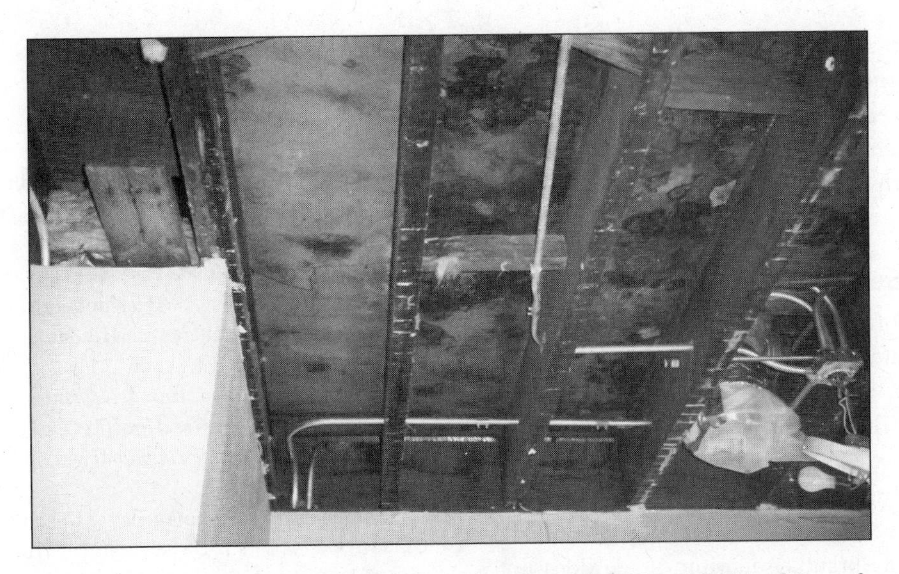

The Problem: A leak in a flat roof has resulted in fungal growth on the underside of the roof sheathing. Recommendation: Roofs should be inspected regularly. Roof leaks should be repaired immediately and rapid drying should be performed to prevent fungal growth. Photo: Restoration Consultants.

Although other solutions are typically more expensive than tar and gravel, you must carefully weigh both lifecycle and health costs when making a roofing choice. Single-ply membranes such as **Brai Roof** contain asphalt and will also outgas to a certain extent during application when heat is applied to fuse the membrane. Once installed, they are fairly stable. These roofs also carry a longer warranty. Brai Roof can be applied in two ways. It can be mechanically fastened, with seams heat welded together. This is the less odorous method and the one we recommend. It can also be glued down with a layer of hot-mopped tar and seams can be sealed with hot tar. We do not recommend this technique. Certain single-ply membranes can be repaired by welding patches onto the existing roof, thereby extending the roof's life for many years. There are also roll-on roofing products that do not require roofing contractors for application or repair.

It is especially important with roofing materials that the manufacturer's instructions for installation and the warranty criteria be carefully followed. Here are some more benign alternatives to tar and gravel roofing for flat-roof applications:

- **AFM Safecoat Dynoflex**: Low-toxic roof coating to replace tar and gravel that can be walked on and remains flexible
- **Brai Roof**: An asphaltic-based single-ply membrane (specify mechanical fastening and torch-down application)
- **Mirrorseal**: A single-ply, fluid-applied roofing system
- **Resource Conservation Technologies, Inc.**: An acrylic polymer paint or roll-on system that uses titanium dioxide with

propylene glycol and contains no toxic dispersants or tints
- **Stevens EP**: A heat weldable, scrim reinforced, single-ply roofing membrane made of ethylene propylene

Joint Sealants

Many solvent-based caulking compounds are formulated with hazardous solvents such as acetone, methyl ethyl acetone, toluene, and xylene. They are toxic to handle and may outgas for extended periods of time. The following are suggested options for exterior use:

- 100 percent silicone aquarium-grade caulk of any brand. Aquarium-grade does not contain any additives that will harm fish and therefore will be safer for humans as well. Be sure to read content labels because some are labeled "pure silicone" but contain other ingredients.
- **AFM Safecoat Caulking Compound**: Water-based elastic emulsion.
- **DAP**: 100 percent **Silicone Sealant** or **Silicone Plus**.
- **GE Silicone II**: Silicone sealant formulated for different types of application; some may contain biocides.
- **Lithoseal Building Caulk**: Urethane modified polymer, inert once cured.
- **Phenoseal Surpass Caulk** and **Sealant, Valve Seal, Vinyl Adhesive Caulk**: Line of water-based sealants and caulks.
- **Weatherall UV Guard Premium Caulking**: A professional strength acrylic-based sealant designed for use in a wide variety of construction applications.

Further Reading

Lafavore, Michael. *Radon: The Invisible Threat.* Rodale Press, 1987.

Lstiburek, Joseph. *Builder's Guides.* Available through The Energy & Environmental Building Association, 10740 Lyndale Avenue South, Suite 10W, Bloomington, MN 55420, 952-881-1098, eeba.org. A series of climate-based field guides with explanations, details, and techniques to effectively implement energy- and resource-efficient residential construction

Lstiburek, Joseph and John Carmody. *Moisture Control Handbook: Principles and Practices for Residential and Small Commercial Buildings.* Van Nostrand Reinhold, 1993.

US Environmental Protection Agency. *A Citizen's Guide to Radon.* 2nd ed., US Government Printing Office, EPA 402-K-92-001, May 1992.

US Environmental Protection Agency. *Consumer's Guide to Radon Reduction.* US Government Printing Office, EPA 402-K-92-003, May 1992.

US Environmental Protection Agency. *Indoor Radon and Radon Decay Reduction Measurement Device Protocols.* US Government Printing Office, EPA 402-R-92-004, July 1992.

US Environmental Protection Agency. *Model Standards and Techniques for Control of Radon in New Residential Buildings.* US Government Printing Office, EPA 402-R-94-009, March 1994.

US Environmental Protection Agency. *Radon Contractor Proficiency (RCP) Program.* US Government Printing Office, EPA 402-B-94-002, September 1994.

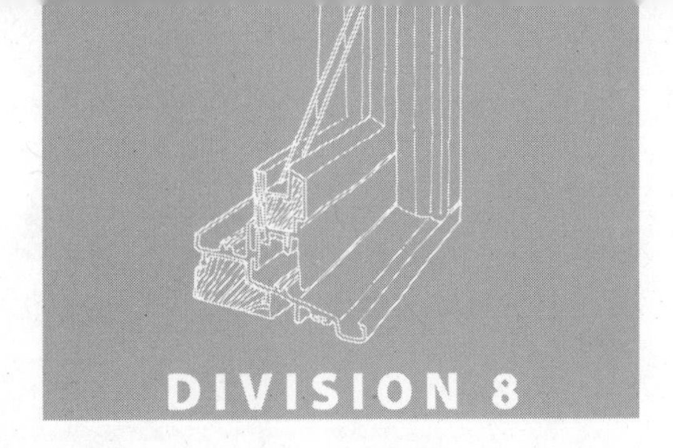

Openings

Wood Doors

Standard Manufactured Doors

Wood doors, both solid and paneled, are typically treated with biocides and manufactured with toxic glues. Paneled wood doors use less glue than solid veneered doors and will therefore outgas less. The face veneer used on flush wood doors is luan, a mahogany commonly imported from the Philippines or Thailand, where it is obtained using forestry practices that damage the environment. Interior fire-rated doors and hollow-core doors often contain a particleboard center that will continuously outgas formaldehyde fumes. Standard manufactured doors should be sealed to lock in harmful vapors. We recommended the following specifications when using standard manufactured doors:

- **All doors shall be thoroughly sealed on all six surfaces.**
- **For a clear finish, seal doors with one of the vapor barrier sealants listed in Division 9. Follow the manufacturer's instructions.**
- **For a painted finish, prime all six sides with one of the primer paints that seals in VOCs, as listed in Division 9.**

Custom Wood Doors

Choosing custom doors allows you to select style, type of wood, and finishes. Some custom door manufacturers will work with you to create a healthier product by using benign glues and less-toxic shop finishes. You can also purchase doors unfinished and have the contractor finish them according to your specifications. Although most custom doors are more expensive, some custom door companies have production or builder lines, which are almost cost competitive with manufactured doors. Paula's chemically sensitive clients who wish to have the warmth and beauty of wood without the terpene emissions of pine doors will often order doors made of harder, less odorous woods such as maple or poplar. For custom doors, specify the following:

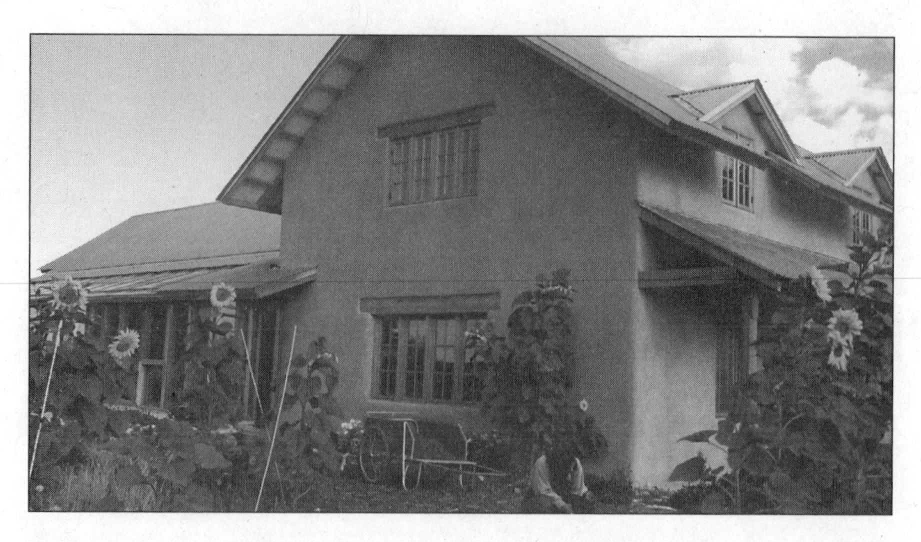

The owner of this ranch home wanted the warmth of wood windows and doors but is extremely sensitive to pesticides. In order to avoid the use of pesticide treated wood all windows and doors were custom made by a local craftsman. Architect: Baker-Laporte and Associates; Builder: Living Structures. Photo: Paula Baker-Laporte.

- **Doors shall be glued with a solvent-free glue such as Elmer's Carpenter's Glue, Envirotec Health Guard Adhesive #2101, or Titebond Solvent Free Construction Adhesive.**
- **Doors shall be finished using the specified low-toxic finish (refer to Division 9 for choices) or with an approved shop-applied finish. Submit a dated sample, MSDS, and product literature for owner's approval of any proposed shop finishes.**

Window and Door Screens

Windows and sliding glass doors generally come with removable screens. Screens for french doors or glass swinging doors usually are not provided by the manufacturer and must be custom made. Aluminum screening was standard in the past but has been almost completely replaced with fiberglass or nylon mesh. These materials are more flexible, more transparent, do not dent, and are easy to replace. Unfortunately, they also can be odorous, especially if they have been treated with insect repellents, pesticides, or other chemicals. When windows arrive onsite the screens should be unwrapped and stacked in a protected environment so they have an opportunity to air out prior to installation in the completed home. If after a substantial airing the screens still have an objectionable odor, they can be replaced with aluminum or copper at a custom screening company. **Andersen** windows are available with aluminum or stainless steel insect screens. **Marvin** windows can be ordered with aluminum screening.

Screens on crank-out casement or awning windows will have more impact on indoor air quality because they are placed on the inside of the glass. Occupants will be exposed to these screens even when the windows are closed. On double-hung windows, the screens are placed outside the glass.

Windows

Moisture Problems Associated with Windows

By far the biggest health concern involving windows occurs when they fail to do their job properly. This job is to let in natural light and allow for ventilation while keeping water out. Windows have drainage channels that are designed to shed water away from the building, but if these are not working properly they can channel water into the building cavity, causing serious water damage.

A simple testing procedure can determine if the windows themselves are shedding water properly (see Division 13 for window testing). Windows can be faulty because of manufacturing defects, mishandling during transport, or improper installation. Windows have a structural weak point where the sill is screwed into the jamb. The seal can break during handling and the tiny gaps can go undetected. Some window manufacturers have added a neoprene gasket at this juncture to make it more secure. If the juncture between the window and the wall contains gaps resulting from incomplete or incorrect application of sealing, air will travel through the gaps. When that air sheds moisture because of temperature differentials, condensation can accumulate. Proper sealing is discussed in the section on insulation around doors and windows in Division 7.

Improper head, jamb, and sill flashing can also result in water finding its way into the wall cavity. (For appropriate flashing materials, see the section in Division 7 on water management at doors and windows.) These water intrusions, which are not readily detectable in the completed building, can eventually lead to structural deterioration and mold problems. In the section on testing for weathertightness in Division 13, we discuss a test that can help determine if there are any installation faults that can lead to future water damage. This test can be performed at a time in the construction when faults can still be easily and inexpensively corrected. All of these potential problems related to windows are exacerbated if the wall cavity does not have a means of drying out once it gets wet.

Because the quality control testing procedures we have referred to are not standard for most residential construction companies, it is unlikely they will be performed unless you specify them in your construction documents. These measures will take a little extra time but can potentially extend the life of a building for many years and prevent mold problems that could be devastating to your health.

Wood Window Frames

Wood windows are routinely dipped in a waterborne fungicide. Unlike wood doors, it can be cost prohibitive to have operable windows custom made. Chemically sensitive individuals will often choose steel or aluminum windows with a baked-on enamel finish to avoid exposure to the fungicide as well as to the terpenes from pine frames. Wood windows can be sealed to avoid these exposures. You may wish to specify the following:

- **Thoroughly seal wood windows on all surfaces exposed to the interior.**
- **Where a clear finish is scheduled, use a clear vapor-barrier sealant as specified in**

the section on clear vapor-barrier sealants for wood in Division 9.

- **Where a painted finish is scheduled, use a primer paint that seals in VOCs, as specified in the section on paints in Division 9.**

Most wood window manufacturers also produce clad windows, which have wood on the inside and aluminum, steel, or fiberglass coating on the outside for weather protection. The cladding provides UV protection so that it is unnecessary to apply protective coatings on the window exterior. If unclad windows are used, you will need to do yearly maintenance consisting of staining and sealing in order to protect the window frames from the elements.

The following products do not contain many of the toxic substances commonly found in exterior wood finishing products and can be used for the preservation of wood window frames and doors:

- **AFM Safecoat DuroStain**: Wood stain
- **Auro Natural Wood Stain No. 160**: Colorless and color finish, good weather resistance
- **BioShield Aqua Resin Stain**: Weather-resistant wood finish with ultraviolet protection
- **BioShield Primer Oil #1**: Undercoat; use finish coat of **Livos Kaldet Stain** or **Livos Vindo Enamel Paint**
- **OS Color One Coat Only**: Weather- and UV-resistant, water-repellent, semitransparent wood stains
- **Weather Pro**: Water-based, water-repellent wood stain

Weatherstripping

Weatherstripping is used around doors to make them airtight and resistant to water leakage. Weatherstripping can also be specified around interior doors where noise or odor control is desired. Most available weatherstrips are made of synthetics, including silicone, urethane foam, polypropylene nylon, and neoprene. Some will outgas. Neoprene, for example, can have a strong odor. Brass and stainless steel weatherstripping are available at many hardware stores. Choose the least odorous weatherstripping that accomplishes the job.

As mentioned earlier, when planning a healthy home the garage and mechanical room should be designed so they do not open directly to the interior because they will introduce harmful byproducts of combustion and odors into the home. A simple breezeway can provide weather protection between a detached garage and the home. However, doors and common walls between home and garage are found in almost all new housing because many people find a detached garage to be an unacceptable inconvenience. Where a door to the garage or mechanical room opens into the living space, it is important to specify that these doors have a threshold sealed with an acceptable sealant. The doors should be fully weatherstripped to prevent harmful fumes from entering the living space through the door openings. In fact, the entire common wall between the home and the garage should be made airtight so that fumes do not seep through the wall from the garage into the home. For the specifics on creating this airtight wall, refer to Division 9.

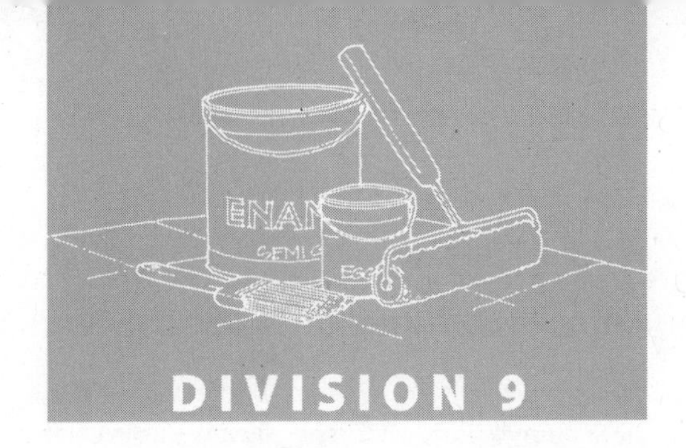

Finishes

Introduction

Finishes include all surface materials and treatments in the home. They are what is seen on a daily basis and, along with furnishings, constitute the personal signature of the owner. Finishes are the predominant source of odors in a new home. They can introduce a multitude of toxic volatile organic compounds into the air and will continue to volatilize, or outgas, for years after the home is completed. However, when chosen carefully, finishes can enhance health and well-being as well as add to the aesthetic value of the home.

Until recently, nonpolluting finishing products were considered specialty items. Fortunately, healthier products are now regularly appearing on the market. Many of these are easily accessible, cost competitive, and comparable in performance to their more toxic counterparts. Some even have the ability to improve air quality by sealing in toxins that may be present in underlying materials.

In some regions, traditional nontoxic finish materials are readily available and widely used. In the Southwest, for example, tile, stone, natural wood, and plaster are commonplace, whereas in many regions of the country they have been replaced even in custom homes by wall-to-wall carpeting, vinyl wall coatings, laminate cabinetry, and other synthetic substitutes. When you build a healthy home, we encourage you to take full advantage of the traditional materials native to your region.

Plaster

Plaster generally provides a healthful interior wall finish. Because of the labor and skill involved in its application it is a more expensive finish, but it is much sought after for its beauty. Plaster has the ability to block the small amount of VOCs present in the gypsum lath and taped joints that it covers in frame construction. Although this dense material works well as an air barrier, plaster will develop gaps due to shrinkage and on occasion will develop

CASE STUDY 9.1

Immune Dysfunction Related to Formaldehyde Exposure in the Home

P.F. is a 54-year-old woman who was in good health until 1981 when she moved into a new mobile home. Shortly thereafter she developed a digestive disorder with gas and bloating, severe insomnia, and a chronic cough with frequent episodes of bronchitis. By the following year she was suffering from persistent fatigue and frequent respiratory infections, including her first case of pneumonia. She became sensitive to most products containing formaldehyde, especially pressboard. She noted that she experienced "brain fog" while shopping at the local mall. Her symptoms continued to worsen, and now included allergies, hypoglycemia, and lethargy.

P. F. consulted with several healthcare practitioners, including a pulmonary specialist, psychiatrist, hypnotist, nutritionist, and acupuncturist. None of them ever questioned her about the air quality in her home. Eventually she received the diagnosis of multiple chemical sensitivity from a physician with similar symptoms, and was finally educated about the underlying cause of her health problems. In 1992, P. F. moved into a house that contained low formaldehyde levels, alleviating some of her symptoms. Her house contained several healthful features such as radiant heat in concrete floors and the absence of pressboard and particleboard in its construction.

However, further modifications were necessary before her health could be stabilized and improved. All gas appliances were removed; filtration was installed for both air and water; and the mechanical room was vented to the outside. By 1996, P. F. had regained her health. However, as is typical in such cases, she still becomes symptomatic on reexposure to toxic fumes and must diligently maintain a "safe" environment for herself.

Discussion

Indoor formaldehyde is gaining recognition as a severe health hazard for occupants of homes and office buildings where chronic exposure occurs. Several organizations, such as the American Lung Association, have recommended that formaldehyde levels not exceed 0.1 part per million. People who have already become sensitized to formal-

minor cracks. To maintain a good barrier, these gaps should be filled with an acceptable sealant. Since most of the initial cracking will take place during the first 18 months while the house is settling, it makes sense to wait and do all of these minor repairs at once. In pumicecrete, clay/straw, and adobe construction, the plaster may be applied directly to the wall material (see Division 4).

Although most plasters are inert, some contain polyvinyl additives that are subject to outgassing and should be avoided. Verify the presence of additives with the manufacturer prior to purchase.

One potential health hazard associated with plaster lies in the method by which it is dried. Because new plaster releases a significant amount of moisture, it is necessary to dry it out quickly so that other building materials are not adversely affected. This is especially problematic in the winter months, when cold temperatures and lack of ventilation slow down the rate of evaporation. The standard solution is to use gasoline or kerosene heaters,

dehyde will have reactions at levels as low as 0.02 part per million. Approximately 50 percent of the population is exposed on a daily basis in the workplace to levels that exceed the 0.1 part per million limit. Mobile homes are notorious for causing health problems because of the extremely high levels of formaldehyde emitted from the plywood and particleboard used in their construction.[a]

Individuals who develop permanent health problems associated with formaldehyde exposure often relate the onset of their symptoms to a flu-like illness, which is diagnosed as a viral infection. However, the affected individual usually does not totally recover from this so-called flu and is left with general malaise, fatigue, and depression. Other symptoms can include rashes, eye irritation, frequent sore throats, hoarse voice, repeated sinus infections, nasal congestion, chronic cough, chest pains, palpitations, muscle spasms, joint pains, numbness and tingling of the extremities, colitis and other digestive disorders, severe headaches, dizziness, loss of memory, inability to recall words and names, and disorientation. Formaldehyde is an immune system sensitizer, which means that chronic exposure can lead to multiple allergies and sensitivities to substances that are entirely unrelated to formaldehyde. This is known as the "spreading phenomenon."

P. F. was typical of people whose multiple chemical sensitivities stem from formaldehyde exposure in that she consulted numerous physicians and specialists in an attempt to obtain a diagnosis. Physical examinations and standard testing usually fail to identify the cause of such health problems. Sometimes it is suggested that the patient is a hypochondriac or in need of psychiatric evaluation. When asked if there might be a connection between the symptoms and formaldehyde, most physicians either do not know or believe that formaldehyde merely causes irritation. As a result, the patient's health continues to deteriorate from continued exposure.

a. Jack Thrasher and Alan Broughton. *The Poisoning of Our Homes and Workplaces: The Indoor Formaldehyde Crisis.* Seadora. 1989, pp. 50–72.

but we do not recommend this practice. The byproducts of combustion generated by this machinery are readily absorbed into the plaster and other building materials. The heaters also create an unhealthy environment for the workers exposed to their fumes. Electric heaters tend to be more expensive to run, with far less BTU output. We recommend a combination of dehumidifiers when necessary and careful scheduling so that the plasterwork is done during a warm, dry period. Although heat may be required for the comfort of the construction team, it is far less significant than dehumidification to the proper drying of wet building materials. In summary, we suggest that the following instructions be included in your specifications:

- **Plaster shall be free of additives.**
- **The use of gas- or kerosene-generated heaters within the building envelope is prohibited.**
- **Turbo high-velocity heaters, other electric heaters, and blow-in heaters with**

combustion sources outside the building envelope are acceptable for adding heat to a building during cold-weather construction.

- **If plaster is applied when weather conditions do not permit the building to remain open and well-ventilated, electric dehumidification should be used. At temperatures under 70 degrees Fahrenheit, moisture levels should be maintained at approximately 45 percent relative air humidity using electric dehumidification until the building is dry enough to consistently maintain this range without the use of this equipment. Interior surface temperatures shall remain above 50 degrees. Refrigerant dehumidifiers may not work well when temperatures drop below 65 degrees Fahrenheit.**

Clay-Based Plasters

From a Building Biology standpoint, clay-based plasters provide a superior wall finish because of the remarkable hygroscopic properties of clay. For more information about mixing your own plasters, we recommend *The Natural Plaster Book* (listed at the end of this chapter). Resources for commercially prepared clay-based plaster are:

- **American Clay Enterprises**: A variety of clay-based plasters for interior finishing, including three texture styles and 42 colors.
- **Japanese Wall**: Several lines of interior and exterior natural plasters imported from Japan. All-natural, nontoxic plasters contain sand, diatomite earth, clay, natural stone chips, and straw.

Plaster Finish

Because of the porous nature of plaster, it will stain and show fingerprints if left unfinished. Plaster walls, which were the norm before the advent of gypsum board or Sheetrock, were commonly painted or covered with wallpaper. Today, homeowners enjoy the organic feel of the color variations in natural plaster and it is fashionable to leave it unpainted. Most people prefer to apply a clear finish over it to protect and enhance its natural beauty, or to leave the plaster unsealed.

Natural beeswax finishes will protect the wall while maintaining its permeability. Traditionally, beeswax was applied with a hot knife and troweled on the wall. There are very few craftsmen who know this art form today. However, we have found that a natural beeswax furniture polish can be applied with a cloth and buffed. As with all plant chemistry products, chemically sensitive individuals may find the scent objectionable and should test a small sample first.

Some synthetic finishes will create a more impervious seal and are less expensive, easier to apply, and more enduring. Synthetic finishes should be carefully evaluated for chemical content and outgassing. Some may be toxic or increase problems with static electricity. Since most make the surface nonporous, they may encourage mold growth on the paper backing of the gypsum lathing behind the plaster if moisture becomes trapped. So, as with gypsum board, if a water accident occurs it should be quickly dried. We have successfully used the following finishes:

- **American Clay Black Soap Finish**: A gelatinous castile soap infused with potash to enrich color and create a soft patina

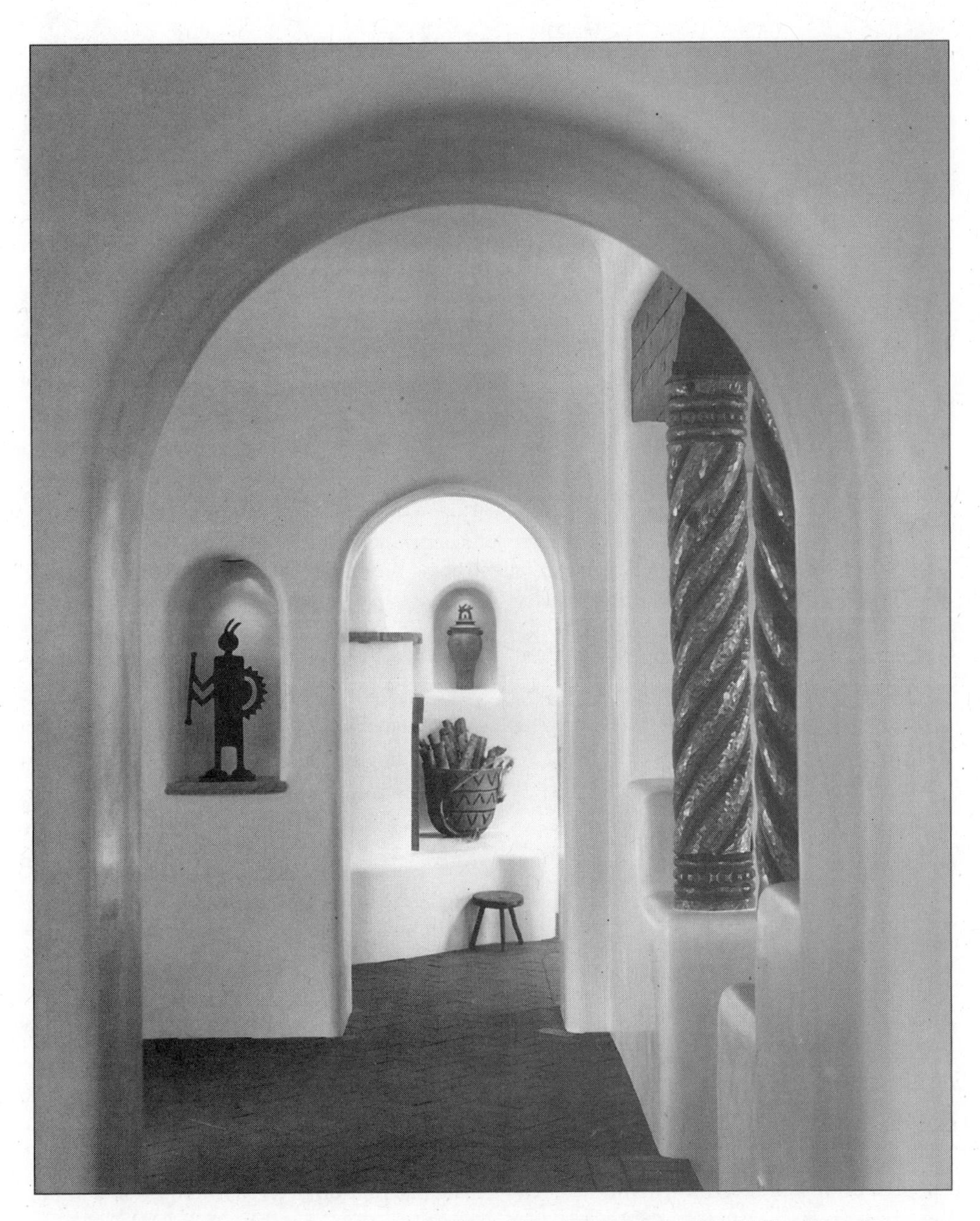

This Santa Fe Style interior combines hard trowelled plaster wall finishes with brick flooring and stone detailing to create a healthy interior. Architect: Baker-Laporte and Associates; Builder: Prull and Associates. Photo: Lisl Dennis.

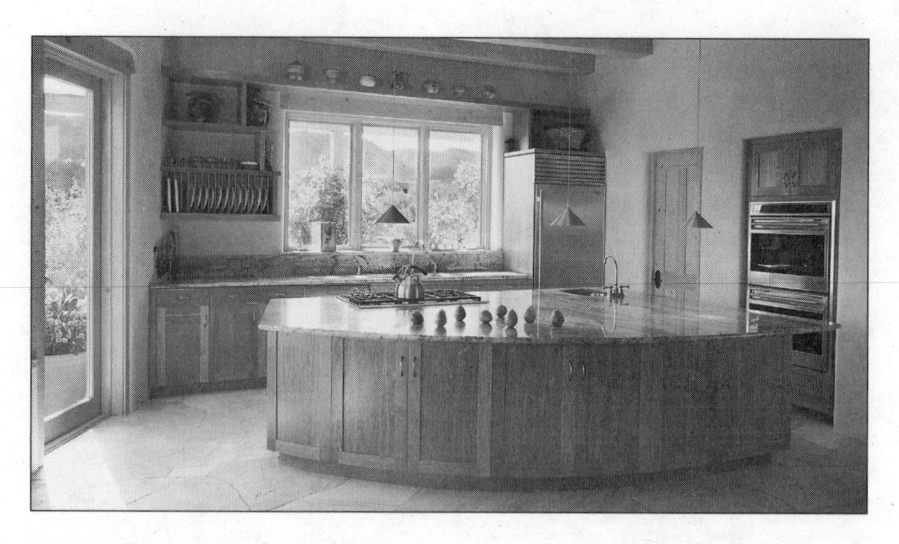

Flagstone floors, granite countertops, solid wood upper shelving, formaldehyde free cabinetry and plaster walls grace this sculptured home. Architects: Baker-Laporte & Assoc. Builders: Prull & Assoc. Photo: Rob Reck.

- **American Clay Gloss Sealer**: Low-VOC product used for high-traffic areas, providing water resistance to walls; easy to clean
- **American Clay Penetrating Sealer**: A low-VOC soy resin/acrylic spray-on sealer that increases durability and water resistance
- **Livos Glievo Liquid Wax**: Apply a thin coat and hand buff
- **Okon Seal and Finish**: For satin gloss

Gypsum Board

Gypsum board, also known as gypboard, Sheetrock, or drywall, is the most common form of interior wall sheathing in modern residential construction. It is considerably less expensive than plaster. The 4- by 8-foot sheets are attached to the studs, then taped, sealed, textured, and painted.

Gypsum board is composed of natural gypsum sandwiched between two sheets of cardboard made from recycled newsprint. This cardboard backing creates problems when water damage occurs because it is a nutrient that encourages mold growth. In his mold investigation work, John Banta has seen many cases where mold has begun to grow less than 72 hours after water damage occurs. Getting immediate help from a remediation specialist with the proper drying equipment is often the key to saving money and health when a water disaster occurs. A skilled specialist will know how to safely remove mold while isolating it so that no further contamination occurs.

Gypsum Board Installation

The installation of gypsum board in standard practice may negatively affect indoor air quality for the following reasons:

- Dust and debris within wall cavities are often enclosed and concealed by the gypboard. If dust and debris are not cleaned out, they can cause problems over time. Dust can eventually work its way back into the living space and become a maintenance problem as well as an air pollutant, and other construction debris can become a breeding ground for mold if it becomes wet.

- Gypsum board itself will outgas because of the inks remaining in the recycled newspaper. To seal in the small quantity of undesirable VOCs generated by the surfacing board, the walls may be primed with a specialty paint or primer. With the printing industry shift to soy-based ink, outgassing may become less of a problem.
- The standard premixed joint compounds may contain several undesirable chemicals, including formaldehyde.
- Like plaster, gypsum board is highly absorbent. In standard practice, gas and kerosene heaters may be used to dry the joint compounds. The byproducts of combustion are absorbed into the walls and will outgas into the building envelope of the completed home.
- Special gypsum boards are made for use in areas that get wet, such as showers, tub surrounds, and countertops. When walls using these products in wet areas are disassembled after several years, the water resistant papers are often moldy, especially at the joints between boards. Cementitious boards without paper backing are made to be used as backerboard in wet locations and do not have the same mold problems that are associated with the paper-backed products.

To avoid these problems, include the following specifications:

- **All wall cavities shall be thoroughly vacuumed and free of debris prior to installation of the gypsum board.**
- **Joint compound shall be a powdered joint cement and texture compound such as Murco M-100 HiPo or approved equal that is formulated with inert fillers and without formaldehyde or preservatives.**
- **Heaters fueled by gasoline or kerosene are prohibited.**
- **If relative humidity rises above 55 percent, electric dehumidification shall be applied until relative humidity remains consistently between 45 and 55 percent without additional dehumidification. Interior surface temperatures shall remain above 50 degrees.**
- **The joint compound must be completely dry before primer is applied.**
- **In wet areas such as showers, tub surrounds, and sink counters, cementitous backerboard without paper backing shall be used. Durock, Hardibacker Board, Permabase, or approved equal may be used for this purpose.**

Creating an Air Barrier with Gypsum Board

In 2x frame wall construction there are often undesirable emissions from materials used in the building envelope. Since, even with the greatest care in choosing materials, there may not be completely inert, cost-effective products available, it often makes sense to create an airtight barrier on the inside face of the building envelope to block the entry of undesirable substances from within the wall cavity itself or from adjoining environments. This also makes great sense from the standpoint of moisture control and energy efficiency. A tightly sealed and taped gypsum board wall, in combination with gasketed or foamed sill and top plates and thorough sealing around all openings (windows, electrical outlets, plumbing penetrations, and recessed lighting), will create an airtight barrier that can perform the same function as an air barrier made of carefully joined plastic sheeting as described in the section on air barriers in Division 7.

This type of airtight assembly will prevent airborne moisture from pouring through cracks into the wall but will allow a small amount of moisture to be carried through by diffusion. In climatic conditions where the building would tend to dry to the inside (i.e., when the inside temperature of the building is cooler than the outside temperature), the gypsum board assembly will also allow moderate amounts of moisture in the wall cavity to dry out instead of remaining trapped. Because gypsum board allows some water vapor to move through it, this is a superior solution for blocking chemical gases out of living spaces. This is especially relevant where air conditioning is used and moisture would tend to condense on a layer of impermeable plastic sheeting (if one were present) and remain trapped in the wall cavity.

Gypsum board can store limited amounts of moisture before it begins to mold. It will not stand up to large amounts of wetting. In hot, humid climates there must be a sufficient vapor barrier on the exterior of the building to prevent excessive moisture from penetrating the wall from the outside and causing the cardboard on the gypsum board to mold. Similarly, in heating conditions it may be necessary to use a paint or primer with a low permeability rating to retard some of the water vapor that would naturally diffuse through the gypsum board. **86001 Seal** is a primer that has a low enough rating to serve as a vapor retardant.

Gypsum board can be purchased with foil backing. Although foil is an excellent vapor blocker, we do not recommend it because it is problematic if water damage occurs. Assessment is hampered because the foil prevents a moisture meter from taking accurate readings. It is also more difficult to dry out a flooded wall cavity when foil-backed gypsum board has been used.

To summarize, using gypsum board in an airtight manner on stud frame construction makes sense in all climatic conditions. However, this is only one part of the moisture control strategy. Developing an overall strategy for the control of moisture in any building must take into account the climatic conditions of the site. The best solution will be different for different locations. While a full discussion of moisture movement and best solutions is beyond the scope of this book, an understanding of moisture movement is essential for the ongoing success of a health-enhancing building in all but the most forgiving dry climates. To this end, we highly recommend the *Builder's Guides* by Joseph Lstiburek, listed at the end of Division 7.

Alternatives to Gypsum Board

Alternatives to paper-backed gypsum board are now available. The following products may be used to replace it and are especially useful in applications where moisture conditions may promote mold growth:

- **DensArmor Plus** is an alternative to regular cardboard-backed panels. It is paperless, faced on two sides with a glass mat, and highly mold resistant.

- Magnesium oxide boards: Currently these products are being manufactured in China. They can be used to replace gypsum board, plywood, cement boards, and oriented strand board (OSB). They resist moisture, bugs, fungus, mold, and fire. Products are available in North America under the product names **Dragonboard**, **MagBoard**, and **Strong-Enviro Board**.

Tile

Tile is generally an inert and healthful floor, wall, and counter surfacing material. We recommend factory-finished tiles that require no further finishing onsite. Many attractive and reasonably priced tiles are rated for commercial and exterior use. This rating almost guarantees a low-maintenance, long-wearing product that will not require onsite refinishing.

The following concerns must be addressed in order to achieve a healthful installation:

- In standard construction, tile is often laid over an unacceptable backing such as particleboard, which contains high formaldehyde levels.
- In wet areas, tile is frequently laid over green board (a gypsum board that has paraffin wax mixed with the gypsum to prevent it from falling apart). However, the paper on the board will still develop mold in the presence of moisture.
- Certain imported tiles contain lead-based glazes or asbestos fillers. Lead content can be simply verified with a lead swab test (see Chart 13.1).
- Certain glazes, primarily imports, have been found to be radioactive, especially cobalt blues and burnt oranges.

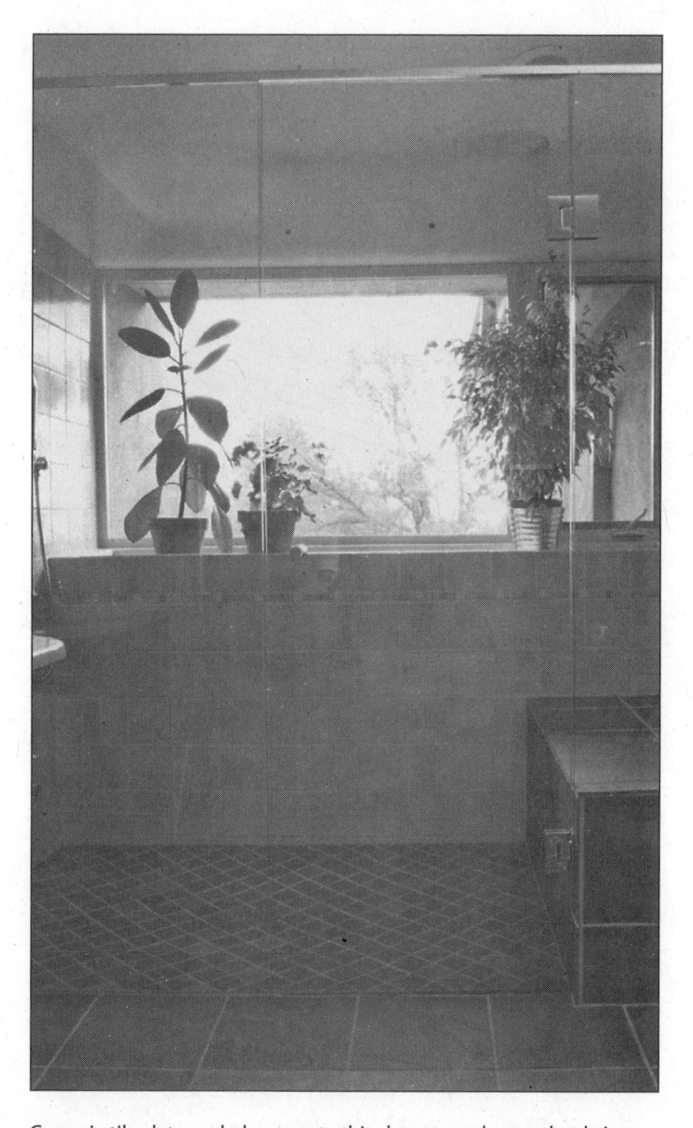

Ceramic tile slate and glass create this shower enclosure that brings views of the beautiful surroundings into this bathroom. Architect: Baker-Laporte and Associates; Builder: Prull and Associates. Photo: Julie Dean.

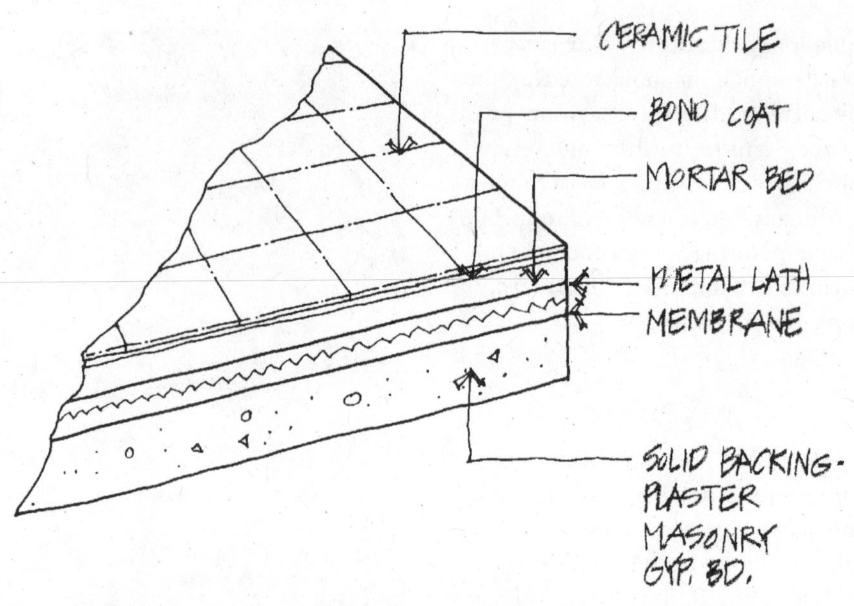

Thick-set tile installation.

- Many tile-sealing products contain harmful chemicals and high levels of VOCs. Selecting tiles with commercially rated finishes and glazes will bypass the need to use tile sealers on the construction site.
- Some standard tile adhesives and mortars contain harmful chemicals.
- Standard grouts usually contain fungicides and latex additives.
- Grouts are porous and can harbor mold and mildew. They should be sealed where exposed to water.

Underlayment for Ceramic Tile

The following are acceptable underlayments for ceramic tile:

- A clean, level concrete slab or gypsum concrete base that has been fully cured.
- Exterior-grade plywood that has been aired out and sealed. Use only where a cementitious underlayment is unavailable. This method will require mastic adhesive and is not recommended for areas that get wet.
- A lightweight, strong, noncombustible, highly water-resistant cementitious board such as **Durock**, **Hardibacker Board**, or **PermaBase**.

Tile Installation

The three basic methods for installing tiles are thicksetting, thinsetting, and adhesion with organic mastics.

Thickset Method

This is the tried and true, old-fashioned way of adhering tiles, prevalent prior to the invention of additives. A thick reinforced bed of mortar consisting of Portland cement, sand, and in some cases lime is floated. While the base is still plastic, a thin layer of Portland cement paste known as the bond coat is spread over it. The tile is adhered to the bond coat and allowed to cure for several days before the tile is grouted.

This method will create the strongest, most durable tile installation available without the use of chemical additives. The following should be specified for this type of installation:

- **Use only additive-free Portland cement, clean sand, lime where required, and potable water. Use the recommended reinforcing and specified cleavage membrane.**
- **For wall, ceiling, and floor installations, follow the method covered by ANSI A108.1 and set the tiles on the mortar bed while it is still plastic.**
- **The cleavage membrane shall be non-asphalt-impregnated, 4 millimeter polyethylene such as Cross Tuff, Tu Tuf 4, or an approved equivalent.**

It is not always possible to use a thickset installation. The 1¼-inch depth required for thicksetting may not be available unless carefully planned from the outset. Tile setters skilled in this method are sometimes difficult to locate. This method is labor-intensive and will be more costly than other installation methods.

Thinset Method

Thinset mortars are powdered sand and cement products mixed with liquid and spread to a thickness of approximately ⅛ to ⅜ of an inch. Once dried they are unaffected by water and can be used in wet applications.

A variety of thinsets are available. Most thinset mortars contain various chemical additives to enhance workability, flexibility, and bonding strength, thus expanding the range of application. Water-mixed thinsets consist of powdered sand and cement. They are available with or without powdered latex and acrylic additives and are mixed onsite with water. Latex and acrylic thinsets consist of powdered sand and cement mixed with liquid latexes and acrylics instead of water. They have higher bond and compressive strength and improved flexibility compared to water-mixed thinsets. Epoxy thinsets develop bonds more quickly than other thinsets. The epoxies emit noxious fumes while curing and these fumes can be absorbed by porous surfaces. The use of epoxies is almost always unnecessary in residential construction. If epoxies are used, workers should wear protective vapor respirators during application and the space should be continuously aired out until all fumes have dissipated. The additive ingredients used in these thinset mixtures are proprietary and not disclosed on the label. When selecting a thinset product, choose one that can do the job at hand with the smallest amount of chemical additives and the least odor.

Thinsets Without Synthetic Additives

The following water-mixed thinsets are available without synthetic additives. They gain their strength through the use of high-quality Portland cement, but are generally considered to be less flexible and more prone to cracking than thinsets with latex additives. They may be used successfully over clean concrete slabs, properly supported cementitious boards, and mortar beds.

- **C-Cure FloorMix 900**, **Thinset 911** (dual purpose), and **WallMix 901**: The "economy" line of C-Cure mortars, which contain no additives other than mineral salts
- **Laticrete Additive Free Thinset**

Low-Odor Thinsets with Vinyl Polymer Additives

The following water-mixed thinsets contain vinyl polymers, which give them greater strength and range of application. They have very little odor and are virtually odorless once cured. However, anyone with sensitivities to vinyl polymer additives is advised to test these products prior to using them.

- **C-Cure MultiCure 905**: A latex-enhanced, dry-set mortar with added bonding strength and flexibility for use over cementitious and plywood substrates
- **C-Cure PermaBond 902**: A dry-set mortar with Portland cement, sand, and additives for use over cementitious substrates

Organic Mastics

Organic mastics are either water- or petroleum-based adhesives that consist of a bonding agent and a liquid vehicle. For petroleum-based mastics, the vehicle is a solvent, usually toluene. These formulations are highly toxic and flammable and are not recommended for use in a healthy home.

Organic mastics enjoy widespread popularity because they are inexpensive, stickier than thinsets, and allow the quickest installations. However, they do not have the strength, flexibility, or water resistance of thinset or thickset applications. Because they are applied in a very thin layer, they do not have leveling capabilities and are suitable only for application over flat surfaces such as plywood or drywall. When they are used over concrete, the vapor emission rate and pH of the slab must be checked to ensure compatibility with the mastic, which can break down if too much moisture is emitted from the slab. If the slab is too alkaline, adverse pH reactions in the mastic can result in a persistent odor that is strong and unpleasant. Refer to Division 13 for more information on calcium chloride moisture testing and pH testing for concrete. Most mastics are not recommended for areas that get wet. Where mastic applications are appropriate, you may wish to choose one of the following water-based products:

- **AFM Safecoat 3 in 1 Adhesive**: Low-odor, low-VOC, water-based mastic for hard composition wall and floor tiles
- **CHAPCO Safe-Set 88** and **Safe-Set 90 Ceramic Tile Adhesives**: Solvent-free, nonflammable, freeze/thaw stable, and almost odor-free ceramic floor tile adhesives
- **Taylor Envirotec 901 Odyssey Ceramic Tile Type I Adhesive**: For ceramic floor and wall tile adhesion

Grouts

As with tile-setting mortars, a number of additives may be used in commercial grouts to impart certain performance characteristics such as improved strength and flexibility, increased water or stain resistance, and improved freeze/thaw stability. Some of these additives, such as epoxies, are quite noxious. In grout applications, they will be exposed to the living space and will continue to outgas until completely cured. Homemade grouts can be mixed on-site by combining Portland cement, sand, lime (optional), and water. They can be colored with the same pigments used to color concrete (see the section on concrete finishes in Division 3). It is important that the person mixing the grout know the proper proportions and sand size for the particular tile application. These applications should be damp-cured for three days. The following commercially available grouts are free of latex additives:

- **C-Cure AR Sanded Grout 922**: A sanded grout available in a limited selection of colors
- **C-Cure Supreme Grout 925**: An unsanded grout for joints less than ⅛ inch and for use with tiles that are easily scratched, such as marble
- **Hydroment**: Ceramic tile grout (sanded) and dry tile grout (unsanded)
- **Mapei 2½" to 1**: For large grout joints greater than ⅜ inch
- **Summitville-700 SummitChromes**: Sanded grout without polymer additives, available in 32 colors

Sealers

Tile Sealers

If an unsealed tile is selected, it is important to specify sealants that are free of harmful chemicals. Many of the commercially available tile sealers are solvent-based, highly toxic products that will emit noxious fumes for a long time after application. If they are used to cover a large floor area, the negative impact can be significant. Consider one of the following specially formulated products:

- **AFM Safecoat MexeSeal**: For sealing previously unsealed tile floors
- **AgriStain for Concrete**: Sealer and stain for concrete, plaster, and porous tiles
- **Zip-Guard Environmental Wood Finish**: A water-based urethane that can be used for sealing very clean, previously unsealed tile floors

Grout Sealers

Sealing grouts will make grout joints easier to clean and more resistant to water penetration and staining. When water penetrates grout joints, it makes them susceptible to mold and bacterial growth. Even grouts containing mildewcides can eventually become moldy. Besides sealing grouts in wet areas, the key to mold-free grout is maintenance. Bathrooms should be kept dry by using exhaust fans, and grout joints should be cleaned regularly. We do not recommend the commercially available grouts enhanced with additives. We have found the following sealing methods to be generally well-tolerated by chemically sensitive individuals:

- **AFM Safecoat Grout Sealer**: A clear, moisture-resistant sealer for porous tile grout to help prevent staining
- **AFM Safecoat Safe Seal**: An odorless, zero-VOC, water-based, low-gloss sealer for highly porous surfaces, it can be diluted in a 50:50 ratio with water and then mixed into the dry grout to form an integral grout sealer

Stone

While stone is generally a healthful and beautiful choice for flooring and decorative accents, it raises the same concerns about proper installation as ceramic tile does. The specifications we have outlined for ceramic tile also apply to stone.

We have tested several stone products for radiation and radon content and found a range of readings from very low to high levels. Although uranium content in construction materials is not usually considered to be a serious concern, John's experience, as shared in Case Study 9.2, leads us to conclude that stone can contribute significantly to ambient radon levels in a home. We recommend that stone, especially granite, be screened for radon prior to installation, even though the Granite Institute has issued a scientific report concluding that granite countertops do not emit radioactivity into the home. Tests are easily performed as described in Division 13.

Stone Installation

Refer to our discussion of the thickset method in the section on tile installation above and to the section on stone countertops in Division 6.

Sealers for Stone

The following finishes are free of petroleum-based solvents and can be used for most stone flooring, shelving, and countertops:

- **AFM Safecoat MexeSeal**: A durable sealer providing water and oil repellency, applied over AFM Safecoat Paver Seal .003, an undersealer for porous materials
- **Lithofin**: Stone sealers
- **Livos Meldos Hard Oil** and **Livos Bilo Floor Wax**: A penetrating oil sealer and a clear, mar-resistant finish wax respectively; can be odorous when first applied and should be carefully tested prior to use by a chemically sensitive individual
- **Naturel Cleaner and Sealer**: Water-soluble flakes that clean, protect, and finish stone surfaces

Flooring

Flooring Installation Over Concrete

Flooring materials such as wood, carpeting, and resilient flooring are often laid over a concrete slab. If the concrete slab has a high moisture content resulting from inadequate curing time or from a high water table, then the perfect conditions exist for mold growth: an environment that is dark, moist, still, and nutritious. Flooring manufacturers publish recommended maximum vapor-emissions levels for installations of their products over concrete slab. When these levels are exceeded, the warranty is void. Unfortunately, slabs are rarely measured for vapor emissions.

Where finished flooring, especially wood flooring, is laid over concrete slab with radiant heat tubing in it, we have encountered an additional problem. A slab that appears to be fully cured will have unacceptably high vapor emissions when the heat is first turned on. Often the heat is turned on only after floor finishes have been applied and the construction is completed.

We consider these to be important quality control issues and suggest the following specifications:

- **Prior to the installation of flooring or subflooring over a concrete slab, a calcium chloride vapor-emissions test shall be performed to verify that the slab meets the manufacturer's maximum vapor-emissions criteria. Testing shall be performed at a rate of one test every 500 feet and at a minimum of once per concrete pour area.**
- **Where adhesives are used to apply a wood floor directly over a concrete slab, the slab should be tested to determine if the pH level in the concrete will be compatible with the adhesive.**
- **Where radiant heat tubing is installed in a concrete slab, heat should be circulated in the floor for two weeks prior to performing a calcium chloride vapor-emissions test.**

CASE STUDY 9.2

A Very Hot Bed

Prior to purchasing a home, a family contacted John to conduct radon testing with electronic monitors, following the EPA's protocol. Closed-house conditions were established 12 hours prior to testing and were maintained throughout the tests. During the testing, one of the electronic monitors located in the dining room indicated 12.5 picocuries of radon per liter of air, while a monitor elsewhere showed close to normal levels. The client was advised that the electronic readings were suspicious and that additional testing was necessary. As the investigation proceeded, it became clear that there was a radon source at one end of the home. In fact, the radon result for a test conducted on a night table in the guest bedroom was 27.0 picocuries, while that for the family room a short way down the hall was 7.0 picocuries. The farther the monitors had been placed from the guest bedroom, the lower the radon value.

Upon visual examination of the guest bedroom, it was noted that the headboards for the two beds were made of rock that appeared to be granite. The headboards were later tested with a small Geiger counter. While normal radioactive background levels away from the headboards were approximately 12 radioactive counts per minute, the counts close to the headboards were over 300. It was clear that the headboards were at least one source of radon in the room.

The headboards were in fact a decorative granite rock imported from Italy. Each headboard weighed several hundred pounds. The floors and walls had been especially constructed to hold the extra weight. It took six strong men to remove each of the headboards to a detached garage. The radon tests were repeated throughout the home with all values now under 1.0 picocurie. The home was given a radon clearance, contingent upon the proper disposal of the headboards.

Discussion

This was the first home John inspected in which a radon source was caused by a building material or furnishing. Although radon from the soil is the most common cause of elevated radiation levels in a home, there are many other possible sources. Since granite rock is sometimes high in uranium, it must be considered a potential source of radon when used in construction. Rock can be a superb building material, but it should always be tested prior to use for the rare possibility of radiation.

Wood Flooring

Wood is a healthful choice for flooring provided that the subflooring, adhesives (if used), and finishes are carefully chosen to be healthful as well. In standard construction, unfinished wood floors are commonly nailed to a formaldehyde-emitting underlayment and then finished with solvent-based finishes that will outgas for many months. Noxious glues may also be used in the installation process.

There are several prefinished engineered flooring systems available that can be applied directly over concrete using a floating floor installation method. When considering a prefinished floor, order a dated sample, product literature, and an MSDS. Manufacturers will publish their underlayment requirements. Most require a vapor barrier of some sort between the underlayment and the flooring product and will state allowable maximum vapor emissions from the subfloor.

In our experience, most factory finishes have proven to be far more durable then any of the more benign finishes available for jobsite application. Furthermore, when a wood floor must be finished onsite the required sanding is a very dusty process, although dust levels can be reduced if you specify that a "dustless" process be used. For "dustless" sanding, a double-filter vacuum called a DCS unit is attached to the floor sander. It can contain up to 90 percent of the dust, making the process less dusty but by no means dustless.

All components of each wood floor application from underlayment to finish must be carefully analyzed. If you can look at both new and older installations that are similar to your proposed application, you will be able to carefully evaluate what the product smells like when it is new and how well it wears over time.

Wood Flooring International offers a complete line of both solid and prefinished engineered flooring using FSC certified wood. Their flooring is engineered to make very full use of the trees harvested. Their American Woods, Monteverde, Pacific Northwest, and Orchard Collections all meet E1 emissions standards (European standards set to limit formaldehyde emissions). These standards would permit up to an estimated 0.14 parts per million of formaldehyde for hardwoods. This is a significantly higher level than is permitted for wood-based products certified by GreenGuard, which sets a limit of 0.05 parts per million.

Prefinished Engineered Wood Flooring Systems

The following wood flooring systems meet stringent European emissions standards:

- **Junckers**: This is a solid wood engineered flooring system from Denmark that can be applied directly over concrete. It has a factory-applied UV-cured urethane finish and comes in a variety of wood species with trim pieces. Wood comes from a source with managed forestry practices.
- **Kahrs**: This is a solid wood engineered flooring system from Sweden with a factory-applied UV-cured multilayered acrylic finish. The wear layer is solid ⅛-inch plain sawn. Available in eleven wood species.
- **Rappgo**: This is a Swedish system manufactured to meet German DIN emissions standards and containing a central layer of low-emissions plywood sandwiched between a top and bottom layer of solid wood. The product is distinctive in that the top wood has long plank length and the flooring holds up well in very dry conditions. It comes with a durable factory processed UV-cured acrylic finish that is fully cured by the time it reaches the jobsite.

Underlayment for Wood Flooring

Interior-grade plywood or particleboard, most commonly used for wood floor underlayment, should not be used anywhere in a healthy house. The following underlayments are acceptable:

- 1- or 2-inch tongue-and-groove wood or rough-sawn lumber laid diagonally.
- Exterior-grade plywood (CDX), if used for underlayment, should be stickered to air

out onsite. When used for chemically sensitive persons, it should be sealed with an acceptable vapor-barrier sealant, as specified in this chapter.

Adhesives for Wood Flooring

Use only solvent-free adhesives or 100 percent silicone. Refer to the section on wood adhesives in Division 6.

Finishes for Wood Flooring

When finishing or refinishing a wood floor onsite, it is advisable to specify "dustless" sanding, as explained above. This technique will help lower the amount of dust generated, but a thorough vacuuming with a true HEPA (high efficiency particulate air) vacuum will still be required.

A wide variety of floor-finishing products are available, some with very toxic ingredients. Because the floor is usually one of the last things to be finished, these emissions can be readily absorbed into other porous finishes and may continue to outgas for weeks or months before the finish is fully cured. It is therefore important to apply a product that is free of harsh, solvent-based chemicals.

Water-Based Sealers for Wood Flooring

- **AFM Safecoat Hard Seal** over **AFM Safecoat Lock-In New Wood Sealer** for medium gloss
- **AFM Safecoat Polyureseal BP** over **AFM Safecoat Lock-In New Wood Sealer**
- **Bonakemi Mega Polyurethane**: An oxygen crosslinking, waterborne polyurethane wood finish
- **Zip-Guard Environmental Wood Finish**: A clear finish

Natural Sealers, Waxes, and Oils for Wood Flooring

A naturally finished wood floor often will require more maintenance than one that is sealed with a synthetic finish, but it will have a nicer feel underfoot. It will not have the electrostatic buildup associated with synthetics and will maintain its "breathability." From a Building Biology standpoint, natural options are preferred. Most naturally derived products have a scent associated with them that many people find to be pleasant but that may be intolerable to sensitive individuals. It is important to test the following natural finishes prior to application:

- **AFM Naturals Oil Wax Finish**: Plant-based hardener and sealer for unfinished wood
- **Auro Floor and Furniture Wax Finish No. 171**: Dirt-repellent, solvent-free wax paste for wooden floors
- **Auro European Furniture Wax No. 173**: High-coverage, dirt-repellent wax paste for wooden floors
- **BioShield Penetrating Sealer #5**: Use by itself, as an undercoat with **BioShield Hard Oil #9**, or as an undercoat with a topcoat of **BioShield Resin Floor Finish #4**
- **Livos Ardvos Wood Oil or Livos Meldos Hard Oil**: Medium to high gloss
- **Livos Bilo Floor Wax or Livos Glievo Liquid Wax**: Plant chemistry or beeswax products
- **OS Color Hard Wax/Oil**: A satin matt oil or wax finish
- **Trip Trap oils**: A range of wood surface flooring treatment oils imported from Denmark and designed to maintain and clean hardwood or engineered wood flooring

Bamboo Flooring

Bamboo flooring has now become a cost competitive and aesthetic rival to wood flooring. The bamboo used for flooring can grow to a height of 40 feet in five years and a bamboo forest will continually renew itself. The bamboo is split into strips and then kiln dried. Bamboo is more dimensionally stable than wood flooring and is 12 percent harder than rock maple. Bamboo flooring is available through the following sources:

- **Bamboo Flooring Directory**: Internet directory of bamboo flooring manufacturers.
- **Bamboo Hardwoods**: Engineered prefinished bamboo floors, sustainably harvested, with a 50-year warranty on finish.
- **Duro Design**: Bamboo flooring supplier.
- **EcoTimber**: Supplier of bamboo flooring, floating floor padding, and sustainably harvested wood flooring.
- **Plyboo**: Hand harvested and grown in managed forests in Asia. Planks are 3-inch-wide tongue-and-groove and come in natural or amber color. Accessories, paneling, and veneer are also available. Plyboo comes unfinished or with an acrylic polyurethane finish. Processing occurs in Asia and an MSDS is not available.
- Hanlite Bamboo, available through **Sustainable Flooring**: Claims to have the lowest formaldehyde in the industry. Sustainably harvested six-year-old bamboo with horizontal, vertical, or strand grain (the newest and most stable bamboo construction), unfinished or finished, 4½ inches wide, 20-year nondelamination warranty. Also extensive line of bamboo millwork.
- **Teragren**: Available unfinished in vertical or flat grain in 12-inch-wide panels or 4-inch-wide tongue-and-groove planks for flooring. A variety of milled trim accessories are also available. Sustainably harvested and grown without the use of pesticides, fertilizers, or irrigation. Available with a very durable German-made UV-catalyzed factory-applied urethane finish.

Resilient Flooring

Although easy clean-up, economy, and a soft walking surface have made sheet vinyl a popular flooring for kitchen and utility areas, vinyl flooring is associated with health hazards. The vinyl chloride fumes it emits are a known carcinogen. In addition, in hot or humid climates requiring air conditioning the vinyl will trap moisture, which can promote delamination and mold growth or rot. We do not recommend vinyl in the healthy home.

Natural linoleum, also known as battleship linoleum, is made from linseed oil, pine resins, wood powder, and jute and is free of synthetic chemicals. When newly installed, this flooring does have a noticeable odor that some people do not tolerate. Cork tile is another natural choice for resilient flooring. The natural smell of the cork is also evident at first unless the cork is presealed. Both linoleum and cork are available with factory-applied acrylic finishes. In hot and humid climates these finishes may impede vapor permeability, causing moisture to be trapped under the surface.

Sources for Natural Linoleum and Cork Flooring

Natural linoleum and cork flooring are available from the following sources:

- **Armstrong/DLW Linoleums**: Natural linoleums in a variety of colors with natural jute backing

- **Bangor Cork Company**: Cork tiles and sheet flooring and linoleum
- **Building for Health**: Cork and battleship linoleum flooring products
- **Dodge-Regupol, Inc.**: Cork tile available unfinished, waxed, or with polyurethane matt or gloss finishes
- **Duro Design**: Cork flooring supplier
- **Eco Design/Natural Choice**: Cork floor tiles and adhesives
- **Forbo Industries**: Natural linoleum flooring products
- **Hendricksen Naturlich**: Cork, natural linoleum, and other natural floor coverings and adhesives
- Jelenik Cork available through **Sustainable Flooring**: A variety of patterns and colors, planks or tiles, and acoustical underlayment
- **Natural Cork Co. Ltd.**: Cork in a variety of colors, patterns, and finishes

Adhesives for Natural Linoleum and Cork Flooring

These adhesives are acceptable for natural linoleum and cork flooring:

- **AFM Safecoat 3 in 1 Adhesive**
- **Auro No. 383 Natural Linoleum Glue**
- **BioShield Natural Cork Adhesive**
- **Envirotec Health Guard Adhesive #2027**
- **Forbo** L910 Linoleum Sheet Adhesive and T940 Linoleum Tile Adhesive
- **Sinan Company No. 380** and **No. 390** for cork flooring
- **Taylor Meta-Tec 2084 Tuff Lok X Link** for cork flooring

Carpeting

Carpeting has been associated with a growing number of health problems. In a typical carpet, toxic chemicals may be found in the fiber bonding material, dyes, backing glues, fire retardant, latex binder, fungicide, and antistatic and stain-resistant treatments. During a 1992 congressional hearing on the potential risk of carpets, the US Environmental Protection Agency (EPA) stated that a typical carpet sample contains at least 120 chemicals, many of which are known to be neurotoxic. Outgassing from new carpeting can persist at significantly high levels for up to three years after installation. Once discarded, carpet is neither renewable nor biodegradable. In major cities, discarded carpeting accounts for 7 percent of the landfill mass.

Synthetic latex, the most common carpet backing, contains approximately 100 different gases, which contribute to the unpleasant and harmful "new carpet smell." Most underpads are made of foamed plastic or synthetic rubber and contain petroleum products that cause pollution at every stage of production and continue to pollute once installed. Felt backings are generally less polluting. We have specified safer carpet backings below. Typically, brands labeled hypoallergenic will be odorless.

Carpet Installation

There are two ways to install wall-to-wall carpeting: tack-down or glue-down. Tack-down installations are preferable because they do not destroy the floor surface and because the carpet is easier to remove and can thus be partially recycled. Tacking strips are nailed, screwed, or glued down around the perimeter of the room. If the strips are glued, it is important to use a low-toxic glue. The carpet and underpad are then stretched and the edges are folded with the underside tacked down.

CASE STUDY 9.3

Toddler Made Severely Ill by Carpet

B. J. is a two-year-old boy who was in excellent health until the age of 10 months, when he suddenly developed seizures. These episodes of rigidity and tremors occurred up to 40 to 50 times a day. The baby was subjected to a series of invasive diagnostic evaluations by many different specialists. The blood tests, brain scans, and electroencephalograms revealed no apparent cause of the seizures. The baby was placed on medication to suppress the central nervous system. The seizures persisted, although their intensity declined.

The baby's grandfather, a building contractor, suggested that the culprit might be the expensive new carpet installed shortly before the onset of the seizures. The parents contacted a representative from the carpet industry, who denied any similar complaints of neurological problems from customers. The parents suspected that this information was incorrect. They sent samples of the carpet to the independent Anderson Laboratories in Vermont for testing. Air was blown across the carpet samples into the cages of mice, whose symptoms were then observed and documented. After a short period of time elapsed, the mice developed tremors, rigidity, and seizures. The parents were horrified by the report. It was clear that their beautiful new carpet had essentially poisoned their son. The carpet and pad were immediately removed from the home, the adhesive scraped off, and the house aired out. The seizures stopped. The child is now off all medication and doing much better, although blood testing shows immune system damage consistent with chemical injury.

Most standard adhesives for carpet installation are solvent-based and contain harmful chemicals. Where a glue-down installation is required, avoid solvent-based adhesives. We have specified several healthier options below. In either installation procedure, seaming tapes will be needed to fasten sections of carpeting together. Safer seaming tapes are also specified below.

There are several untreated natural fibers available for wall-to-wall installations, including wool, coir, and sisal. When these are installed with low-toxic or nontoxic backing and either tacked-down or using low-toxic glue, they will provide a safer solution than most standard installations. Warning: Wool carpets are often treated with highly toxic mothproofing pesticides. Therefore, an expensive 100 percent wool carpet is not necessarily a safer carpet.

Wall-to-wall carpeting, whether standard or natural, serves as a reservoir for dirt, dust, mold, bacterial growth, and toxins tracked in from outside, even when it is regularly vacuumed and shampooed. It is also highly absorbent and will readily acquire odors. Typical cleaning agents for wall-to-wall carpets contain harmful ingredients, including perfumes, chemical soil removers, brighteners, and antibacterial agents.

Although we strongly recommend the use of throw rugs of natural fibers, which can be removed and cleaned, instead of wall-to-wall carpeting, we offer the following guidelines for selecting the least-toxic carpeting for those who choose to use it:

- Verify with the manufacturer that wool carpets have not been mothproofed.
- Of the synthetic carpets, 100 percent nylon is considered one of the safest.
- Choose carpeting that has little or no odor. Even the slightest odor on a small sample will be magnified many times in a fully carpeted room and can result in a very prominent, unpleasant, and unhealthy smell.
- Choose your carpeting as early as possible so it will have the most time to air out prior to installation. Buy carpeting from a supplier who will agree to warehouse it for you. This means that the carpet will be unrolled and aired out in the warehouse prior to shipping.
- Avoid carpeting that contains antimicrobial agents such as fungicides and mildewcides.
- Avoid carpeting containing permanent stain-resistance treatment.
- Avoid carpeting or pads containing styrene-butadiene rubber.
- Carpeting with woven backing is preferable to rubberized backing.
- Follow underpad and installation recommendations in these specifications.
- Use nontoxic and odor-free shampoos, and maintain carpets regularly to prevent mold, bacteria, dust, and pesticide buildup.
- To prevent moth infestations in untreated wool carpets, vacuum the carpets on a regular basis, moving furniture if necessary to reach all areas where larvae may hide. A vacuum cleaner that is equipped with a true HEPA filter is a must if you have carpet. It is the only type that collects very tiny particles such as dust mite feces and mold spores. Portable vacuums that are not equipped with HEPA filtration will spew dust into circulation, often leaving a room with more ambient dust than was there prior to cleaning.
- Establish a no-shoes policy for your home.
- If the carpet or pad gets wet, dry it as quickly as possible to prevent microbial growth. Warning: Never use wall-to-wall carpet in bathrooms, kitchens, laundry rooms, or mechanical rooms. Carpeting in these areas inevitably becomes damp, inviting mold and bacterial infestation.

In new construction, homeowners are typically given an allowance and asked to choose the carpeting. This allowance can also be used toward the purchase of healthier floor coverings.

Sources for nontoxic underpadding include:

- **Endurance II**: Synthetic jute pad in 20- or 32-ounce weights
- **Enertia Padding**: Wool-based carpet padding without dyes, fire retardant, mothproofing, or adhesives
- **Hartex Carpet Cushion**: Available in three weights
- **Hendricksen Naturlich**: Recycled felt underpadding, heat bonded with no chemical additives
- **Ultra Touch**: 29-ounce carpet cushion of recycled fibers

Acceptable adhesives and seaming tapes for carpet installation include:

- **AFM Safecoat 3 in 1 Adhesive**
- **Auro No. 382 Floor Covering Adhesive**
- **CHAPCO Safe-Set 3 Premium Fast Grab Carpet Adhesive**
- **Envirotec Health Guard Adhesives:**

CASE STUDY 9.4

EPA Takes a "Stand" on the Carpet Controversy

In October 1987, the EPA installed carpet at its headquarters in the Waterside Mall in Washington, DC. A total of 1,141 complaints were received regarding adverse health effects related to the new carpet.[a] These complaints included decreased short-term memory, loss of concentration, confusion, anxiety, headaches, joint and muscle pains, rashes, digestive disorders, reproductive abnormalities, asthma, insomnia, chronic fatigue, and multiple chemical sensitivities. Dozens of workers remained permanently disabled. After the EPA investigated these carpet complaints from its headquarters building, it published a report showing a positive correlation between the EPA worker complaints and the new carpet.[b]

Despite the results of its own study, and the removal of 27,000 square yards of carpet from the headquarters building in 1989, the EPA published a public information brochure that stated, "Limited research to date has found no links between adverse health effects and the levels of chemicals emitted by new carpet."[c]

EPA's Director of Health and Safety told the *Washington Times* that "the freshly manufactured carpet clearly caused the initial illness." Within a few weeks of making that statement he was removed from his job. EPA management expressed concern that testing and regulation of carpet emissions could potentially cost the carpet industry billions of dollars.[d]

Discussion

The Consumer Product Safety Commission (CPSC) has received hundreds of complaints about carpets causing respiratory and neurological problems.[e] Toxic emissions from carpets include fumes from formaldehyde, benzene, xylene, toluene, butadiene, styrene, and 4-phenylcyclohexene (4PC). These chemicals can potentially cause cancer, birth defects, reproductive disorders, respiratory problems, and neurological damage such as anxiety, depression, inability to concentrate, confusion, short-term memory loss, and seizures. In spite of overwhelming evidence to the contrary,

Several different adhesives for carpeting (refer to manufacturer)

- **Envirotec Health Guard Seaming Tapes**: Several different seaming tapes for carpeting (refer to manufacturer)
- **Hendricksen Naturlich Manufacturer's Adhesive**

Carpet Treatment

The following carpet treatment will help remove pesticides, formaldehyde, and other chemicals from the carpeting and pad and will seal in chemicals to prevent outgassing: **AFM SafeChoice Carpet Shampoo**, **AFM SafeChoice Carpet Seal**, and **AFM SafeChoice Lock-Out**. Follow the manufacturer's instructions. Test a small sample of carpet with these products for shrinkage and color fastness prior to full application.

The treatment is not suitable for carpets with a large wool or cotton content because the wet application can cause shrinkage.

Wet-Applied Finish Materials

Paints, stains, and sealers are all wet-applied finish materials that will have a significant impact on indoor air quality as they are drying.

the carpet industry has consistently denied adverse health effects of carpeting.

In 1992, in response to public concern, the carpet industry announced its Green Tag program, which has lured consumers into a false sense of safety. The program tests only a small sampling of carpets once a year. The testing is based only on volatile organic compound emissions, not biological health effects.[f] In fact, some carpets from the Green Tag program tested at the Anderson Labs have caused death to the mice exposed to their fumes.[g]

a. Bill Hirzy. "Chronology: EPA and Its Professionals: Union Involvement with Carpet." 1992. Cited in "Carpet: Trouble Underfoot." *Informed Consent.* November/December 1993, p. 31.
b. US Environmental Protection Agency. "Indoor Air Quality and New Carpet: What You Should Know." EPA/560/2-91/003. US Government Printing Office, March 1992.
c. Bill Hirzy. "Chronology: EPA and Its Professionals: Union Involvement with Carpet." 1992. Cited in "Carpet: Trouble Underfoot." *Informed Consent.* November/December 1993, p. 31.
d. Susan E. Womble. "Evaluation of Complaints Associated with the Installation of New Carpet." Memorandum, Consumer Products Safety Commission (CPSC) Chemical Hazards Program, August 13, 1990.
e. Ibid.
f. Carpet and Rug Institute. "Carpet Industry Program Steps Out Front on Indoor Air Quality: Labeling for Consumers Now Underway." Press release, July 17, 1992.
g. Anderson Laboratories. "Carpet Off-gassing and Lethal Effects on Mice." Press release, August 18, 1992.

Once thoroughly cured, they will no longer release VOCs. While some materials will have very low odor and/or will dry almost instantly, others may be odorous for months. Because of the large surface area that these materials cover, their impact can be significant and they must be carefully chosen. Consider the following:

1. *Performance:* A product that is more durable will not need to be reapplied as often. A product that is more odorous initially but has time to completely cure during the construction period may well be worth considering if it is more durable than the alternatives. However, adequate ventilation for the construction team during the curing period must be included in this strategy.
2. *Application Procedure:* Manufacturer's instructions must be strictly followed. If applications are not sufficiently dried between coatings, they may remain tacky and odorous indefinitely. This same problem can occur if underlying joint compounds or plasters are not sufficiently cured.
3. *Construction Protocol:* Good ventilation during the application of wet products will not only speed drying time but will

also (along with the use of recommended safety gear) help assure the well-being of the construction team. Furthermore, good ventilation at the time of application will reduce the impact of these odors on porous materials that can acquire odor easily. Planning for and specifying a flush-out period at the end of all construction is a good way to allow outgassing prior to occupancy. Where weather permits, fans can be used with open windows to speed this process. Air filters and ventilation equipment may help during inclement weather.

4. *Factory applied finishes:* Some materials come with an optional factory-applied prefinish. Wood, bamboo and cork flooring, and ceramic tiles are some examples of materials that are commonly offered prefinished or unfinished. Factories often have facilities for safely and fully curing the finishes before the products are shipped out. These factory-applied finishes are often more durable than the lower-VOC finishes that would be suitable for onsite application. Prior to approving a factory-applied finish it is prudent to have a dated sample sent to you to examine along with an MSDS. On occasion, samples may still have persistent odors or the MSDS may reveal the use of unacceptable toxins.

Paints

Because paints cover such large surface areas, careful selection is crucial. Paints are commonly a source of indoor air pollution. Certain paints and coatings, on the other hand, can improve indoor air quality by sealing out odors in subsurfaces so that they do not outgas into the living space.

All paints and wet-applied coatings have three major components: pigment, binder, and carrier, also known as the vehicle. Water-based (latex) paints use water as the carrier whereas oil-based (alkyd) paints use a variety of much more volatile solvents as the carrier. In the past, oil-based paints were considered to be more enduring than latex paints. However, with recent improvements in latex paint technology, oil-based paints can be entirely eliminated from residential construction. Among the thousands of latex paints available, there is a wide range of volatility, toxicity, and performance. Since the previous edition of this book was published, many more low- to zero-VOC water-based paints have become available from commercial manufacturers. In addition, some of the original commercial "environmental paint" products have been reformulated for higher performance in the areas of hideability, wearability, and scrubability.

Low VOC is not the only measure of a paint's effect on human health. Both synthetic binders and various additives can cause negative reactions for some people, and paints often contain substances that are environmentally undesirable. Finding out about the presence of these ingredients can be challenging. Additives such as biocides are often proprietary or are present in such small amounts that they are not required to be listed on an MSDS.

Several independent nonprofit organizations have arisen internationally to set environmental standards for consumer products. **Green Seal** is a US-based organization that has created evaluation standards for architectural coatings that have low-VOC emissions and exclude five heavy metals and 21 toxic organic compounds. The commercially available paints listed below have, according to the manufacturers, met these Green Seal criteria.

A more extensive list can be obtained through Green Seal.

Individuals with chemical sensitivities should test paints to determine the best choice for them. Our experience has shown that sensitivities vary and that none of the paints has a perfect track record with everyone. In some cases, paints with acrylic rather than vinyl or vinyl acrylic binders have been better tolerated. Below are several low- to zero-VOC content paints that you may wish to consider for your project.

Commercially Available Interior Zero- and Low-VOC Paints from Conventional Manufacturers

Following are widely distributed low emission paints. Please note that the product names shown in bold type are the paint line being recommended for each manufacturer. These manufacturers also make paint lines that we do not recommend.

- **Air Care Odorless**: Solvent-free eggshell and flat by Coronado Paints
- **American Pride 100 Line**: Green Seal certified zero-VOC paints by Southern Diversified Products
- **E Coat** and **Enviro-Cote**: Paints by Kelly-Moore
- **Enviro-Pure**: Green Seal certified zero-VOC paints by M.A. Bruder & Sons
- **Genesis Odor Free**: Paints by Duron
- **Harmony**: Paints by Sherwin Williams
- **Lifemaster 2000**: Paints by ICI Dulux/Glidden
- **Premium Interior Paint Zero VOC**: Green Seal certified zero-VOC paints by Olympic
- **Pristine Eco Spec**: Green Seal certified paints by Benjamin Moore
- **Yolo Colorhouse**: Green Seal certified zero-VOC interior paints by Yolo Colorhouse.
- **Z-coat (59-Line)**: Green Seal certified zero-VOC interior paints by General Paint

Specially Formulated Paints from Alternative Manufacturers

Although generally more expensive, the following paints have been specially formulated and often better meet the needs of chemically sensitive individuals:

- **AFM SafeCoat Enamel Low VOC and Safecoat Zero VOC**: Formulated with propylene glycol instead of ethylene glycol and free of ammonia, acetone, formaldehyde, and masking agents
- **Ecological**: Odorless, formaldehyde-free, water-based terpolymer paint
- **Enviro Safe**: No fungicides, low-biocide, and custom mixed to order
- **Miller Acro**: Specify low-biocide, no-fungicide
- **Murco GF1000** and **Murco LE1000**: No fungicides and only "in-can" preservatives that enhance shelf life but become entombed in the dry paint

Paints Derived from Natural Sources

The following paints, which are derived from natural sources, contain few or no petrochemically derived ingredients and may be more environmentally sound choices. Some may not be suitable for the chemically sensitive. Products that contain d-limonene may have vapors that are more toxic than those of petroleum distillates or turpentine and should be used with proper ventilation.[1] They are often harder to work with, but when skillfully used can render a more lively wall surface:

- **AGLAIA Natural Paints**: Plant-based natural paint products, free of petrochemicals and artificial resins
- **Auro Natural Paints**: Made exclusively from natural sources by Sinan Co., with efforts made to support ecological diversity
- **BioShield Clay Paint #12**: Zero-VOC paint made from naturally occurring clays
- **BioShield Solvent Free Wall Paint** and **BioShield Casein Milk Paint**: Very low VOCs, made from natural or minimally toxic synthetic materials
- **Green Planet Paints**: Zero-VOC clay-based paints utilizing soy resin and mineral pigments
- **Livos Naturals**: Low-toxic paints, all ingredients listed on label, many organically grown; both water- and oil-based products available
- **Milk Paint**: Made from milk protein, lime, earth pigments, and clay, petrochemical-free, biodegradable, nontoxic, odorless when dry; not recommended for damp locations because it is susceptible to mildew. Milk paint can sour in liquid form. Comes in powder form in 16 colors (see **Clear Coat** as recommended topcoat).
- **Minerva Finishes**: Line of all-natural lime-based paints for interior and exterior applications (refer to product literature for specific application and use)
- **Sinan Company**: Several natural water-based and casein-based paints (refer to Resource List for various products)

Vapor Retardant Paints

The following paints are vapor retarders that can be used to block unwanted outgassing from vapors found in a material:

- **86001 Seal**: A clear, water-reducible primer sealer and vapor retarder
- **AFM Safecoat New Wallboard Primecoat HPV**: Specially formulated to cover the uneven porosity of new gypsum board and other surfaces with a high recycled content
- **AFM Safecoat Transitional Primer**: For use on various previously treated surfaces; seals and reduces outgassing
- **BIN Primer Sealer**: A white pigmented shellac sealer used as an undercoat/primer/sealer, free of biocides, effectively seals in odors from drywall, and should be used in a well-ventilated space since the alcohol base is strong smelling during application (available through most paint and hardware stores)

Stains and Transparent Finishes

Many standard sealers for wood are solvent-based and contain several highly toxic chemicals that outgas for long periods after application. Several more healthful water-based products are now available. Since water-based products tend to raise the grain on wood or absorb unevenly, many installers who are inexperienced with their use have been disappointed with the results. We have found several good installers who have overcome their initial reluctance and now insist on using less-toxic, water-based products, knowing that in doing so they are safeguarding themselves, their employees, and their clients. Natural, more healthful oils, lacquers, shellacs, and waxes are also available.

Clear-Seal Water-Reducible Wood Finishes

- **AFM Safecoat AcriGlaze**: Clear mixing medium and finish, ideal for restoring old finishes, sealing, and preserving painted work

- **AFM Safecoat Hard Seal**: Used in conjunction with **AFM Safecoat Lock-In New Wood Sealer**
- **AgriStain**: Bio-based interior and exterior stain for metal, wood, gypsum, and cement
- **Aqua-Zar**: Water-based nonyellowing polyurethane in satin or gloss finish
- **Clear Coat**: Nontoxic acrylic coating for use over painted and wood surfaces; may be used in conjunction with **Extra-Bond**, which will promote adhesion on surfaces other than bare wood
- **Hydrocote Hydroshield Plus**: Water-based polyurethane for interior and exterior use
- **Zip-Guard Environmental Wood Finish**: Clear finish for interior woodwork (the same company makes a product called Zip-Guard, which is solvent based)

Natural Oil, Lacquer, and Shellac Wood Finishes

- **AFM Naturals Clear Penetrating Oil**: Plant-based sealer for interior and exterior wood applications
- **AFM Naturals Oil Wax Finish**: Plant-based hardener and sealer for unfinished wood, bamboo, and cork
- **Auro No. 123 Natural Finishing Oil**: Oil primer, sealer, and protective treatment
- **Auro No. 143 Organic Linseed Oil Finish**: Interior and exterior penetrating, protective, and conditioning treatment for wood
- **Auro No. 251 Clear-Coat Paint Glossy**: Oil-based transparent finishing lacquer for use on indoor surfaces; can be tinted
- **BioShield Primer Oil #1**: An oil-based sealer that creates an elastic and breathable grain-enhancing prime coat for priming and sealing hardwoods and softwoods
- **BioShield Resin Floor Finish #4**: Breathable and elastic finish that will create depth and dimension in flooring substrates of all types
- **BioShield Penetrating Sealer #5**: Crafted from linseed oil, plants, and other less hazardous materials, a high-solids primer that excels at sealing cork, dry and absorbent woods, slate, stone, and brick
- **BioShield Hard Oil #9**: Specially recommended for high-moisture and high-traffic areas, this is one of the most durable low-VOC oils suitable for hard and softwood floors
- **Block Oil**: Natural finish for any wooden food preparation surface; may be used to treat any unsealed interior wood surface
- **Sinan Company No. 143 Linseed Oil**: Organically grown, for plain oiled-rubbed finish
- **Sinan Company No. 251 Natural Clear Varnish, Clear, Glossy**: **Clear, Glossy #251** or **Clear, Satin #261** varnish with good covering qualities for indoor wood use only
- **Sinan Company No. 253 Natural Undercoat Enamel, White, Water-Based**: Suitable for priming or intermediate coats for interior and exterior use on wood
- **Sinan Company No. 260 Natural Enamel, White, Water-Based, Interior, Satin**: Low-gloss lacquer for interior use only, to be used after one undercoat of No. 253; can be tinted

Wood Stains

- **AFM Safecoat Durostain**: Interior and exterior

- **BioShield Aqua Resin Stain**: Zero-VOC, resilient wood stain finish for interior and exterior applications
- **BioShield Earth Pigments #88**
- **Hydrocote Danish Oil Finish**: Stain that colors and protects in one step
- **Livos Kaldet Stain, Resin & Oil Finish**: Satin, semi-flat, water-resistant finish, interior and exterior, strong surface hardening capacity for wood cabinets, doors, and windows
- **OS Color One Coat Only**: Natural oil-based stains
- **PureColor**: Two-stage stain formulation of pure mineral ions and oxygen catalyst with no solvents, oils, VOCs, odors, acids, or bleaches

Clear Vapor-Barrier Sealants for Wood

These products are used to help lock in noxious fumes so they do not escape into the air. In fact, since no seal is ever perfect, vapor-barrier sealants generally serve to decrease the amount of outgassing at any one time while increasing the overall time it takes for any substance to completely volatilize. We recommend that all efforts be made to speed up the outgassing time prior to application of vapor barrier sealants.

Outgassing can be accelerated by using filtration or adsorbers indoors or by doing the application outdoors in a weather-protected area whenever possible. VOCs readily release noxious vapors in heat. Harmful chemicals can thus be dissipated more quickly if they are exposed to elevated temperatures. This can work well in controlled factory conditions but is not recommended for products in the home. Adsorbers are substances such as zeolite or aluminum silicate to which VOCs adhere. When adsorbers are placed in a room, they help remove VOCs from the ambient air.

Although most coatings seal to some degree, and will be more effective when applied in several layers, the following products are advertised by their manufacturer as recommended specifically for locking in noxious fumes. The manufacturer's instructions for application must be followed in order to achieve an optimum seal.

- **AFM Safecoat Hard Seal**: Clear sealer for low-moisture areas
- **AFM Safecoat Safe Seal**: Clear sealer for porous surfaces; also an effective primer

Further Reading and Services

Anderson Laboratories, PO Box 323, West Hartford, VT 05064, 802-295-7344. For evaluation of toxic effects of selected carpets, insulation, and other building materials through testing on mice. Consultations are available by phone for a fee.

Carpet and Indoor Air: What You Should Know. June 1993. Available free of charge from New York State Attorney General, 120 Broadway, New York, NY 10271.

Environmental Access Research Network (EARN). 315 W. 7th Avenue, Sisserton, SD 59645. For a list of carpet-related articles, studies, and reports available from EARN's photocopying service, send $1.00 and request "carpet list."

Foster, Kari et al. *Sustainable Residential Interiors.* John Wiley and Sons, 2007. A guide to sustainable principles and practices that can be applied to every level of interior design.

Guelberth, Cedar Rose and Dan Chiras. *The Natural Plaster Book.* New Society Publishers, 2003. A step-by-step guide for choosing, mixing, and applying natural plasters.

Thrasher, Jack and Alan Broughton. *The Poisoning of Our Homes and Workplaces: The Indoor Formaldehyde Crisis.* Seadora, 1989.

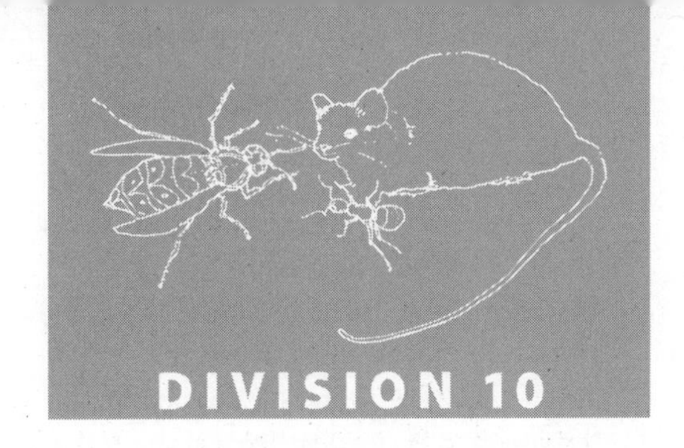

Specialties

Integrated Pest Management

All creatures have their rightful place in nature. However, for most this place is not within the walls of human habitations and hence the need for humans to exercise pest control. While many pest control companies advocate regular prophylactic spraying of homes with toxic chemicals, this approach can have devastating consequences for the health of all living beings, including the occupants of the home. Although pests are effectively eliminated, they eventually return because the underlying structural problems that created the conditions inviting to them have not been addressed.

Integrated pest management (IPM) offers a holistic approach to controlling pests. IPM differs from standard pest management in that the emphasis is on prevention and on the least toxic methods of pest control. The goal is to work effectively with nature to alter conditions without harming the environment. IPM precepts can be summarized as follows:

- Accurate identification of a pest is necessary so that its modus operandi may be understood and incorporated into a pest management plan.
- Careful consideration is given to whether any action at all is required. Entomophobia (fear of insects) is rampant in our culture. For many, the first reaction upon seeing an insect is to kill it. Pesticide commercials persuade us that panic and lightning speed action are necessary. In contrast, IPM encourages an attitude of tolerance to creatures that do no harm. It also encourages rational determination of when intervention will be necessary.
- If a pest must be eliminated, the first step is to see if its current access to nourishment and habitat can be limited. In the case of ants, for example, this might mean cleaning up crumbs from the floor and counters and caulking cracks.
- If a pest must be trapped or killed, the most environmentally benign methods

are considered first. Least toxic chemicals are employed as a last resort.

- If a chemical must be used, then toxicity, risk, and exposure must be carefully evaluated. (Refer to Northwest Coalition for Alternatives to Pesticides, listed at the end of this chapter, for fact sheets on the various pesticides.)
- Careful observation and record keeping are an essential part of an integrated pest management program.

In new home construction you have the opportunity and responsibility to prevent infestations before they occur. An integrated approach to pest management in new construction would include the following:

- identification of potential pests found in the building site area
- research on identified pests, including eating habits, reproductive cycles, habitat, and common routes of entry into the home
- use of construction strategies that will create inhospitable and inaccessible conditions for pests

In general, a well-constructed home will also be pest resistant, incorporating the following features:

- weathertightness
- appropriate grading and drainage
- provisions for the prevention of excess moisture buildup from within, including extraction fans and windows that allow cross-ventilation
- selection of dry wood without rot or infestation for use in construction
- appropriate treatment of exterior wood for prevailing climatic conditions
- screening of all openings such as basement and soffit vents
- removal of all ground cover, leaves, chip and wood piles, and other potential insect habitats from around the building

Throughout the book we have specified techniques for the prevention of pests where appropriate. If you are building in an area with a particularly difficult pest problem, you may need to take measures beyond the scope of this book. For example, if your home is near a shipyard or a row of poorly constructed grain elevators, you may wish to incorporate more rat control techniques into your construction than would generally be specified. We heartily recommend *Common Sense Pest Control* by William Olkowski et al. (listed at the end of this chapter) as a comprehensive guide to specific pest problems. The following chart provides an overview of major household pests and construction techniques that discourage them.

Further Reading and Services

Biointegral Resource Center (BIRC), PO Box 7414, Berkeley, CA 94707, 510-524-2567. Useful source of information on pesticides and alternative pest treatments.

Moses, Marion. *Designer Poisons: How to Protect Your Health and Home from Toxic Pesticides.* Pesticide Education Center, 1995. A sobering exposé of specific pesticides and the chronic health effects that can result from their use, with useful information on safer alternatives.

National Coalition Against Misuse of Pesticides, 701 E. Street SE, Suite 200, Washington, DC 20003, 202-543-5450, info@beyondpesticides.org. Provides useful information about pesticides and nontoxic alternatives.

Northwest Coalition for Alternatives to Pesticides (NCAP), PO Box 1393, Eugene, OR 97440, 541-344-5044, pesticide.org. Provides a comprehensive information service on the hazards of pesticides and alternatives to their use. Maintains an extensive library of over 8,000 articles, government documents, videos, and other reference materials, and offers information packets, fact sheets, and the quarterly *Journal of Pesticide Reform*.

Olkowski, William et al. *Common Sense Pest Control: Least-Toxic Solutions for Your Home, Garden, Pets, and Community.* Taunton Press, 1991. Comprehensive, well-documented information on integrated pest management and least-toxic control for all kinds of pests.

Schultz, Warren. *The Chemical-Free Lawn: The Newest Varieties and Techniques to Grow Lush, Hardy Grass.* Rodale Press, 1989. Techniques for growing lush and hardy grass without using pesticides, herbicides, or chemical fertilizers.

Chart 10.1: Common Pests and Management Strategies

Pest	Types of damage	Modus operandi	Recommendations
Termites (subterranean)	• Structural damage • Tunnels created in wood	• Require moist conditions • Termites must be able to get from the soil into the wood structure via earthen tubes; they do not live in wood	• Control moisture • Seal off wood from ground contact • Use termite shielding, sand barriers, and/or termite-resistant sill plates
Termites (drywood)	• Structural damage • Tunnels created in wood	• Can access house through walls • Live in wood	• Tight construction • Caulked joints • Boric acid in framing
Rats	• Carry disease • Destroy food supply • Breed quickly	• Require hole ½" wide to enter	• Screen all points of entry, including openings along pipes and wires • Make home weathertight • Ground floors should be elevated 18" above grade • Subterranean concrete floors should have a minimum thickness of 2" • Use wire mesh under wood floors • Use noncombustible cement stops between floor joists
Mice	• Chew through electrical wires, causing fire hazard • Transmit pathogens • Breed quickly	• Require dime- size openings • Feed on dry foods, grains, clothing, paper • Usually seek indoor habitat when outdoor climatic conditions become severe	• Seal all holes and crevices, especially where pipes and wires protrude through surfaces

Chart 10.1: Common Pests and Management Strategies (cont'd.)

Pest	Types of damage	Modus operandi	Recommendations
Ants (carpenter)	• Create nests inside walls and ceilings, under siding, and where wood and soil are in contact near foundations • Infest both hardwood and softwood	• Require wood with high moisture content (minimum 15%)	• Use kiln- or air-dried lumber and keep it dry • Prevent contact between structural wood and earth • Allow for proper ventilation of damp areas
Bees (carpenter)	• Chew on wood • Burrow into structural members and exposed wood elements	• Enjoy untreated exposed wood (especially softwoods)	• Paint or varnish exposed wood (sills, trim, etc.) • Fill in holes and indentations in wood
Beetles (wood-boring)	• Bore through wood	• Require moisture content in wood to be 10 to 20%	• Prevent moisture changes and temperature fluctuations • Allow for good ventilation in attic spaces • Keep roof frame and sheathing dry • Use air- or kiln-dried lumber • Seal wood
Cockroaches	• Invade food storage areas such as kitchens and cupboards • Can carry disease-causing organisms	• Most species prefer warm, moist areas	• Avoid moisture and decayed organic buildup in or near home • Use boric acid in framing in areas prone to infestation • Use screens on vents and windows
Fungus (wood decay)	• Attacks and weakens wood, leaving it susceptible to invasion by wood-boring and wood-eating insects	• Grows best at temperatures between 50 and 95 degrees F • Requires a minimum of 20% moisture	• Allow for proper roof insulation and ventilation to prevent condensation • Seal wood joints at corners, edges, and intersections • Prevent moisture accumulation near pipes, vents, and ducts • Do not use wood containing mold in construction • Seal all wood exposed to the elements • Use proper ventilation strategies to control moisture buildup generated by human activity • Use building products and procedures that allow moisture vapor to escape rather than being trapped

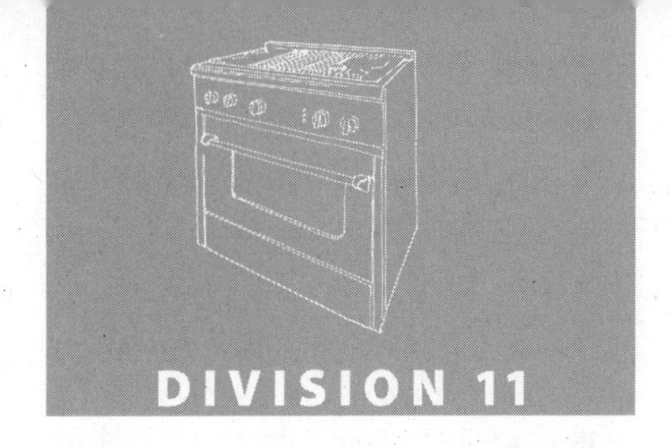

Equipment

Water Treatment Equipment

Water Purification in Standard Construction

Poor indoor air quality is not the only form of pollution that affects human health. Our water sources, both public supplies and private domestic wells, have also become increasingly contaminated. Public concern about water quality has increased dramatically. In late 2005, the Environmental Working Group (EWG) found in an analysis of more than 22 million tap-water quality tests (most of which were conducted to meet EPA compliance) that 260 contaminants were detected in water served to the public.[1]

Of the contaminants identified in the EWG study, the EPA has set enforceable health limits for 114 contaminants and nonenforceable, recommended standards for five. More than half (141) of the total contaminants identified are unregulated and without safety standards. The statistics reported by EWG are believed to represent an underestimate of the exposure of American consumers to unregulated contaminations in the nation's tap water. Not considered in the study were unregulated pharmaceuticals and personal care product chemicals, which, surprisingly, were found in the tested water. The good news is that EWG's analysis found over 90 percent compliance with enforceable health standards.

Water Quality Parameters

Water purification is not standard in home construction, and unless you specify water testing and purification they will not be included. Although water purification is usually considered an "extra," whole-house systems are best planned for and installed at the time of construction. But before you can contemplate options for water quality improvement, you need to know what is in your water.

This is relatively easy to determine if you are on a city or other public water system, but water in private wells is not regulated. The Safe Drinking Water Act (SDWA), passed in 1974 and amended in 1986 and 1996, gives the

Environmental Protection Agency (EPA) authority to set drinking water standards for public water systems that provide water for human consumption through at least 15 service connections or regularly serve at least 25 individuals. To find out more about regulated water contaminants and to learn about the potential health effects and the sources of these contaminations, consult the EPA's Drinking Water Contaminants website.[2]

There are two categories of EPA drinking water standards: primary and secondary. Primary standards (NPDWRs) are legally-enforceable standards that apply to public water systems and are classified into the following categories: microorganisms, disinfectants, disinfection byproducts, inorganic chemicals, organic chemicals, and radionuclides. Primary standards protect drinking water quality by limiting the levels of specific

Improving Drinking Water Quality with Reverse Osmosis

WARREN CLOUGH

Pure water is one of the three essentials of life. The Bau-Biology approach is always to look first to nature. For water, we can look to the seagull. In 1969, Steven Sourirajan, professor of environmental studies at the University of California, discovered that the seagull has a special membrane in its throat that enables it to drink salt water. The membrane allows water to be absorbed and the extra salt is then spit out through the nasal passage.

This observation allowed Sourirajan to develop the first reverse osmosis water purifier. Today reverse osmosis has been developed into a marvel of modern water purification technology and is being used all over the world. It has become the most effective method ever invented for water purification. It out-performs flocculation, distillation, carbon filtration, and other methods. Entire city-wide reverse osmosis units have been put into production, sometimes costing hundreds of millions of dollars for a municipal system.

Reverse osmosis units are also being installed in homes. These units need annual servicing for several reasons:

- Filters need cleaning as they collect dirt.
- Reverse osmosis membranes can deteriorate.
- Bacteria can develop in the system.

The reverse osmosis membrane is only one part of this system. For truly pure water, there are multiple other filters and steps before and after the reverse osmosis membrane. Reverse osmosis membranes have openings that are too small to be called holes. These pores allow water molecules to pass through but prevent the passage of contaminants. If the filters become plugged with trash, the flow of water is slowed down, reducing the pressure of the water stream, which should be around 60 pounds per square inch. Ideal pressure produces the maximum water purity and best flow and extends the longevity of the components.

In addition to salts, other contaminants are frequently found in water and can be effectively reduced by a reverse osmosis system:

- Heavy metals such as lead, cadmium, mercury, and arsenic, found in all water to varying degrees, are removed by the reverse osmosis membrane.
- Volatile contaminants such as chlorine, am-

contaminants that can adversely affect public health and are known or anticipated to occur in water.

Secondary standards (NSDWRs) are nonenforceable guidelines for contaminants that may cause cosmetic effects (such as skin or tooth discoloration) or have aesthetic effects (such as taste, odor, or color) in drinking water. The EPA recommends secondary standards but does not require water systems to comply. States may choose to adopt them as enforceable standards.

The EPA Consumer Confidence Rule requires public water suppliers that serve the same people year round (community water systems) to provide a consumer confidence report (CCR) to their customers. These reports, also known as annual water quality reports or drinking water quality reports, summarize sources used (rivers, lakes, reservoirs, or aquifers), any detected contaminants, compliance efforts, and educational information. The reports are due to customers by July 1 of each year. To find the CCR for your municipal

monia, and trihalomethanes are also found in public water supplies and can be removed with pre- and post-filter activated carbon. The carbon also helps remove other volatile industrial and agricultural residues such as pesticides and herbicides.
- Bacteria are another important concern, but these will typically be killed by the chlorine found in most municipal water systems. Prefilters will then remove the dead bacteria along with other types of sediment. For purification of water supplies that are not chlorinated, ultraviolet purifiers can be added to the system to kill bacteria.

Reverse osmosis units should be tested and serviced on a regular basis. Annual testing of water quality is a good indicator of how well the unit is functioning and when the reverse osmosis membrane needs to be replaced. Poor water quality in some parts of the country means that membranes and filters need to be replaced more frequently there.

Servicing includes not only replacing filters as necessary but also cleaning and disinfecting the unit. The procedure involves disassembling the reverse osmosis system, cleaning the unit, flushing it with hydrogen peroxide, replacing the filters, and checking the unit's performance.

Laboratory water quality tests are only as good as the person doing the evaluation. This means water testing should be performed by a qualified water testing laboratory that specializes in water purification and not just testing. It is of little value to know what is in your water if you do not have a way to remove it.

Warren Clough is a chemist, Certified Water Specialist, and Bau-Biologist with 50 years' experience analyzing water quality and making water purification system recommendations. His company offers free initial telephone consultations and charges minimal fees for water testing to evaluate reverse osmosis units. It can be reached six days a week during normal business hours at Ozark Water Service and Air Services, 114 Spring Street, Sulphur Springs, AR. 72768, 800-835-8908, ozark waterandair.org.

CASE STUDY 11.1

Bath Water Found to be Culprit in Copper Toxicity Case

When F. W. was 63 years old she was seen by Dr. Elliott for a chronic vaginal discharge that had persisted for five years. She had been previously evaluated by several healthcare practitioners for this problem. Although her gynecologist had been unable to find evidence of a yeast or bacterial infection, the patient was nevertheless placed on a variety of antibiotics, which seemed to exacerbate the problem.

During the interview, it was discovered that the patient's symptoms seemed to improve when she traveled. She went on to disclose that a rash she had all over her body also improved while she was away from home. She concluded that her symptoms were probably related to stress, although there were no obvious new stressors in her life that could have accounted for this peculiar reaction. When questioned about events in her life that took place around the time of onset of her symptoms, she revealed that she had moved into a new home. Dr. Elliott suspected that the source of the patient's problem could be the bath water, since water was the only substance in contact with her vagina.

A water sample was sent to a laboratory for analysis. The results showed extremely high copper levels. Upon further inquiry, it was discovered that many water samples from the same part of town were also showing high copper levels. Apparently, the carbon dioxide in the water created enough of an acidic environment to dissolve the copper in the water supply piping.

The patient decided to install a whole-house water filtration system that could be customized to remove carbon dioxide in the household water.

system, consult the National Tap Water Quality Database.[3]

Remember, however, that water leaving the treatment plant may be further contaminated by the time it reaches your tap. During its journey, treated water can pick up lead from solder or old pipes and copper from pipes. Pipes made of PVC, the most common type of new piping, release chlorinated compounds and other chemicals into the water. Pipes that have breaks can suck in mud and silt and are prone to bacterial contamination.

Municipally treated water is usually low in biological contaminants because of chlorination, but it is not well-screened for industrial and hazardous waste. The chlorine with which almost all municipal water has been treated often reacts with naturally occurring organic compounds, creating potentially harmful trihalomethanes. Water experts in your area will know the range of contaminants found in your municipal system and the best strategies for eliminating them.

Private well-water quality is not governed by EPA regulations, but primary and secondary standards for public systems are useful guidelines for the treatment of water in private wells. EPA recommends testing private water supplies annually for nitrates, coliform bacteria, total dissolved solids, and pH levels to detect contamination problems early. Your local water specialist should be able to make general recommendations for well-testing in your area.

Before consumption begins on a private water well, samples should be submitted for

Within a few days after installation, her rash and vaginitis disappeared. Because of evidence of excess copper stored in her body, she underwent a program of vitamin and mineral supplementation and heavy metal chelation. She is currently doing well and is without complaints. In a follow-up visit, she stated that the greenish ring that had been present on the bathroom fixtures also had disappeared.

Discussion

Copper is essential to human life, but in high doses can cause anemia, rashes, liver and kidney damage, and gastrointestinal irritation. While the need for filtering the household drinking water may be obvious, this case study illustrates that bath water may be an unrecognized source of toxic exposure. Because the skin is a large surface area, it allows for significant absorption of substances into the body from bath water. We do not suggest that you avoid tub bathing, which can be both pleasurable and therapeutic. Instead, we recommend that your water be filtered at the point of entry into the house. Filtration systems are most effective when they are customized to fit both the homeowner's personal needs and the local water conditions. These conditions can vary greatly from one location to another. Whether or not you decide to install a whole-house water filtration system, we recommend that you have your water tested periodically.

a comprehensive laboratory test by an EPA-approved laboratory. In addition to determining what is in the well water, the test will help establish a baseline for future changes in water quality. Every well should be tested individually as even adjacent wells may have highly variable water chemistry because of different depths or geological variance of the aquifer.

Types of Water Purification Systems

We recommend a whole-house water purification system as an essential feature of the healthy home for most locations. Choosing the proper system will depend on several factors including location, budget, water use, and taste preference. No single filtration medium can remove all contaminants from all water. Because water quality and individual needs vary, no single combination of systems will provide a universal solution.

Choosing a system can be a complex and confusing process. The average homeowner typically does not know the right questions to ask in order to get accurate information. Water filtration systems have become popular internet marketing products and many people selling them are not much more knowledgeable than potential customers about the range of needs and possibilities. We recommend that you consult with an individual who has the following credentials:

- a broad-based, longstanding experience with water quality in your area
- a wide variety of equipment from several manufacturers

- the ability to provide you with several options at various prices
- the ability to explain the pros and cons of each system

Water Conditioning

Water conditioners are used to improve the aesthetic quality of water, including color, corrosiveness, clarity, and hardness. They use a process of ion exchange to eliminate from the water undesirable substances (such as calcium and magnesium) that may precipitate scale on fixtures, laundry machines, hot water heaters, dishwashers, shower stalls, sinks, and skin. Water conditioners can also be effective in removing sediment, chlorine, and certain metals, such as low levels of manganese and iron (both of which can cause stains) as well as odor from hydrogen sulfide. Flow rate is affected by both the size and the design of the water softener and must be appropriately specified on an individual basis. Conditioned water is often referred to as "soft" water.

In the ion exchange process, calcium or magnesium ions are exchanged with either sodium or potassium. Sodium chloride is the more common regenerate for water conditioning, but many water treatment companies have switched to potassium chloride, which is widely believed to be a healthier and more ecologically sound choice. Potassium chloride is essentially a refined potash, and when returned to the ground water it can serve as a fertilizer for many plants. The small amount ingested daily from water conditioned with potassium is about equivalent to what you would gain by eating half a banana and can be a positive addition to your diet.

For those with a medical condition affecting electrolyte balance, blood pressure, or kidney function, we suggest you consult a physician before you consider purchasing a water-conditioning system with salt-based regenerates. Potassium chloride may also contain traces of naturally occurring gross beta radiation.

Because of chloride discharge into city systems and the subsequent impact of chlorides on rivers and agriculture, some municipalities are moving to ban new salt-regenerating water conditioners and give rebates to customers who switch to salt-free systems. Municipal water and sewer systems are not configured to remove chlorides. This issue is of particular concern in dense metropolitan areas, but since the ion exchange process is also commonly used to remove water contaminants in private domestic wells, chlorides also are discharged into septic systems and ultimately into shallow aquifers.

One of the most promising developments in water treatment is the advent of chemical-free, nonelectrical, nonbackwashing, salt-free systems to treat hardness as an alternative to softening. In one system, which uses template-assisted crystallization, hardness minerals are attracted to a media nucleation site, which then sloughs off seed crystals that travel through the plumbing system in a molecular configuration not prone to accumulation as scale.

The single best source for verifying a manufacturer's claims about any water treatment product is National Sanitation Foundation International (NSF), which is the industry's gold standard for the testing and certification of water treatment systems and components. Before buying water treatment equipment, we recommend that you visit nsf.org and look up individual products and manufacturers to verify certification for efficiency and contaminant reduction.

Chart 11.1: Water Filtration Methods

Type of system	How it works	What is eliminated	What is not eliminated	Comments
Carbon filters: There are countless varieties of carbon filters. The two most commonly used filters in water purification are described here. Granulated activated carbon (GAC) has an amazingly large surface area (up to 1,000 square meters per gram) for adsorptive activity. Carbon filters are not bacteriostatic and will become contaminated with use. Inexpensive sediment prefilters will extend life. Inexpensive chlorine tests can indicate when to change the filter if it is used with chlorinated water. These filters can themselves become a source of contamination if not changed frequently enough. Locate the tank away from inhabited areas when used to filter radon. Although carbon filters are less expensive than aeration systems, they can collect radioactivity and may require special methods of hazardous waste disposal. Aeration is preferable to carbon filtration for radon removal.				
GAC (granulated activated carbon)	Carbon is steam-treated so that the surface becomes pitted, thereby increasing surface area and adsorption capacity.	Trihalomethanes, dissolved gases including chlorines, most pesticides, many chemical pollutants, radon gas	Heavy metals, sediment, fluoride, viruses and bacteria, dissolved solids, and particulates, including radioactive particulate matter	Requires that water have sufficient contact time with the filter. Because GAC can breed bacteria, it is most effective when used with treated municipal water.
Carbon block	Powdered carbon is glued together to form a matrix structure that adsorbs contaminants.	Trihalomethanes, dissolved gases including chlorine, most pesticides, many chemical pollutants, radon gas, particulate matter; can be used for heavy metals under some limited conditions	Fluoride, nitrates, viruses, and bacteria	Considered more effective than GAC if water conditions are within certain parameters. Will remove heavy metals only for a limited time. Periodic retesting is essential. Not recommended for most heavy metal removal. Glue content is a concern. Whole-house or point-source available.
Reverse Osmosis (RO) RO involves forcing water through a semipermeable membrane with extremely fine pores from a more concentrated solution (ultimately becoming the reject water) to a more dilute solution (the product water). The water's direction of movement is the opposite of what would be experienced during osmosis and is achieved by applying water pressure to the solution on the more concentrated (contaminated) side of the membrane. RO will remove a variety of ions and metals as well as some bacterial contaminants (cysts), but not coliform bacteria. RO systems will remove some arsenic (arsenic V but not the more toxic arsenic III). Reverse osmosis is well documented in the literature and in post-treatment testing proves to be effective in removing uranium, but NSF does not certify for uranium reduction. RO membranes eject the bulk of almost any dissolved and suspended contaminant including ionic, organic, and silica compounds. One criticism of reverse osmosis-filtered water is that it is stripped of essential minerals. Although this is true, it is a tradeoff for overall water quality. Most consumers do not depend on water for their nutritional needs but elect to take vitamin supplements or remineralize their RO water. Savvy water treatment companies use a crushed limestone (calcite) post-RO filter to impart a pleasant taste to the water. Parents sometimes express concern that RO removes fluoride added to municipal water for dental health purposes. This is true, but water fluoridation in general is a controversial issue and today most children under professional dental care receive whole-mouth fluoride treatments.				

Chart 11.1: Water Filtration Methods (cont'd.)

Type of system	How it works	What is eliminated	What is not eliminated	Comments
The most valid criticism of RO is that anywhere from 3.5 to 5 gallons of water are rejected for every gallon of purified water produced. Many inexpensive, noncertified RO systems have much higher rejection rates, are extremely wasteful, and still do not deliver verifiable contaminant reduction, the primary reason for using reverse osmosis. While reject water is routed to the drain, it is not lost but reenters the hydrologic cycle. In many cases, the RO reject water may be collected and redirected for irrigation purposes. Seek out a five-stage RO system. Plastic parts can be problem for individuals with petrochemical sensitivities. When selecting a reverse osmosis system, look for certification by National Sanitation Foundation (NSF) International (www.nsf.org) to ensure materials quality, system performance, and contaminant reduction. Be wary of self-proclaimed lists of contaminant reduction and verify the certification for the specific unit you are considering on the NSF website under Drinking Water Treatment Units.				
CTA (cellulose triacetate) RO membrane	Water is forced under pressure through a fine membrane that screens out dissolved solids.	Dissolved solids (60 to 90%), heavy metals, asbestos, radioactive particles, some bacteria; NSF certified under-counter RO removes 99.99% of cysts	Dissolved gases, some biological contaminants, sediment	Most suitable for pre-treated municipal water in which biological contaminants are already low. Filter requires chlorinated water supply to prevent bacteriological decay.
TFC (thin film composite) well membrane	Same as above.	Dissolved solids (60 to 98%), heavy metals, asbestos, radioactive particles, some bacteria, limited amount of biological contaminants	Dissolved gases, sediment	Cannot be used with chlorinated water supply unless prefiltered with carbon.
Sterilization				
Ultraviolet (UV) purification	UV radiation penetrates membrane of microbe and inactivates it.	Biological contaminants	Dissolved gases, sediment, radiologicals (note that protozoan cysts such as *Giardia* and *Cryptosporidium* may not be completely eliminated if there is any shadowing effect caused by hardness or sediment)	Does not provide residual disinfection. Sediment, hardness, minerals, iron, manganese, or turbidity will make system ineffective because a shadowing effect shields bacteria from UV.
Oxidation with ozone, hydrogen peroxide, chlorine, or injected air	Oxidation can change the valence state of water contaminants so that they can be physically filtered.	Clarifies, deodorizes, and precipitates metals; oxidizes and eliminates bacteria, viruses and organic matter	VOCs, pesticides, chlorine; does not remove anything from water	Use of chlorine as oxidizing agent not recommended from ecological and health standpoints. Post-system carbon filtration is recommended.

Chart 11.1: Water Filtration Methods (cont'd.)

Type of system	How it works	What is eliminated	What is not eliminated	Comments
Others				
KDF (kinetic degradation fluxation)	Zinc/copper alloy causes chemical transformation of contaminants as they pass through KDF, which disrupts metabolic function of bacteria.	Controls bacterial growth; removes some heavy metals, chlorine, and biological contaminants	Trihalomethanes, bacteria, radiologicals	Very effective when used as prefilter, followed by carbon filter and then reverse osmosis. Does not work well in all pH conditions; requires 150 ppm of total dissolved solids (TDS) to be effective. Is bacteriostatic but not a bactericide. Suitable for water with very low bacteriological count. Works best on hot water. Testing after installation is advised.
Shower-head filters	Small filter/shower head combination that threads into existing plumbing.	Chlorine. Some filters may have other properties. Verify contaminant removal potential at www.nsf.org.	Radiologicals, pesticides, gasoline, bacteria. Do not remove trihalomethanes, pesticides, or VOCs because of lack of contact time. Not considered effective treatment for most biological contaminants or chemical contaminants of health concern.	Very inexpensive and often very limited in scope. Do not require plumber to install. See May 2007 *Consumer Reports* for reviews of shower head, pitcher, carafe, and other inline filters.
Distillation	Water is turned to vapor, condensed, and then collected.	Dissolved solids, microorganisms, nitrates, heavy metals, sediment, radioactive particulate matter	VOCs, dissolved gases, including chlorine	Effective when used with carbon postfilter. High maintenance, low production, and high energy consumption. Flat taste. Metal-bodied distillers may add aluminum or other heavy metals to water.
Sediment filters	Can be a filter medium in cartridge or tank applications. Can be a settling tank where water is siphoned off the top after particulates sink.	Particulate matter, sand, dirt	Remove only particulate matter; strictly a physical process	Most often used as prefilter for other systems. Backflushing models use additional water for self-cleaning.

Chart 11.1: Water Filtration Methods (cont'd.)

Type of system	How it works	What is eliminated	What is not eliminated	Comments
Aeration	Water is run over a series of plates, where it is depressurized and blown with a fan so that gases and odors can escape. It is then repressurized.	Radon, odors, dissolved gases	Bacteria, solids, heavy metals, and dissolved radiologicals	Aeration is the EPA-preferred method for radon removal.
Centralized Water Purification				
Ultrafiltration	Water pressure pushes water molecules toward the hollow center of fiber membrane tubes. Large particles and microorganisms are trapped within the fiber and then flushed out during automatic backwashing.	Removal of chlorine by activated carbon and physical blocking of bacteria, parasites, and viruses greater than 0.02 microns	Heavy metals, radioactive particles, arsenic, and nitrates	Ultrafiltration is touted as eliminating the need for bottled water, but it is far less effective for contaminant removal than RO. Ultrafiltration systems do not soften water and do require water backwashing.

Authors' note: This table has been created by Steven Wiman of Good Water Company for this edition of *Prescriptions for a Healthy House.*

Residential Equipment

Much has been written about the energy efficiency of appliances. Since appliances account for as much as 30 percent of household energy usage, choosing wisely can greatly reduce energy consumption. Because many sources of information are available on appliance energy values, we have limited discussion in this book to health issues related to appliance selection. (See the end of this chapter for books about reducing appliance energy consumption.)

Appliances and Magnetic Fields

All motorized equipment found in homes will generate magnetic fields when in operation. Some epidemiological studies have linked exposure to these magnetic fields with increased incidence of cancer, Alzheimer's disease, and miscarriage. Magnetic fields from properly wired appliances drop off very quickly in an exponential relationship to your distance from them. These fields can be easily measured with a small handheld instrument called a gaussmeter, which allows the user to determine the safe distance from an appliance.

The US government has not yet set reasonable standards for safe exposure levels, nor has it taken a strong position regarding the health effects of magnetic fields. However, various government documents and public utility disclosures state that if you are concerned, you can practice "prudent avoidance" of these fields. Recommended safe exposure limits set by various experts have ranged from 0.5 milligauss to 1,000 milligauss. The Swedish National Energy Administration has recommended that children should not be subjected to magnetic field levels greater than 3 milligauss. The

Bau-Biologie Institute in Germany considers readings above 0.2 milligauss to be a deviation from naturally occurring conditions.

In Division 16 we include information and recommended specifications for designing and building a home in which magnetic fields transmitted by household wiring do not surpass 0.5 milligauss. You can follow the simple guidelines below to limit your exposure to magnetic fields from appliances:

- Design your home so that major appliances are located at a safe distance from sitting and sleeping areas. In doing so, remember that magnetic fields travel with ease through walls made of common building materials, and that areas located out of sight behind an appliance are also exposed. For example, placing a refrigerator back-to-back with a bed, even though separated by a wall, will continually expose a person in that bed to an elevated magnetic field.
- Duration and strength of exposure are both factors. A low-level exposure for long periods of time may be more harmful than a brief, high-level exposure. For this reason, pay particular attention to fields that may be generated around sleeping areas.
- We suggest that you buy and learn to use a gaussmeter. With this device, you can measure the fields emanating from appliances. For more information on choosing and operating a gaussmeter, see Division 16.
- Check your home and appliances regularly with the gaussmeter to determine whether field levels have increased. Elevated fields can sometimes indicate that an appliance has developed dangerous ground faults or is about to fail. Early detection of these fields will also decrease the risk of fire or electrocution.

Appliances and Electric Fields

Whereas magnetic fields exist only when appliances are being used, electric fields are present as long as the appliance is plugged in. Unfortunately, few appliances are manufactured in a manner that results in low electric fields. It is possible to rewire appliances so that they operate with reduced electric fields, but this requires the services of an electrician familiar with electric field shielding. Electric fields from appliances are relatively easy to control by following these suggestions:

- Keep appliances unplugged when they are not in use, especially in the bedroom. Not only will this eliminate the electric field but it will also reduce the risk of fire. Although this practice is much more common in Europe, the American Association of Home Appliances and Underwriters Laboratories has also issued a warning stating that small appliances should be unplugged as a fire prevention measure.
- Avoid using extension cords around beds or areas where your family spends a lot of time. They tend to emit high electric fields when they are plugged in.
- Use a battery-operated or wind-up clock next to the bed.
- Wire your bedroom so that the circuitry can be conveniently shut off when you go to sleep, thus eliminating the electric fields. Refer to Division 16 for details.

Appliance Selection

Microwave Ovens

Microwave ovens emit high electromagnetic fields (EMFs). These ovens are designed to heat food by creating enough microwave energy to vibrate molecules in the food until heat is produced. When microwave ovens are in use, magnetic fields extend out as far as 12 feet. The actual microwaves produced during operation are supposed to be contained in the oven by internal shielding, but leaks can occur. If you decide to use a microwave oven, the following suggestions will make using it safer:

- Maintain a distance of four to 12 feet from the microwave oven while it is in use. This is especially important for children, who might enjoy watching the food as it is cooking.
- Have your appliance professionally checked for microwave leakage on an annual basis. You can check it yourself on a more frequent basis with a less precise do-it-yourself tester. (One is available through **Professional Equipment**, a mail order catalog.) Any detected leakage is unacceptable. Microwave leakage standards in the US are much less stringent than in some parts of Europe. Unfortunately, differences in the power supply prevent the use of European microwave ovens in North America.
- Do not use a microwave that appears to be malfunctioning. Signs of this would include sparks flying, funny noises, fires, or the unit turning on or cycling when the door is open. If any of these occur, evacuate the area immediately. Do not take time to try to unplug the unit. Instead, shut off the circuit breaker to the microwave. If you do not know which one it is, shut them all off. Only then is it safe to return to the room to unplug the microwave oven.
- The shielding on a microwave is delicate. A very small amount of damage can cause a complete shielding failure. Even a paper towel stuck in the door is enough to cause the microwave shielding to fail.
- Do not microwave food in plastic containers. Chemicals from the plastic can leach into the food. Some of these chemicals are known to disrupt the endocrine system.

Trash Compactors

Trash compactors are now commonplace in new homes. They can be convenient, but they can also be difficult to clean. When choosing a trash compactor, examine it carefully to be sure you will be able to reach into it easily for cleaning. Verify that accidental liquid spills inside the unit will be contained and not run under or behind the unit. You may want to have the trash compactor installed in such a way that it can be easily removed for cleaning.

Some trash compactors come with a deodorizer chamber. With the exceptions of baking soda and zeolyte, most deodorizers contain phenols, formaldehyde, or paradichlorobenzene, all of which should be avoided.

Refrigerators and Freezers

There are many styles of refrigeration units available. Self-defrosting models have a drip pan located somewhere under the unit. Some units have drip pans located in the back or mounted internally, where they are inaccessible. When purchasing a unit, make sure the drip pan is easily accessible from the front and has adequate clearance underneath for easy cleaning. The pan should be cleaned monthly to prevent odors or the growth of microorganisms. It is also important to keep the cooling coils clean of dust. Not only will this improve your air quality but it also will save energy because the unit will not have to work as hard to stay cold.

Cook Tops, Ovens, and Ranges

All electric cook tops, ovens, and ranges

produce elevated magnetic fields. Surprisingly, it is frequently the built-in electric clock that is the largest source, regardless of whether the equipment is gas or electric. Use a gaussmeter to determine the distance of the field.

The act of cooking generates significant amounts of indoor air pollution through vapors and airborne particulate matter such as grease. In addition, food particles left on burners are incinerated and release combustion byproducts.

Gas-fueled appliances are a significant source of indoor air pollution as they can release carbon monoxide, carbon dioxide, nitrogen dioxide, nitrous oxides, and aldehydes into the air. In *Why Your House May Endanger Your Health,* Alfred Zamm describes how gas kitchen ranges have been the hidden culprit in many cases of "housewives' malaise." According to Zamm, "A gas oven operating at 350°F for one hour, because of the inevitable incomplete combustion, can cause kitchen air pollution, even with an exhaust fan in operation, comparable to a heavy Los Angeles smog. Without the fan, levels of carbon monoxide and nitrogen dioxide can zoom to three or more times that."[4]

For chemically sensitive individuals, any combustion appliance may be undesirable and we recommend choosing electric over gas for a range/oven. Many cooks, however, prefer to cook with gas because it allows for better timing and temperature control. If you choose a gas range, the following measures will help reduce the amount of pollution:

- Have flames adjusted to burn correctly. They should burn blue. A yellow flame indicates incomplete combustion and the subsequent production of carbon monoxide.
- Choose an appliance with electronic ignition instead of a pilot light. Any model built in the US after 1991 will be equipped with electronic ignition.
- Follow the guidelines for proper ventilation discussed below.

If your preference is to cook with gas, consider purchasing a gas-fired cook top with an electric oven, since it is not necessary or even desirable from a chef's standpoint for the oven to be a combustion appliance.

Various smooth cook top surfaces are available, including magnetic induction and halogen units. Because they are much easier to clean than coiled elements, they produce less pollution from the burning of trapped food particles. These units should be tested with a gaussmeter to determine the extent of their magnetic fields while in operation.

Oven cleaning is another source of pollution generated in the kitchen. Continuous-cleaning ovens contain wall coatings that continuously outgas noxious fumes. Self-cleaning ovens produce polynuclear aromatic hydrocarbons, which are a source of air pollution. Most brand-name oven cleaners are toxic. The safest way to clean an oven is with baking soda and elbow grease. If baking soda is poured over the spill shortly after it occurs, the spill can be easily cleaned up after the oven has cooled.

Kitchen Ventilation

Because the kitchen generates significant indoor pollution and moisture, the ventilation of this room should be given special consideration above and beyond general home ventilation. Range hoods must be vented to the outside. There are models available that simply circulate the air through a carbon filter and

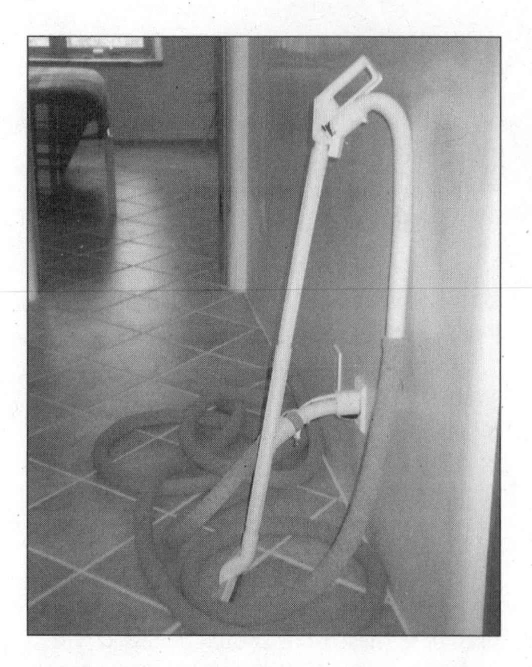

A central vacuum system is convenient and dust free. Photo: Paula Baker-Laporte.

back into the room. These do not remove cooking pollution sufficiently, but unfortunately many kitchens come equipped with them because they are inexpensive and do not require a roof penetration.

We recommend the largest range hood available, with variable speed control so that you can adjust speed according to your requirements. Some models come equipped with remote fans, which are quieter. When ventilation fans are in operation, especially at higher speeds, it is important that make-up air be supplied. If a home is not equipped with a whole-house supply system, you should open a window to supply make-up air. If a clean source of air intake is not provided by design, the exhausting of air can create enough negative pressure that air will then be sucked into the house through the path of least resistance. This path could be through a chimney flue for a furnace or water heater, causing dangerous backdrafting of air many times more polluted than that being replaced.

Laundry Appliances

Washers and dryers with porcelain-on-steel or stainless steel interiors are preferable to those with plastic interiors. Although gas dryers are more energy efficient than electric dryers, they cause the same pollution problems as gas ranges. By planning a laundry room with easy access to a drying yard, you can take advantage of the most energy efficient of all dryers: the sun.

Dryers should be vented directly to the outdoors. Some heat recovery devices are available that recirculate the hot air from the dryer back into the house. We do not recommend these because they do not sufficiently filter fine particles and, if a gas dryer is being used, combustion gases can be released into the indoor air instead of being vented outdoors.

Vacuum Cleaners

Conventional portable vacuum cleaners suck air through a filter bag and then pump the "cleaned" air back into the room. The air that is returned is only as clean as the filtering mechanism is efficient. In fact, conventional vacuuming can stir up dust and pollen to such an extent that the ambient air is more polluted with small particulate matter than it was before the cleaning. Several brands of HEPA vacuums are available and are far superior to conventional vacuum cleaners. Their "high-efficiency particulate air" filter effectively traps microscopic particulate matter. Water-filter vacuums were popular before the availability of HEPA vacuums. They can become a reservoir for mold and bacteria unless thoroughly dried after each use.

If you are building a new home, you have the opportunity to install a central vacuum system. When the motor and dirt receptacles are located remotely in a basement, garage, or utility room, central vacuums avoid the pollution problems associated with most portable models. Although more expensive than conventional portables, central vacuums cost only slightly more than a good HEPA or water-filter model. They are convenient and easy to operate. The hose is simply plugged into a wall receptacle and there is no machinery to lug around. We recommend central vacuums that exhaust air directly to the outdoors as this will prevent any small particles missed by the collection bag from being exhausted back into the home.

Further Reading and Services

American Institute of Architecture, Denver Chapter, and Architects/Designers/Planners for Social Responsibility. *Sustainable Design Resource Guide*. AIA/ADPSR, 2005. See aiasdrg.org. Information about energy efficiency and appliances.

A'o, Lono Kahuna Kapua. *Don't Drink the Water: The Essential Guide to Our Contaminated Drinking Water and What You Can Do About It.* Kali Press, 1998.

Bower, Lynn Marie. *The Healthy Household.* Healthy House Institute, 1995. Has a useful section on household cleansers.

Conacher, Duff. *Troubled Waters on Tap: Organic Chemicals in Public Drinking Water Systems and the Failure of Regulation.* Center for Study of Responsive Law, 1988.

EPA Safe Drinking Water Hotline, 800-426-4791, epa.gov/safewater.

Goldbeck, David. *The Smart Kitchen: How to Design a Comfortable, Safe, Energy-Efficient, and Environment-Friendly Workspace.* Ceres Press, 1994.

The Good Water Company, Stephen Wiman, 2778 Agua Fria, Bldg. C, Ste. B, Santa Fe, NM 87501, 800-471-9036, 505-471-9036, goodwaterglobal .com. Water filtration and consultation.

Hague Quality Water International, 4343 South Hamilton Road, Groveport, OH 43125, 614-836-2115. Excellent whole-house water purification system.

Ingram, Colin. *The Drinking Water Book: A Complete Guide to Safe Drinking Water.* Ten Speed Press, 1991. A guide for safe drinking water.

National Testing Laboratories, Inc., 6555 Wilson Mills Road, Cleveland, OH 44143, 800-458-3330, watercheck.com. Comprehensive water testing.

Ozark Water Service and Air Services, 114 Spring Street, Sulphur Springs, AR 72768, 800-835-8908, ozarkwaterandair.org. For air and water testing and consultation regarding toxic gases, molds, asbestos, volatile organic compounds (VOCs), pesticides, gas leaks, EMFs, and radon.

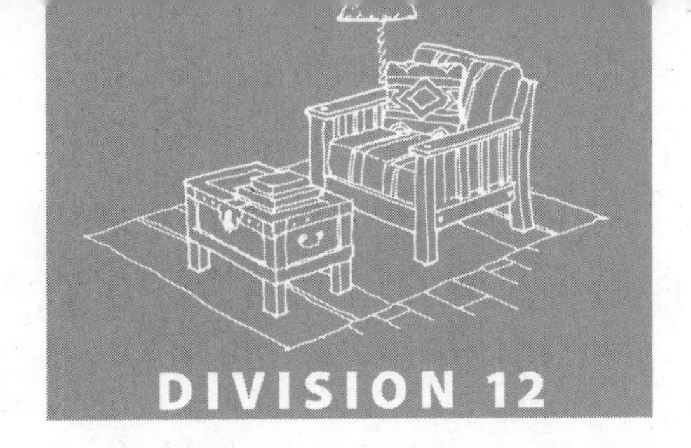

Furnishings

Residential furniture is rarely included in the construction contract. The owner will typically select the furniture and have it installed on her or his own or with the guidance of an architect or interior designer. Nevertheless, we are including some guidelines and resources for the selection of healthful furniture because new furnishings can have a major impact on indoor air quality.

Most standard furniture is built like most standard housing. It is mass-produced with little or no thought about the health of the buyer. For those of you who have gone to great effort to create a healthy home, shopping wisely for healthy furnishings is the next logical step. Once again you will find yourself in the role of a pioneer. Most furniture salespeople will not understand what you mean when you speak of healthy furniture. Yet formaldehyde and other chemical levels can soar when new furnishings are brought into the home. The furniture can continue to pollute the environment throughout its life.

As with the production of building materials, there are many broader environmental concerns pertaining to the manufacture of furniture. These include the use of endangered wood species, toxic waste produced at the manufacturing facility, factory workers' exposure to hazardous chemicals, wasteful packaging, and the exploitation of exporting countries. These factors are discussed in depth in other publications. We will concentrate on health concerns for the homeowner.

Wood Furniture

Most newly constructed wood furniture is actually veneered wood attached to a core of particleboard or plywood. These manufactured sheet goods are often bound with urea-formaldehyde glues, which will outgas for many years. Even so-called solid wood pieces may contain hidden plywood or particleboard components in order to save on production costs. When selecting wood furnishings, keep the following recommendations in mind:

- Purchase solid wood furniture that does

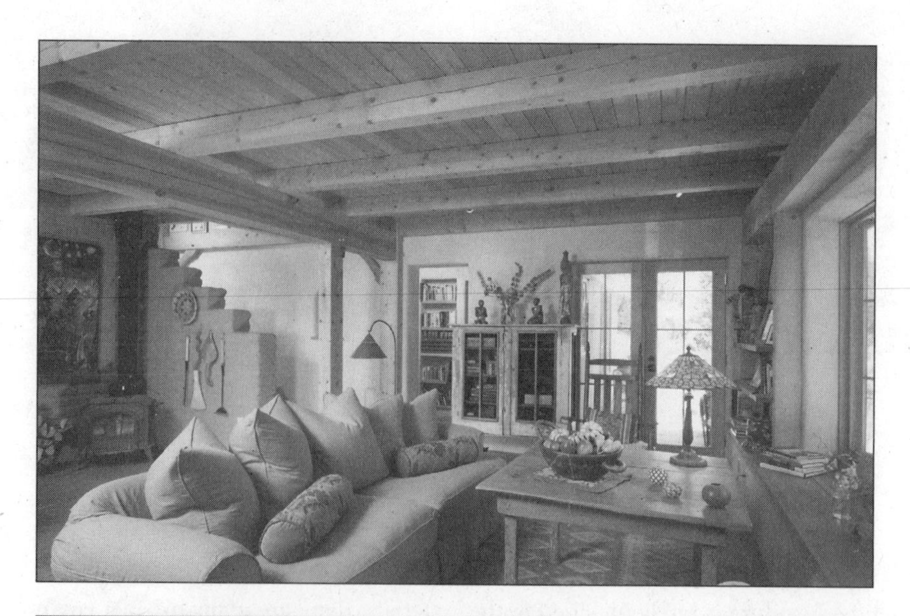

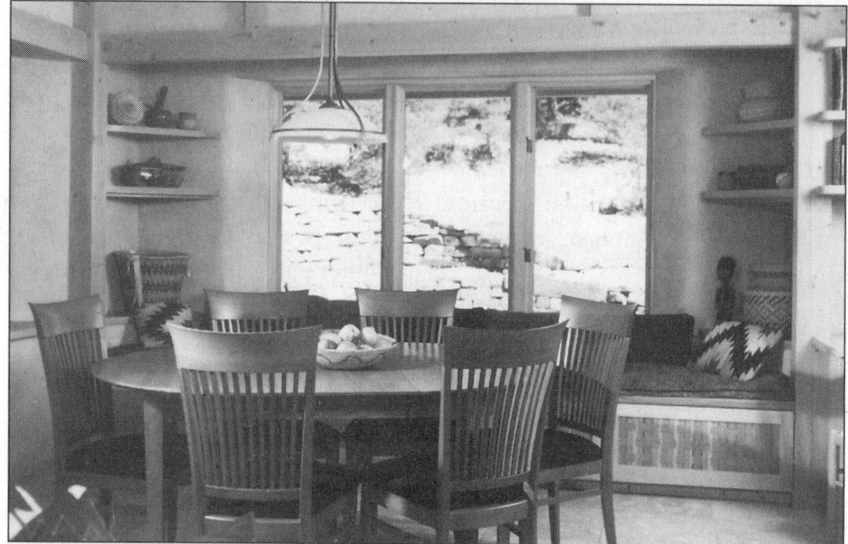

Above: Interior of Daryl Stanton Residence features solid wood antique furniture, custom made organic cotton and wool upholstered furniture and area rugs. Kitchen has solid wood cabinets and open shelving. Architect: Baker-Laporte Associates; Builder: Econest Building Co. Photo: David Hoptman.

Below: Interior of Baker-Laporte Residence features solid wood furniture — formaldehyde free built-in window seat and custom made cotton uphostery with organic cotton stuffing. Photo: Lisl Dennis.

not make use of veneers or sheetgoods. Hardwoods are preferable because they emit fewer terpenes than softer woods. Numerous farmed hardwoods are available. Old-growth forest need not be destroyed by your furniture selection. Although the initial purchase price for solid wood furniture may be higher, you will be investing in heirloom quality.

- If veneered wood is all your budget will allow, consider sealing all surfaces and edges with one of the low-VOC vapor-barrier sealants listed in Division 9. In addition, consider materials such as wrought iron and glass for tables and wicker or rattan for seating. Examine cane furniture prior to purchase to make sure it is free of mildew and mold.
- Furniture imported from tropical countries is often sprayed with pesticides while in transit. Furniture imported from Europe will meet E1 emissions standards and is often constructed with low-emissions sheetgoods. Look for furniture that meets GreenGuard emissions standards, which are more stringent. This furniture must achieve formaldehyde emission rates of less than 0.05 part per million. Chemically sensitive individuals should test for individual tolerance to these amounts of formaldehyde.

Following are sources for solid wood or low-emissions furniture:

- **Casa Natura**: Solid wood furniture
- **Ikea**: Solid wood and veneered wood furnishings sourced from sustainably managed forestry operations and meeting E1 emissions standards
- **Pacific Rim**: Handcrafted, solid western maple furniture made from wood grown in managed forests in Washington and Oregon
- **Pottery Barn**: Solid wood furniture
- **Smith and Hawken**: A variety of sustainably harvested teak and cedar solid wood furniture
- **Eco-terric**: Green and healthy furnishings for the home
- **H3 Finishes** for wood furnishings

Durability, not health, is the criterion used by manufacturers when choosing finishes for wood furniture. The majority of commercial wood sealers are solvent-based and will outgas harmful chemicals. We offer the following suggestions:

- Look for furniture with low-VOC, water-based natural oil or wax finishes.
- Buy unfinished furniture and finish with low-VOC finishes.
- If you purchase furniture with a standard finish, air it out before placing it in your living space.

Upholstery

Most commercially available upholstered furniture is stuffed with synthetic foam or latex. Many foams will initially have a strong odor. They will break down over time and emit fine particles of chemical dust into the air. Polyurethane foams are extremely hazardous when burned. Furniture stuffing can be made with natural ingredients such as wool, natural latex, down, kapok, and organic cotton batting. Although these alternatives are not widely available in readymade form, you may find an upholsterer in your vicinity who is willing to work with you. A hardwood frame made for a futon, or solid hardwood benches, can be turned into healthy couches with the addition of custom-made pillows. Down and kapok stuffings can be allergens for some people.

Upholstery textiles are often synthetic and treated with toxic chemicals to improve stain resistance. Look for natural, untreated upholstery fabrics such as organic cotton, wool, or silk. **AFM Safe-Choice Lock Out** can be used on some fabrics to help repel dirt and stains. Materials must be tested for shrink resistance and color fastness prior to application.

Some sources for all-natural upholstered furniture are:

- **Cisco Brothers**: FSC certified furniture with water-based glues and environmentally friendly manufacturing processes
- **Eco-terric**: Green and healthy furnishings for the home, healthy-home consultation, and interior design
- **Furnature**: Manufacturer of natural, organic furniture line, mattresses, and bedding for people with multiple chemical sensitivities

Window Dressings

Most window dressings are made of synthetic fabrics treated with chemicals to make them wrinkle resistant. The recommended

Developing an Ecologically Sound Upholstered Furniture Line

ROWENA FINEGAN

While I was studying to become a certified Bau-Biologist, I was captivated by Bau- Biologie's philosophy. After much soul searching, I realized I wanted to incorporate its principles into the world of interior design, which had been my business for fifteen years.

To create healthy homes, I needed to be able to offer my clients healthy furniture, and at the time there was virtually nothing available. So in the fall of 2003 I approached Cisco Pinedo, owner of Cisco Brothers Corporation, a furniture manufacturer in Los Angeles, with the idea of producing a totally clean and healthy line of furniture. He readily agreed and we embarked on the lengthy journey of finding materials that would pass our stringent standards, based on the principles of Bau-Biologie. I would do the research and present options for Cisco to make the final choices.

Cisco was already using sustainably harvested alder wood produced specially for the furniture industry, so wood for the frames was not a problem. He has since made the change to using Forest Stewardship Council (FSC) certified wood for his entire line. All the glues and finishes are toxin-free, which means they do not leave irritating chemical residues in the air after use and they help reduce the toxic soup that results from chemical-laden finishes mixing together in today's tight houses. Only stainless steel screws are used in the construction of the frame and the legs are constructed from reclaimed wood, including teak harvested from rescued heirloom homes in Myanmar.

Chemical-free pure latex rubber was chosen as the main body of the upholstery for its superior qualities. It is flexible yet stable, lasting longer than petrochemical-based materials. It is absor-

dry-cleaning process further contributes to the chemical load. Natural fabrics can also be problematic on windows because ultraviolet light breaks down the fabric, creating dust and the need for frequent replacement. **Homespun Fabrics and Draperies** offers draperies of nontoxic 100 percent cotton fabrics.

Naturally finished wood shutters, louvers, metallic venetian blinds, or bamboo roll-downs can be attractive solutions that avoid the problems associated with fabric window dressings. **Pella Corporation** produces a line of windows with retractable shades sandwiched between double windowpanes. New on the market, Eagle Window and Door Company offers the **Eagle System 3** tilt-and-raise blind system. Blinds are sandwiched between insulating glass for dust-free and odorless

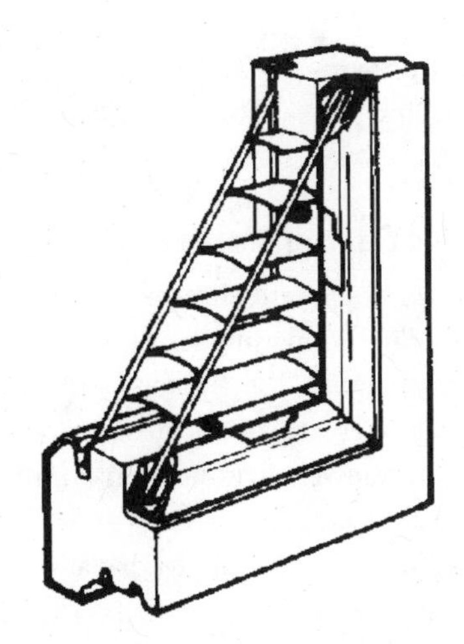

Cutaway view of narrow slat blinds between window panes. Credit: Pella Corporation.

bent and resilient, contributing to excellent heat and moisture regulation, and contains no harmful chemicals. Surprisingly, many people are not aware that latex is a natural product of the Para rubber tree. Its extraction does no harm to the trees, thus making it a sustainable material. And of course the latex used in our line is harvested from environmentally friendly rainforest trees.

Jute webbing eliminates the need for metal springs and avoids the health problems that may result from electromagnetic fields. Jute cording is used in place of polyester or cotton piping cord. The wool batting used to wrap the latex comes from regions where the soil is continually turned, pesticides and other chemicals are forbidden, and sheep are still herded using guardian dogs. Sheep-dip pesticides are consistently linked to nerve damage in farm workers, and low-dose exposure is believed to aggravate anxiety and depression. There is also a concern that antibiotics used on sheep may leach into groundwater and could compromise the effectiveness of antibiotics for humans.

All our fabrics are laundered in chemical-free vegetable-based laundry detergent and are either certified organic or produced using chemical-free base cloth and vegetable or low- impact dyes. Each furniture piece is available either upholstered or with washable slipcovers. We recommend the use of slipcovers as another way to keep our homes healthy.

After two and a half years of collaboration, Cisco Brothers launched a line of healthy and sustainable furniture "for people who live responsibly and who are committed to protecting our planet." This line is the first to combine cutting-edge

window dressing in four blind colors and six shade styles.

Shower Curtains and Liners

New PVC liners and shower curtains have a strong odor from outgassing toxins. Many shower curtains are treated with harmful chemicals to create mildew resistance. Cotton duck cloth shower curtains are naturally water repellent, wrinkle resistant, and attractive but they take a long time to dry and must be treated to resist mildew growth. They can be machine washed and dried. They are available through several mail order companies including **Gaiam** and **Heart of Vermont**. Natural hemp curtains are now available through **Real Goods**. A glass shower enclosure, although more expensive to install, will be a permanent, low-maintenance, and healthy solution.

Beds and Bedding

The most important furniture decision with regard to health is the choice of beds and bedding. We spend approximately a third of our lives in bed. Infants and children spend even more time there. While we sleep, our noses are in close contact with our bedding.

Standard mattresses are made of synthetic fabrics and padding and treated with petrochemical fire retardants. A bed that promotes health should have many of the same characteristics as a home that promotes health. The bed should be:

- nontoxic

design and green and healthy practices. This was a natural progression for Cisco Brothers, a company that has always been socially responsible, providing employment through apprenticeship programs to underdeveloped communities in South Los Angeles since the early 1990s.

Simultaneously, I set about trying to find suitable fabrics produced without the chemicals used in standard agriculture. Cotton is the world's most important fiber crop and one of its most important cash crops. It is also one of the most intensively sprayed field crops. In the United States, according to the US Department of Agriculture, more than 53 million pounds of pesticides and 1.6 billion pounds of synthetic fertilizers were applied to cotton fields in 1996. In California, cotton production ranks second for the total amount of pesticides used.

Organic farmers practice soil building with cover crops and composting, crop rotation, and safe and effective pest and disease control. Weed management means hoeing by hand, and instead of using defoliants organic farmers rely on a hard freeze to defoliate the cotton.

Eco-terric's exclusive collection of organic Kalamkari fabrics comes from a small fair-trade village operation in the southwest of India. This is an ongoing endeavor in conjunction with the artisans, and features organic cotton dyed with 100 percent natural dyes. All solids are hand-woven, and all prints are block-printed by hand. The natural beauty of these fabrics, combined with the timeless art and craftsmanship of the Kalamkari tradition, has made this collection the perfect complement to our mission of bringing natural beauty with color to the home.

- able to absorb and dispel moisture without supporting mold or mildew growth
- easy to clean and sanitize
- nonconductive of electricity (free of metal)
- highly insulative

The following futon bedding system fulfills these characteristics. The mattress is made of layers. One or more 1- to 4-inch-thick untreated organic cotton futons are topped with a 1- to 3-inch wool futon. The layers rest on a slatted frame raised above the floor to a comfortable seating height. The cotton futon provides firm back support, while the wool futon adds resilience. Varying the thickness and the number of layers will accommodate different firmness preferences.

To properly maintain a futon, it should be aired weekly in sunlight to sanitize it and then fluffed and replaced in a rotated position so it will wear evenly. A bed made of thin futons has an advantage over a single thicker mattress because the layers can be easily lifted and carried. It is important that air be allowed to circulate under the futon to facilitate evaporation of moisture, thereby preventing mold or mildew growth. A slatted platform will hold the futon firmly in place and permit air circulation around it.

Since the first edition of this book was published, many organic, metal-free mattress options have become available. These mattresses often are made of a combination of natural latex, wool, and organic cotton. This combination system conforms to the body shape and comes in a variety of firmnesses offering

I have been saddened on many occasions by stories of cotton farmers in India whose lives are made virtually unbearable by health problems resulting from constant contact with pesticides and by huge debts owed to the giant chemical companies. It was tremendously exciting to receive the news that Srinivas Pitchuka, owner of Bundar Kalamkari House and Syamala Arts and Crafts, with whom I have worked on our collection over these past years, was the recipient of an award for being the first company in his province to produce organic textiles.

I will continue to search for ways to produce furnishings and textiles that not only enrich our health and our homes but also care for our planet and those who work on it.

Rowena Finegan, BBEC, owner and founder of Eco-terric, strives to create beautiful, colorful, and environmentally friendly living spaces using healthy materials that are also socially responsible. After studying Bau-Biologie, Rowena was inspired to open her first Eco-terric store in Bozeman, Montana, in 2005. The newest location is at The Green Home Center on Polk Street in San Francisco. She collaborated with Cisco Brothers of Los Angeles to create the Inside Green furniture collection. She is also creating a line of organic textiles suitable for use in home decor. Rowena is a contributing writer to *Green*Light* magazine and has been featured in the *San Francisco Chronicle, Furniture Today* and *Helena Lifestyles*. See eco-terric.com.

CASE STUDY 12.1

The Bedroom as Sanctuary

When J. D. was 51 years old he consulted Dr. Elliott complaining of insomnia, asthma, and fatigue. It became clear from an exhaustive environmental history that J. D.'s symptoms began during the time he lived downwind from a location where aerial spraying was carried out seasonally for pest control. The repeated pesticide exposures apparently had left the patient feeling debilitated, without his usual zest for life, and with multiple medical problems, including allergies and sensitivities to a wide range of substances.

As part of his treatment program, J. D. was advised to reduce his exposure to toxins in his home. Since he was on a limited budget owing to his decreased earning capacity, he concentrated his cleanup efforts primarily on the bedroom, intending to focus on the rest of the house later. Given the time he spent in bed, J. D. realized that his bed should be the healthiest place in the house. He had recently purchased a mattress made of artificial foam. The synthetic fibers were emitting formaldehyde fumes as the mattress aged, probably contributing to the tight feeling in his chest upon waking. Fortunately, J. D. was able to sell his boxspring mattress and purchase an organic cotton futon, which he placed in an untreated wooden frame. His formaldehyde impregnated, wrinkle-free sheets and polyester bedding were exchanged for 100 percent organic cotton pillows, sheets, and blankets. Because of his concern about possible dust mites in the mattress, he used an organic cotton barrier cloth, woven so tightly that it was impenetrable to these insects. He laundered his bedding frequently in unscented, nonchlorinated detergent.

After J. D. recovered financially from replacing his bedding, his next project was to pull up the old carpet in the bedroom. Although the carpet was several years old and no longer outgassed toxic fumes, it was still a reservoir for dust, dirt, and microorganisms in spite of frequent vacuuming. J. D. wanted a floor that was attractive, health enhancing, and easy to clean. He chose to install presealed cork flooring because it resembled wood yet felt soft to the bare foot. On the floor he placed two untreated wool scatter rugs that could be easily taken up and cleaned.

The heating system in J. D.'s house is forced

good support and absorbency in a chemical-free environment. Untreated wool will repel dust mites, mold, and mildew. The mattress base should be a European-style wood-slat foundation, which allows the natural mattress to breathe and gives the same height and look as a conventional box spring. People with sensitivities to natural latex would need to test a mattress with latex before making a costly purchase as most mattresses are nonreturnable.

Permanent-press bedding is treated with formaldehyde that remains in the fabric after washing. Wool blankets may be mothproofed with harmful chemicals. Even pure cottons, unless organically grown, are heavily sprayed with pesticides. Healthy choices for bed sheets include organic natural fibers in cotton, cotton flannel, silk, hemp, or linen. Blankets, duvets, and comforters are available in organic down, silk, wool, or cotton.

air. The ductwork had been cleaned on a regular basis and electrostatic air filters were used on the return air ducts. Nevertheless, J. D. decided to close off the vents to his bedroom and use an electric ceramic heater. In addition, for the bedroom he bought a portable air filter that contained a HEPA filter for dust, mold spores, and pollen and a charcoal filter for fumes. The electric motor in the air filter was sealed to avoid toxic emissions and the unit itself was housed in a metal box.

J. D. did not know whether he was sensitive to electromagnetic fields. Since there would be little time or expense involved, he decided to take the necessary measures to reduce EMFs. He discarded his electric blanket, replaced his digital alarm clock with a battery operated one, moved his telephone into an adjacent room, and plugged in his television at the other side of the bedroom so that the screen was more than eight feet from his head.

The curtains on the windows were replaced with naturally finished wooden louvers, which were handsome and easy to clean. The room was cleaned once a week with a simple solution of vinegar and water. He was careful not to introduce toxic odors such as air fresheners, fabric softeners, colognes, and other artificially scented household products. When he occasionally needed to dry-clean his clothes, he left them on the back porch for a few days to air out the toxic chemicals found in dry-cleaning fluid. He was careful to remove his shoes before entering his sanctuary.

J. D.'s efforts paid off. He noted a definite improvement in his overall health. He was now able to get a full night of uninterrupted sleep and awake feeling refreshed, without the tight sensation in his chest. His energy increased and he was able to think more clearly. J. D. gradually regained his enthusiasm for life and has become a great proponent of the benefits of bedroom sanctuaries.

Discussion

We spend an average of eight hours a day in our bedrooms. Sleep is an important time for rest and recovery for all of us, whether we are sick or in the best of health. Designing our bedrooms with special care can create a healing environment where our bodies can mend from the daily barrage of exposures we all experience to varying degrees.

There is some confusion about the various terms used to describe cotton products. According to the Pesticide Action Network, conventionally grown cotton accounts for nearly 25 percent of the world's insecticide use. Organic cotton is grown without the use of synthetic pesticides or fertilizers and with farming practices that increase soil fertility. Natural or green cotton products use conventionally grown cotton but are free of harsh chemical bleaches, dyes, and sizing elements such as formaldehyde. "100% cotton" indicates that no other fibers have been used in the fabric but does not mean that the fabric is organic or naturally processed.

Sources for organic beds and bedding include:

- **Casa Natura**: Consultant and retail source for natural and organic beds, bedding, and linens

A Checklist for Choosing a Healthy Mattress

MARY CORDARO

Our homes are places for rest, retreat, and regeneration. If designed, built, and furnished simply and intelligently, they can help us restore our balance and our connection with nature. For most of us, however, creating a healthy home environment is unfamiliar — and sometimes overwhelming — territory and it is hard to know where to begin. Even if you can't make every detail in your home healthy, be sure your bedroom is as healthy as possible. It's the most important room in the house. And the most important piece of furniture in the house is your bed, where you spend a third of your life. We are most vulnerable when we sleep. Our bodies let down, shed metabolic waste, and regroup. A healthy, natural, and well-designed mattress can provide the right conditions for all the important processes of the body's natural electrical system, internal organs, and subconscious mind to work smoothly and without interference.

Our entire body is in close, direct contact with the materials we sleep in and on. And for eight hours a night we literally inhale, at very close range, whatever is in those materials. Most ordinary mattresses are made almost entirely of raw ingredients from the petroleum industry that are made into synthetic components such as viscoelastic and polyurethane foams, including Dacron, whose formulations may contain TDI (toluene discarnate, which OSHA labels as a hazardous material) and other toxic chemicals. To meet federal flammability regulations, they may also contain synthetic chemical fire retardants called organophosphates. Mattresses containing natural materials, such as conventional cotton and wool, may also contain pesticide residues. The older a mattress gets, the more toxic it becomes if it contains organophosphate flame-retardants and/or pesticide residues because, as the breakdown progresses with age, the rate of release of those toxins increases. They are released as chemical molecules that never completely outgas and that bind to house dust, which is then inhaled or ingested. Even mattresses marketed as "natural" may still contain toxic ingredients. Mattress layers can also be held together with glues and their fabrics may be treated with chemicals and harsh dyes. These materials are then wrapped in a quilted surface layer of synthetic fabric stuffed with polyester. These ordinary mattresses trap moisture, dirt, and dust, creating a dust-mite haven that can exacerbate allergies.

But there's good news. Thanks to a fast-growing sustainable lifestyle industry, you can now choose beautiful bedding, linens and textiles made from organic natural materials, and comfortable mattresses that are healthy for the back and for those who suffer from allergies. Here is a checklist of things to consider when buying your new bed.

First, narrow your search by limiting your choices to mattresses made only of high-quality natural components such as pesticide/chemical-free or organic wool, organic cotton, and natural latex, which comes from the rubber tree. Let's look at each of these components in more depth.

Mattresses and bed systems made with high-quality certified organic wool or locally produced pesticide- and chemical-free wool batting are my preference because both are healthy and highly fire retardant. Since mattresses made without chemical fire retardants still have to pass federally mandated burn tests, you can be sure your family is safe. Furthermore, wool cushions the joints and muscles, wicks and dries moisture away from the body, and is naturally dust mite resistant, so you don't need synthetic barrier covers. Since the average body loses about a pint of moisture vapor into the bed every night, it's important that the battings used in beds and bedding efficiently and effectively wick and dry to eliminate conditions favorable for mold and dust mites. Wool is also a temperature and humidity regulator, which means you'll sleep not only drier but also warmer in the winter and cooler in the summer, even in very humid climates. Except for rare individuals with severe wool allergies, even most people who can't wear wool clothing have no reaction to wool inside a mattress because it is chemical-free and encased under the mattress ticking.

Some plusher organic mattresses also contain organic cotton batting placed under the wool layer to keep out dust mites. Organic cotton batting is a much healthier choice for you and the environment than conventional cotton batting because standard cotton is farmed with high levels of pesticides and herbicides. Not only is standard cotton a toxic burden for the earth and for farm workers but pesticides residues also can remain in the cotton batting throughout the manufacturing process. Even if these residue levels are low, you don't want to spend eight hours a night with your face next to them.

Natural fabrics such as organic cotton sheeting and ticking are free of the chemicals used in conventional fabric manufacturing. Organic fabrics that are undyed, or dyed with natural and low-impact pigments, are free of the volatile organic compounds (VOCs) that outgas in low levels from conventional fabric finishing, synthetic dyes, and permanent fabric treatments. Natural fabric coverings also eliminate a subtle type of electromagnetic field called electrostatic charge. The result is a more healing bed, with natural surfaces that because of the absence of static don't attract as much dust as synthetic ones.

Natural latex is a comfortable and contouring alternative to synthetic memory foams and mattresses imbedded with metal coils. Natural latex mattresses avoid the chemical stew found in typical foam mattresses and need no coils, or innersprings, that might sag or protrude and can prematurely age your mattress. High-quality natural, sustainably produced latex does not sag over time, does not need metal springs to keep its shape, and can offer continuous support for as much as 20 years or longer, depending on the quality of the latex and an individual's changing support and comfort needs. Make sure that the mattress manufacturer uses only 100 percent natural latex and no synthetic rubber blends.

Second, when choosing your mattress it is important to note that mattresses with metal coils may pose other challenges for your body. Metal bedsprings (as well as metal bed frames) can act as antennas for human-made frequencies, especially those from FM radio, providing subtle, long-term exposures to a variety of low levels of electromagnetic fields (EMFs). Metal also becomes magnetized, which may interfere with our bodies' natural orientation to magnetic north.

Finally, pay special attention to the facility where the bed is made. To avoid cross-contamination from other types of materials, your organic bed should be made in a facility that produces

- **Coyuchi**: Organic cotton bedding
- **Eco-terric**: Green and healthy furnishings, beds and bedding, and accessories for the home
- **Gaiam**: Organic bedding and home accessories
- **Heart of Vermont**: Organic futons, mattresses, and bedding
- **Janice's**: Natural and organic bedding
- **Mary Cordaro Collection**: Natural, healthy beds and bedding
- **Natural Home**: Natural beds and bedding
- **Nirvana Safe Haven**: Organic and natural beds, bedding, futons, and home accessories for the health-minded and chemically sensitive

only organic beds and bedding, or at the very least isolates its organic facilities from areas where synthetics may be used and does not run any synthetic or conventional fiber or fabric through machines used for organic materials.

Ask if the factory does its own sewing, quilting, and garneting. (Garneting is a mechanical process whereby short fibers are combed into a specific orientation and formed into thin webs, which are then layered to create the batting used in a mattress.) If the manufacturer tends to outsource these and other steps in the manufacturing process, the chances greatly increase that your "organic mattress" has been cross-contaminated by synthetic materials in manufacturing plants that make both conventional and organic products.

Find out if the raw materials such as the cotton or wool used in your mattress are domestically produced. Transporting them from other countries in containers may add to the cost and will certainly increase the chance that the materials have been exposed to contamination from pesticide sprays and other synthetic materials. Long-distance transportation also greatly increases the product's environmental footprint.

Ask the manufacturer if its mattresses have passed the federal open flame test, certified by a third party, without the use of synthetic materials. Although wool is a very important component, it is not the only ingredient necessary for a mattress to meet federal flammability regulations. Natural wool, in the right weight and properly garneted, along with correct construction of organic and natural materials, will be an effective fire retardant provided there are no synthetic materials in the mattress.

If the mattress and bedding products are certified with an environmental label, make sure to inquire what that label actually certifies. Check that the certification process includes testing not only for VOCs but also SVOCs, or semi-volatile organic compounds, including pesticides, flame retardants, biocides (chemicals that kill bacteria and mold), and plasticizers.

There are many beds on the market today that claim to be made of natural materials and to offer significant health benefits. Because your health and the health of your family are so important, and because you have so many natural beds to choose from, be sure to do your homework and take this checklist with you when you shop for the right mattress.

Mary Cordaro is a certified Building Biology Practitioner. She is president and founder of H3Environmental, a healthy bedroom products company, and has been consulting/educating on the healthy home since 1989. Mary is the creator of The Mary Cordaro Collection, a luxury line of healthy, organic beds and bedding. See h3environmental.com.

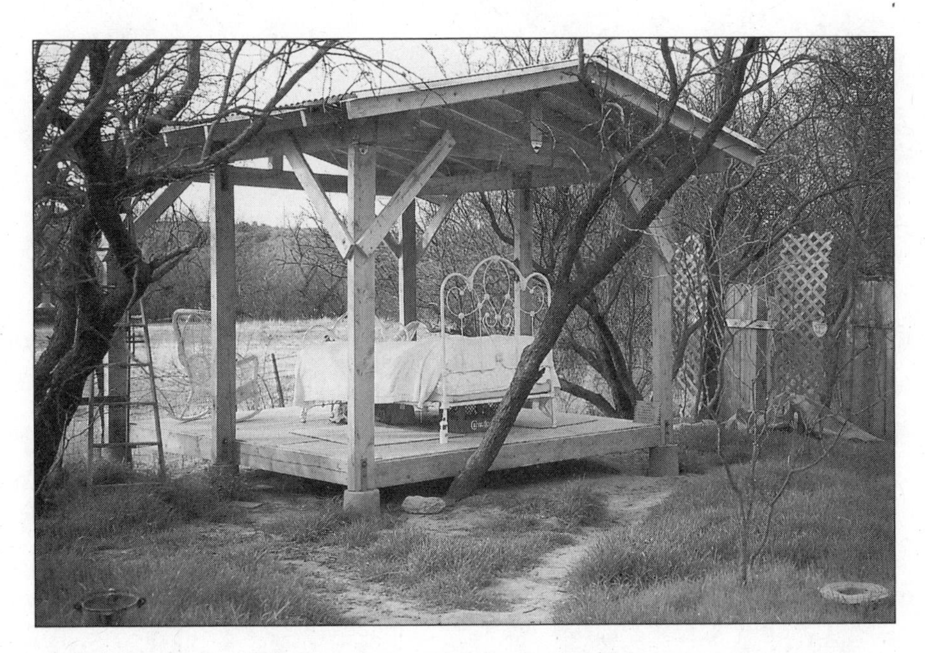

This bedroom, found in Arizona, provides its owner with an abundance of fresh air! Photo: Robert Laporte.

- **Sachi Organics**: Manufacturers of organic cotton beds and futons and retailers of organic bedding and linens
- **Shepherd's Dream**: Custom-made wool mattresses, solid wood bed frames, and organic linens
- **Sleeptek Oasis Collection**: Custom-made organic mattresses and bedding sets

Further Reading

Leclair, Kim and David Rousseau. *Environmental by Design*. Hartley and Marks, 1993. Overview of larger environmental concerns related to furniture manufacturing

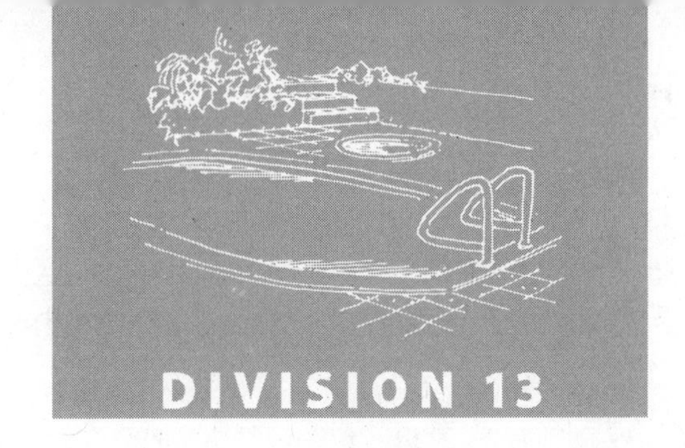

Special Construction

Swimming Pools and Hot Tubs

If you wish to include a swimming pool or hot tub inside your home, the two major health concerns to consider are water sterilization and humidity-related mold infestation. The standard disinfectants used to kill microbes and algae in swimming pools are chlorine or other halogenated compounds, which are easily absorbed through the swimmer's skin as well as inhaled into the lungs. There are several alternatives to chlorination. Ozonation is a popular method used in Europe for sterilizing water. Other methods include electrolysis, ultraviolet light, and filtration through charcoal and pesticide-free diatomaceous earth. Pools using these alternate methods need to be frequently monitored for the presence of bacteria. Occasionally a small amount of harsher chemicals may be required.

Nonchlorine-based systems for pool disinfection include:

- **AquaRite Saline Generator**: Uses common salt and converts it to free chlorine with none of the side effects of standard chlorination
- **ClearWater Tech, Inc.**: Ozone generator system for pool disinfection
- **DEL Industries**: Water ozonation for pools, wells, and spas
- **Real Goods**: Source of the Floatron, a solar-powered pool purifier combining solar electric power with mineral ionization and reducing chlorine usage up to 80 percent

Enclosing a large body of heated water within a living space will create a humid microclimate, which is an invitation to mold growth and can result in damage from condensation. Design measures can prevent mold growth and condensation damage. The following features should be integrated into the design:

- fitted covers that remain in place to prevent evaporation when the pool or hot tub is unoccupied

CASE STUDY 13.1

Asthma from a Chlorinated Swimming Pool

When B. W. was a five-year-old boy he came with his parents to consult with Dr. Elliott about his asthma. The most recent flare-up had occurred during a school field trip to the local swimming pool. Upon further questioning, a pattern emerged revealing a relationship between water and the triggering of the child's asthma. Dr. Elliott suspected that the chlorine in the water was acting as an irritant to his airways. She suggested that the family swim in a public pool that had switched to ozone for water purification. In that particular pool, chlorine was used as a supplement, but only in very small quantities. They were happy to note that their son could now swim comfortably with his friends without difficulty breathing. The family went on to purchase filters for their showerheads that effectively removed chlorine from their showers. They also removed all chlorinated cleaning products from their home. Now that there was one less triggering agent for the asthma, Dr. Elliott could more effectively focus on strengthening the boy's lungs.

Discussion

Chlorine is a poison used to kill bacteria in water. It is absorbed through the skin, inhaled into the lungs, and ingested. At room temperature, chlorine is a gas with a pungent smell. It is very reactive, combining readily with most elements to form compounds, many of which, such as chloroform, trihalomethanes, and organochlorines, are known to be carcinogenic. Symptoms commonly resulting from swimming in chlorinated water include runny nose, red eyes, cough, asthma, joint pains, swelling, nausea, urinary discomfort, rashes, and hives. We suggest that you use a less toxic disinfectant for your pool.

- adequate mechanical ventilation and dehumidification
- a watertight enclosure around the pool area that retards vapor diffusion to prevent water damage to the surrounding structure
- surface finishes that are impervious to water and easily cleaned
- a rigorous maintenance program to remove condensation and mold growth as soon as they appear

Because of the intensive upkeep required to maintain a pool or spa so that it does not negatively impact indoor air quality, we do not readily recommend including an enclosed body of water inside a healthy home. However, if an indoor pool is planned for the home, consider taking advantage of the large body of heated water as part of the design for a comprehensive climate control strategy. The water can act as a reservoir for solar heat storage and humidification.

Environmental Testing

It may be desirable to conduct diverse quality control tests or product analysis while selecting materials and throughout the construction process. This testing can help ensure that materials and installations are as specified. Planning in advance for many of these tests is recommended. Waiting until the last minute will result in costly construction delays since many of these procedures will require that you order test kits, hire specialists, or wait for laboratory results.

Materials Testing

In choosing healthy materials, you and your architect will base decisions on information supplied by the manufacturer, such as product literature and an MSDS, as well as on the appearance and smell of the products. While certain hazardous substances, such as lead, asbestos, mercury, and polychlorinated biphenyls (PCBs), are no longer a concern for products manufactured in North America, precautions may be required if you are using recycled or imported materials. Available tests are included in Chart 13.1. Materials tests you may want to consider are discussed below.

pH Testing for Concrete Slabs

Concrete must be properly cured to ensure its strength and durability. Improperly cured concrete may exhibit a strongly alkaline pH, which can cause adverse chemical reactions when certain adhesives and flooring materials come into contact with the concrete. The pH of cured concrete must be under 9 to be considered acceptable. A pH test is performed by dampening an area of concrete with distilled or deionized water. The dampened area is then tested with pH paper or with a special pH test pencil available from the **Sinak Corporation**. The color change that the paper or pencil mark indicates is the pH level.

Formaldehyde Testing

Although many manufacturers are now using less formaldehyde than they once were, it is still a common additive in many products. The cumulative effect of several products containing only moderate amounts of formaldehyde can cause severe health consequences. Our approach is to avoid this chemical whenever formaldehyde-free substitutes can be located.

A simple do-it-yourself spot test can be used to ensure that products containing formaldehyde are not used. A drop of test solution is placed on the material in question and allowed to stand for two minutes. If the drop changes from clear to purple, formaldehyde or other harmful aldehydes are present. The shade of purple can range from a faint pink to a dark plum, depending on the concentration of aldehydes. The test must be read at exactly two minutes because the drop will eventually turn purple even if no aldehydes are present. The solution leaves a purple stain on porous materials and should be used in a place where will not be visible.

Surface Sampling for Fungus

Materials damaged by mold growth should be rejected, but not all stains are from mold. Laboratory analysis will probably be required to determine if mold is a problem, but there are several do-it-yourself methods for collecting mold samples.

Bulk Sampling

Collect a small amount of the material in question in a doubled plastic bag and send it to the laboratory. A teaspoonful of the suspected material is probably enough.

Tape Sampling

Press a piece of clear cellophane tape onto the surface to be tested. The best place for sampling is at the edge between the stained area and the clean area. Then stick the tape to a plastic bag

Bau-Biology Standard SBM 2008: A Unique Indoor Environmental Assessment Tool

PETER SIERCK

The professional Bau-Biology Standard SBM 2008 provides a unique and comprehensive assessment and evaluation system consisting of over 30 indoor environmental parameters. The Standard uses an unorthodox approach because it is not based on single threshold limit values derived from medical dose responses. Instead, the Standard uses a gradient scale with four different levels based on the concentration levels normally encountered in nature or non-problem buildings. The evaluation criteria are determined by the deviations from this normal state and are expressed as categories of change. The categories are: normal environment, slight change, significant change, and severe change. The table below defines the four categories used in the Standard and provides an example for carbon dioxide (CO_2) levels.

Normal Environment	Slight Change	Significant Change	Severe Change
Reflects normal environmental conditions or common and inevitable background levels in our civilized environment	Slightly higher levels; following the precautionary principle, long-term mitigation is recommended, especially with sensitive or ill individuals	Likely to present an elevated risk; short-term mitigation is recommended	Call for immediate action and mitigation; in many cases international guidelines for occupational exposure limits may be reached or exceeded
CO_2 <500 ppm	CO_2 500-700 ppm	CO_2 700–1000 ppm	CO_2 >1000 ppm

The Bau-Biology Standard is based on the precautionary principle. It is derived from studies based on long-term exposure during the human regeneration phase (while sleeping) and was established over decades of experience. The reference values are designed for sleeping areas, not for commercial or industrial workplaces. All other standards in North America are based on the workplace and do not directly address health at home. The Bau-Biology Standard itself is divided into two sections: Evaluation Guidelines and Standard Testing Methodology. These are further differentiated into three groups of environmental parameters:

- Group A. Indoor Air Climate and Environmental Toxins
- Group B. Fungi, Bacteria, and Allergens
- Group C. Physical Fields and Radiation

A comprehensive assessment of potential biological environmental risk factors and their reduction to achievable levels are the basis of the Standard.

The Institute for Bau-Biology and Ecology (IBN) was founded in 1976 by Anton Schneider of Germany. The German word "Bau" means building, habitat, or shelter. "Biology" refers to the study of living things. The institute studies and addresses the impact buildings have on human health and promotes healthy, environmentally and ecologically friendly construction techniques.

The Standard was developed between 1987 and 1992 by the consulting firm of Baubiologie

Maes in conjunction with the IBN, environmental consultants, physicians, and scientists. The document was initially published in the German journal *Wohnung und Gesundheit* (Living Spaces and Health) in 1992. A ten-member Standard Committee reviews and revises the document periodically. The latest update was in 2003. In the meantime, the Standard has been internationally accepted as a comprehensive tool for independent indoor environmental assessments in Europe, Australia, and New Zealand and is available in the United States through the International Institute for Bau-Biologie & Ecology in Clearwater, Florida.

The three groups of environmental parameters and categories of change are outlined in a condensed version in the following tables. The Baubiology Evaluation Guidelines are proposed for sleeping areas and are not directly related to work areas.

Group A: Indoor Air Climate and Environmental Toxins

A	Parameter	Normal environment	Slight change	Significant change	Severe change
1	Carbon dioxide concentration in air (ppm)	600	600–1000	1000–1500	>1500
2	Relative humidity (%)	40–60	<40 / >60	<30 / >70	<20 / >80
3	Formaldehyde concentration in air (ppm)	0.02	0.02–0.05	0.05–0.1	>0.1
4	Total volatile organic compounds in air (µg/m³)	<100	100–300	300–1000	>1000
5	Total pesticides concentration in air (ng/m³)	<1	5–25	25–100	>100
6	PCP, lindane, permethrin in wood (mg/kg)	<1	1–10	10–100	>100
7	Dichlofluanid, chlorpyrifos in dust (mg/kg)	<0.5	0.5–2	2–10	>10
8	PCBs, chlorinated fire retardants in dust (mg/kg)	<0.5	0.5–2	2–10	>10
9	Polyaromatic hydrocarbons in dust (mg/kg)	<0.5	0.5–2	2–20	>20
10	Plasticizer in dust (mg/kg)	<100	100–250	250–1000	>1000
11	Small air ions (per cm³)	>500	200–500	100–200	<100
12	Electrostatic charge in air (V/m)	<100	100–500	500–2,000	>2,000

Group B: Fungi, Bacteria, and Allergens

B	Mold counts (spore counts or colony forming units)	I. Mold counts should be less or similar when compared to surrounding outdoor environments or non-problem buildings.
		II. Mold types in the indoor air should be similar to those present in the outside air.
		III. Particular toxic species such as *Aspergillus* or *Stachybotrys,* yeast-like fungi such as *Candida* or *Cryptococcus,* and coliform bacteria should be present only in low concentration levels.
		IV. Any suspected microbial colonization (water damage, odors, material deterioration, high RH, or building history) should be investigated.

Group C: Physical Fields and Radiation

C	Parameter	Normal environment	Slight change	Significant change	Severe change
1	AC electric fields in air (V/m)	<1	1 –5	5 –50	>50
2	AC electric fields on body (mV)	<10	10 –100	100 –1000	>1000
3	AC magnetic fields, flux density (mG)	<0.2	0.2 –1	1–5	>5
4	Microwaves in power density (uW/m^2)	<0.1	0.1–10	10–100	>100
5	DC electrostatic charge, surface (V)	<100	100–500	500–2,000	>2,000
6	DC electrostatic charge, discharge time (s)	<10	10–30	30–60	>60
7	DC magnetic fields, deviation (μT)	<1	1–2	2–10	>10
8	DC Magnetic fields, deviation (degree)	<2	2–10	10–100	>100
9	Ionizing radiation (increase in %)	<50	50–70	70–100	>100
10	Radon gas in air (Bq/m^3)	<30	30–60	60–200	>200
11	Terrestrial radiation, deviation (nT)	<100	100–200	200–1,000	>1000
12	Terrestrial radiation, deviation (%)	<10	10–20	20–50	>50

The Standard Testing Methodology for these environmental parameters was developed in conjunction with the Evaluation Guidelines to provide consistent and repeatable measurement results. Bau-Biology building investigations and assessments are unique because they examine a large number of environmental factors and look to nature, our planet Earth, for guiding principles.

The Standard makes a quantum leap by abandoning the traditional dose response-based threshold and action levels. It provides information on normally encountered background levels and establishes gradients that enable the environmental consultant to put measurement values into a real-life, proactive perspective.

Most indoor environmental testing in the United States focuses on a very few factors such as mold, asbestos, formaldehyde, and lead. Rarely does it address the electromagnetic spectrum, which has changed so significantly over the last decades. The knowledge of how to test, assess, evaluate, and heal our habitats and structures empowers us to improve our health, safety, and well-being in a lasting way.

For a copy of the actual standards or more information on testing, assessment, and Bau-Biology concepts, contact the author or the institutes and associations listed below:

- Peter Sierck, President, Environmental Testing & Technology, Inc., 5431 Avenida Encinas, Suite F, Carlsbad, CA 92008, 760-804-9400, PSierck@ETandT.com, Baubiology.com
- Institut für Baubiologie & Ökologie Neubeuern IBN, baubiologie.de
- International Institute for Bau-Biologie & Ecology (IBE), Clearwater, Florida, buildingbiology.net
- Berufsverbad Deutscher Baubiologen (VDB), baubiologie.net
- Verband Baubiologie, verband-baubiologie.de

Peter Sierck, CMC, CMRS, REA, BBEI, founder of Environmental Testing and Technology, Inc. (ET&T) in 1986, pioneered indoor air quality testing methods and procedures for residential and commercial buildings. Peter is a naturopathic physician, industrial hygienist, and Bau-Biologist. He has surveyed and helped remediate over 3,000 buildings and is a member of the Bau-Biology Standard Committee.

or glass slide and ship it to the laboratory. The lab technicians will stain the tape sample to make the fungal growth easier to view and then examine it under a microscope.

Culture Collection

Special moist, sterile swabs called culturettes are good for this type of sampling. The culturette is presterilized and comes with a fluid-filled glass ampoule to provide just the right amount of moisture. The ampoule and swab are housed in a sterile plastic tube. About one minute before collecting the sample, squeeze the area of the tube over the ampoule to break the ampoule and release the fluid, which then soaks the cotton swab. Slide the moistened swab from its sterile tube and use it to wipe one square inch of the area to be tested. Then insert the swab back into the sterile plastic tube for shipment to the lab. Since this method uses liquid, the fungal spores will be hydrated and begin to colonize. It is important to ship the specimen to the lab via overnight delivery service or the test may be invalid.

Vacuum Dust Collection

A filter designed to fit on a domestic vacuum cleaner is used. Since the filter's pores are smaller than mold spores, any mold spores present are collected. The filter canister is then shipped to a laboratory for analysis.

Other Mold Test Methods

The practice of testing for molds by letting spores settle on an open culture dish is now discouraged by knowledgeable specialists. Since certain harmful molds such as *Aspergillus* and *Penicillium* are very light and have a tendency not to settle on culture dishes, they are underrepresented in the analysis. Other methods of testing for airborne fungal spores and contaminated materials are available but require a trained technician with sophisticated equipment.

Radioactivity Testing

Although radioactivity in building materials is rare, John Banta's home inspections have revealed radioactive stone and tile glazes. Highly radioactive materials can be tested simply by holding a radiation detector next to the material.

For lower levels of radiation, measurements of longer duration should be performed. Place at least one pound of the material in question in a glass container with an instrument for measuring radioactivity. A useful instrument designed for this purpose is **Radalert 100**, whose small size allows it to fit easily inside a one-gallon glass pickle jar along with the material to be tested. Set the meter for total counts and leave it to measure for a timed period of 12 to 24 hours. As a control, the test must also be performed in the same way, in the same location, but with the jar empty. Repeat both tests several times to be sure a radiation-emitting solar flare or short-term cosmic event did not interfere with the results. To obtain an average count per minute, divide the total number of counts recorded for each test by the total number of minutes the test ran. A substance that measures less than 10 percent higher than the control test is considered to be free of radiation. Readings more than 20 percent higher than the control test are considered to be significant.

Moisture Testing

Ensuring that materials are dry is essential in healthy building. Building materials can be ruined by moisture damage. The following four building practices can cause warping, deterioration of materials, and microbial growth:

1. Application of finish flooring materials over insufficiently cured concrete slabs
2. Failure to quickly and thoroughly dry out precipitation that enters an unfinished structure
3. Installation of wood members with a moisture content greater than 17 percent
4. Enclosure of walls containing wet-applied insulation systems, such as cellulose or spray foams, before they are properly cured

It is not always possible to detect by visual inspection whether a material is wet. A variety of test procedures have been developed to assist in determining if a material is dry.

Moisture Meters

There are two general types of moisture meters. The first uses sharp pin probes that are pushed into the material to be tested. The pin probe meter detects moisture by electrical conductivity, since wet materials conduct greater amounts of electricity than dry materials. This meter leaves pinholes in the materials being tested. The second type of meter sends an electronic signal into the material. The degree of moisture determines how the meter will register the returning signal.

Both types of moisture meters are battery operated and can be used repeatedly. The meters range in cost from about $200 to over $1,000 and can require some technical experience. For example, damp wood is measured with a different setting and scale than damp concrete or brick. Companies that specialize in fire and flood damage restoration are likely to have this equipment and be experienced in its use. If you decide to purchase or borrow a moisture meter, plan on spending some time becoming familiar with it and thoroughly reading the owner's manual and instructions. Keep in mind that hidden metals or salt deposits may falsely indicate that materials are wet when in fact they are dry.

Testing for Weathertightness

All homes are supposed to be weathertight but many are not. One simple method for testing is to literally water the house. You can specify that the exterior of the house shall be weathertight before any interior construction begins. Once the exterior is complete and the doors and windows are installed and caulked, spray the house with a hose so that every part of the house gets soaked for at least 15 minutes. Then inspect all areas inside the house for leaks. A moisture meter will be useful for this task.

This test should be performed only prior to the installation of interior sheathing or insulation so that leaks can be easily detected, dried out, and remedied. The test will be much more effective if a negative pressure can be created in the house while the test is being performed, as this will more accurately simulate pressure conditions that exist during a storm. A blower door is an excellent way to create a known negative pressure for this test. (See the section on blower doors below.)

Window Testing

Water infiltration caused by faulty windows or installation procedure is a common source of building failure leading to mold infestation and water damage. Because water infiltrating through window assemblies will often leak directly into the wall cavity, a problem can go undetected for a long time and once it is discovered the damage is often extensive.

Such problems can be avoided if the proper testing protocol is carried out at the time of installation. Some windows are designed with drainage channels and weep holes that allow water to drain to the outside of the building and not into the wall. One way to test the effectiveness of a window's drainage capacity is to temporarily block the weep holes with putty and then fill the drainage channel with water. If the window is properly manufactured and installed, the water should not drain out of the drainage channel when the weep holes are plugged. This test should be performed on each window for a minimum of 15 minutes. Be sure to remove the putty from the weep holes when the test is complete.

Humidity/Temperature Testing

Newly constructed buildings generally have higher humidity levels caused by the moisture inherent in building materials and processes. It is important to dry enclosed buildings out quickly to levels that will not support mold growth and to verify that acceptable levels have been reached and are maintained. Humidity should be monitored and controlled from the time the building is enclosed until all wet-finish materials have been applied and dried. Humidity controls are especially important in humid climates or when massive wet materials such as concrete or plaster are used. Inexpensive meters for determining temperature and relative humidity called thermohygrometers can be purchased at most electronics and hardware stores.

Relative humidity (RH) varies depending on temperature. Warmer air will have a lower RH than colder air with the same amount of water vapor. With a special chart called a psychrometric table, a trained consultant can convert readings from the thermohygrometer to determine the actual amount of water in the air or at surfaces at various temperatures. These figures are used to determine if a structure is dry enough. At 70 degrees Fahrenheit, mold will not grow at an RH level of under 60 percent measured at the surface. One way to measure the surface humidity is to affix the thermo hydrometer to the surface with a sheet of plastic sealed over it. After a few minutes the meter will stabilize and the RH can be read. If it is determined that humidity levels are too high, we recommend electric dehumidification. Note that if you can see condensation continuously on the windows for two days in a row, the building probably has areas that are wet enough to support microbial growth.

Certified water-loss technicians are trained and equipped to measure and dry buildings that have excessive levels of moisture. There are two associations that certify technicians and can help you locate qualified people in your vicinity. These are the **Restoration Industry Association (RIA)** and the **Institute of Inspection, Cleaning and Restoration Certification (IICRC).**

Calcium Chloride Moisture Testing

Large quantities of water are present in cement, gypsum concrete, aircrete, and other poured masonry materials. These materials must be adequately dried before finishes are applied. It is common in new construction for a carpet or other floor finish to be laid on a slab before the slab is thoroughly dry. Further drying is inhibited, allowing microbial spore levels to climb as mold growth invades these damp areas.

Kits for testing moisture in masonry are available (see Chart 13.1). They contain calcium chloride salts, which absorb moisture from the air at a known rate. A kit contains a plate that holds the calcium chloride salt, a plastic dome, and an adhesive material. Weigh the calcium chloride to the nearest hundredth of a gram. (You can find scales for weighing the salts at your local pharmacy.) Then place the calcium chloride test plate on the floor area to be tested and cover it with the plastic dome, which is sealed to the slab with the adhesive material. After 60 to 72 hours, remove the plastic dome and reweigh the calcium chloride. Based on the weight gain and the number of hours that have passed, you can determine the material's water vapor emissions rate. The kit instructions also contain a chart that will help you determine when the slab is dry enough for the application of various finishing materials. If a scale is unavailable, the sealed exposed kit can be shipped back to the manufacturer for weighing and calculations.

Thermal Imaging

Thermal imaging using infrared cameras has rapidly become an affordable tool for diagnosing moisture problems. This versatile tool is also used for energy conservation audits (see the next section) and can detect overloaded electrical circuits, poor electrical connections, and "hot spots" on electrical equipment that may indicate a potential failure or fire hazard.

Infrared cameras are sophisticated devices that are used to examine the spectrum of energy just outside our visual range. They "see" heat. We see the colors of the rainbow: violet, blue, green, yellow, orange, and red. Infrared is the portion of the spectrum just beyond red, which we can't see but can certainly feel with our skin in the form of heat.

Thermal imaging can frequently diagnose moisture from leaks and condensation because damp surfaces are subject to evaporative cooling, resulting in cooler surface temperatures. Since thermal imaging uses surface temperature differences to indicate potential issues, moisture and missing insulation may appear the same. Thus moisture problems generally must have further diagnosis using moisture meters to confirm and identify the source of the moisture, but as a first screening step thermal imaging can help tremendously.

Energy Efficiency and Airflow Testing

Thermal Imaging for Energy Conservation Audits

When used by a knowledgeable, trained thermographer, an infrared camera can detect heat loss from missing insulation, air infiltration, and leaking ductwork. The US Department of Energy's Office of Energy Efficiency and Renewable Energy is now recommending that anyone purchasing a home have it scanned as part of the escrow. They advise: "Even new houses can have defects in their thermal envelopes. You may wish to include a clause in the contract requiring a thermographic scan of the house."[1]

For thermal imaging to be most effective, there needs to be a temperature difference. In evaluations of ductwork and heating or air conditioning systems, the temperature differential is provided by the equipment being evaluated. In evaluations of energy efficiency from thermal insulation and of air infiltration, there needs to be a sharp temperature

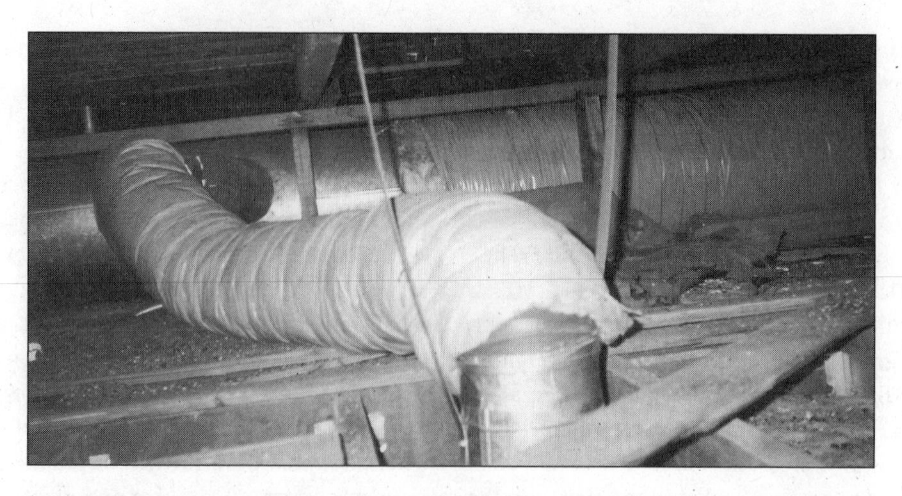

The Problem: This furnace ductwork, located in an attic, was not firmly connected to the supply register. As a result heat is being lost in the living space and insulation fibers are being blown into the air resulting in poor indoor air quality. Recommendation: ductworks must be well sealed and tested for air leakage. Photo: Restoration Consultants.

difference between the inside and outside environments. Inspections of this type will be most effective when performed during the hot summer or cold winter months when there is at least a 20-degree Fahrenheit temperature difference between the inside and the outside of the building.

Blower Doors

Blower doors consist of a sophisticated fan set in an adjustable frame. They are used to test airflow and pressure in a home. There are many uses for blower doors, such as detection of leaks in walls and in heating, ventilation, and air conditioning (HVAC) system ductwork. You can also determine if the ventilation is adequate and identify the location of energy leaks in the structure.

Since the equipment requires extensive training to use, we recommend that you hire a technician to carry out blower door testing. For most new homes this testing will cost several hundred dollars. Dollars saved in energy conservation from identified and corrected leaks may soon offset the cost of testing.

Theatrical Fog Machine

Certain parts of the home, such as garages, attics, and crawl spaces, should be completely sealed from the rest of the house in order to prevent the passage of contaminated air into living spaces. One easy way to test for leaking airflow is to use a theatrical fog machine. This is the same equipment used onstage and in movies to create fog for special effects and can be rented from most theatrical supply companies. Place the unit in the area to be tested, turn it on to fill the space with fog, and then observe the adjoining areas for signs of fog that indicate where leaks must be sealed.

When testing the garage, seal the door and the open vents with tape and plastic to prevent the fog from escaping. The same can be done for attic and crawl-space vents and other intentional openings to the outdoors. Common air-infiltration points revealed by the fog test include electrical outlets, the juncture where the gypsum board meets the floor, and around poorly sealed plumbing, electrical, and ductwork penetrations. Theatrical fog testing is especially helpful when performed in conjunction with a blower door. This will allow simulation of a variety of adverse weather conditions that may create unusual indoor air quality problems during inclement weather. Be sure to notify the fire department before you begin this type of test; otherwise a well-meaning neighbor who sees the smoke might dial 911 and set the fire trucks in motion.

Testing for Leakage in Air Distribution Systems

A consultant can test for leakage in air distribution systems in a manner similar to blower door testing for a whole house. Doing this testing while the ductwork is still accessible, before it is covered with finishing materials, will simplify repairs. Supply and return registers are sealed off so that the system can be depressurized using a blower door or calibrated fan. The combined airflow through all leakage openings can then be determined. Ideally, leakage should be less than 3 percent. If a small amount of excess leakage is revealed, a theatrical fog machine can be used to trace the sources. If leakage is extensive, it will be necessary to examine all junctures and reseal where required prior to retesting.

Radon Testing

In Division 7 we discussed radon gas and mitigation. There are several acceptable methods currently being used to measure radon in air and in water. Some test kits are available through local hardware stores (see Chart 13.1). It is important to follow the manufacturer's instructions precisely.

Radon Testing in an Existing Structure

The general procedure for radon air testing, regardless of the type of kit used, is:

- Close the home for a minimum of 12 hours before beginning the test and keep it closed throughout the testing period. You may enter and leave the house as long as the doors are not left open.
- Place the sampler about 30 inches above the floor and at least two feet away from the wall in the area being tested. Keep the sampler away from doors, windows, fireplaces, outside walls, corners, and any other places where drafts or stagnant air may exist. These precautions are necessary to ensure that the sampler is exposed to a representative sample of air.
- Accurately record the starting and stopping time. This information, along with the date, must be included with the sample when it is returned to the lab. Without precise recording information, the results cannot be considered valid.

A typical radon test kit costs less than $25. After each individual test, the kit must be returned to a laboratory for analysis. Multiple testing or continuous monitoring can be carried out with electronic radon monitors.

Radon Land Test

Radon mitigation is most effective and least costly when incorporated into the construction of the home. If you are building a new home and there is reason to suspect a radon problem, a land test is advisable. Although the test will not provide a definitive answer as to what the radon levels will ultimately be in the finished home, it is nevertheless an indicator that will help you decide whether mitigation measures should be included in your construction plans.

The test kit available for measuring radon in the soil requires placing a special collection box with its open side over the soil to be tested. Mound soil around the lip of the box to form a tight seal and keep the box in place. Radon gas is trapped and concentrated in a carbon medium and can then be measured by a testing apparatus. Record the starting time and date. After the prescribed period of time (usually 48 hours), push the soil away, retrieve the tester, and return it to its foil pouch. Record the stop time and send it with the other information and materials to the lab for analysis.

Radon Water Testing

Radon found in water poses a health threat when released into the air and inhaled. Hot, steamy baths or showers with water that has high radon content can be a serious source of exposure. Since the EPA requires municipal water sources to screen for radon, it is necessary to test only well water. Small amounts of radon can be removed with special carbon filters. A high radon content (5,000 picocuries per liter or greater) is more difficult and costly to remove. (See Chart 13.1 for test kits for radon in water.)

Testing for Chemical Fumes

A barrage of chemical odors often assaults new homeowners as they enter their newly constructed home. Many people who have never before been affected by chemical sensitivities find they are bothered or made chronically ill by prolonged exposure to the fumes in their new home. Sniffing finishing materials such as upholstery, carpets, and paint before they are installed will reveal important information. However, even if a building product or material passes the sniff test when sampled, the odor can become unbearable once the product is installed because chemical fumes accumulate inside the house and are emitted from a much larger surface area than that of the sample.

If you are unsure how you will tolerate a product once it is applied or installed in your house, we recommend that you test the product before purchase in a manner that will simulate the level of concentration in the home. One method is to place a sample of the product in question in a large glass jar with the top screwed on tightly to allow fumes to accumulate. The following day, open the jar and sniff the contents for unacceptable fumes. If the sample is too large to be placed inside a container, keep it next to your pillow while you sleep. Pillow testing should be done only if you are reasonably sure you will not have a severe reaction with prolonged exposure.

For some products it is important that the samples be new. For example, a carpet swatch that has been in a showroom for three years will not provide an accurate indication of what a freshly unrolled carpet will smell like in your home. Samples of other products — such as wet-applied finishes like paints, sealers, and adhesives — should be applied to an inert surface such as glass or foil and then be allowed to air out in an uncontaminated location for a few weeks to better simulate the cured or semi-cured state that the product will be in on move-in day.

This type of testing, although somewhat

helpful, has obvious limitations. While the test gives information about the product in question, it does not indicate cumulative effects or synergistic effects with other chemicals. Since you cannot predict these effects in advance, the goal is to choose products with the lowest levels of odor and toxic emissions.

Further Reading

Floor Seal Technology, Inc. *Concrete Vapor Emissions and Alkalinity Control.* Available from 800-572-2344, 800-295-0221.

Institute of Inspection, Cleaning and Restoration Certification. *ANSI/IICRC S500-2006 Standard and Reference Guide for Professional Water Damage Restoration.* 3rd ed., IICRC, 2006. Available from 2715 East Mill Plain Blvd., Vancouver WA 98661, 800-835-4624, 360-693-5675, iicrc.org.

Institute of Inspection, Cleaning and Restoration Certification. *IICRC S520 Standard and Reference Guide for Professional Mold Remediation.* IICRC, 2003. Available from 2715 East Mill Plain Blvd., Vancouver WA 98661, 800-835-4624, 360-693-5675, iicrc.org.

Chart 13.1: Test Kits and Equipment

Manufacturer	Product	Contact points
Indoor air quality	AQS commercial building IAQ test kit for VOCs, formaldehyde, and mold	Air Quality Sciences, Inc. Laboratory Services 1337 Capital Circle, Marietta, GA 30067 770-933-0638 info@aqs.com aqs.com
Formaldehyde, microwaves, radon	A variety of home test kits for radon, formaldehyde, and microwaves	AirChek Inc. 1936 Butler Bridge Rd., Fletcher, NC 28732 800-247-2435 radon.com
Lead	Lead Check Swabs #K910 turn pink if lead is present and can be used on ceramics, paint, soil, and solder	Professional Equipment PO Box 5197, Janesville, WI 53547 800-334-9291 professionalequipment.com
Mold	Easy-to-use mold test kit #K2400	Professional Equipment PO Box 5197, Janesville, WI 53547 800-334-9291 professionalequipment.com
Mold	Do-it-yourself mold test units with online instructions and telephone consultation for result interpretation and remediation advice	RCAnalytical RestCon Environmental 3284 Ramos Circle, Sacramento, CA 95827 888-617-3266 916-736-1100 rcanalytical.com restcon.com
Pesticides	Agri-Screen Ticket, a do-it-yourself pesticide testing kit for various surfaces	Neogen Corporation 620 Lesher Place, Lansing, MI 48912 800-234-5333 neogen.com
Pesticides in water	Watercheck water test kit that detects up to 20 pesticides	The Cutting Edge Catalog PO Box 4158, Santa Fe, NM 87502 800-497-9516 cutcat.com

Chart 13.1: Test Kits and Equipment (cont'd.)

Manufacturer	Product	Contact points
pH testing	Calcium chloride moisture and alkali test kit for concrete slabs	Taylor Tools 303-371-7667 taylortools.com
pH testing	pH test pencil for measuring the alkalinity of concrete slabs	Sinak Corporation 1949 Walnut Ave., San Diego, CA 92101 800-523-3147 sinakcorp.com
pH testing	Surface pH test kit for concrete slabs	Vaprecision, Inc. 3211 W. MacArthur Blvd., Santa Ana, CA 92704 800-449-6194 kits@vaportest.com vaportest.com
Radioactivity	Radalert 100 device for measuring radioactivity	International Medcom 6871 Abbott Ave., Sebastopol, CA 95472 707-823-0336 medcom.com
Radon	Test kits for radon in water and long- and short-term test kits for radon in air	Professional Discounts Supply 1029 S. Sierra Madre, Suite B, Colorado Springs, CO 80903 719-444-0646 radonpds.com
Thermal imaging cameras	Thermal imaging cameras and training in their use	Restoration Consultants Inc. 3284 Ramos Circle, Sacramento, CA 95827 888-617-3266 916-736-1100 moistureview.com
Vapor emissions testing	Reusable calcium chloride moisture and pH dome test kit for concrete slabs	Sinak Corporation 1949 Walnut Ave., San Diego, CA 92101 800-523-3147 sinakcorp.com
Vapor emissions testing	Calcium chloride moisture and alkali test kit for concrete slabs	Taylor Tools 303-371-7667 taylortools.com
Vapor emissions testing	Anhydrous calcium chloride vapor emissions test kit for concrete slabs	Plaza Hardwood, Inc. 219 W. Manhattan Ave., Santa Fe, NM 87501 800-662-6306 505-992-3260 plzfloor.com
Vapor emissions testing	Anhydrous calcium chloride vapor emissions test kit for concrete slabs	Vaprecision, Inc. 3211 W MacArthur Blvd., Santa Ana, CA 92704 800-449-6194 vaportest.com

Although do-it-yourself tests may indicate that a problem is present, consultation with a remediation specialist is often required for accurate diagnosis and safe, effective remediation.

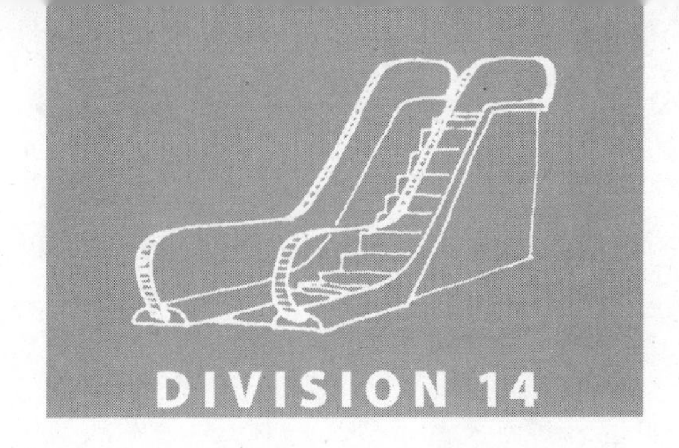

Conveying Systems

This division is not used in most residential construction.

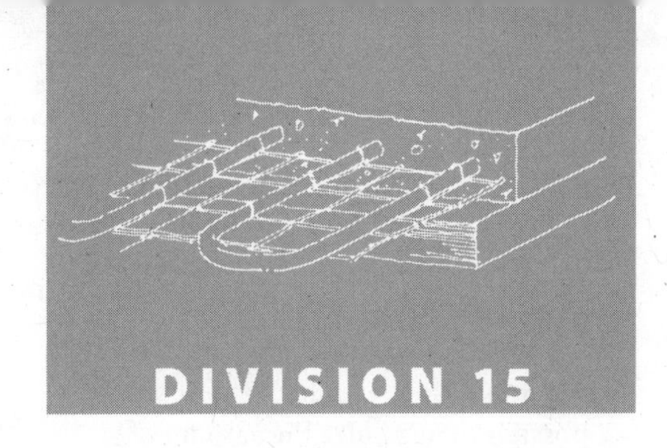
DIVISION 15

Mechanical

Water Supply and Waste

Polyvinyl chloride (PVC) is the standard for residential supply and waste piping. PVC plastic piping has been shown to outgas diethyl phthalate, trimethylhexane, aliphatic hydrocarbons, and other harmful gases. It should not be used for water supply piping in a healthy home. Because of the pollution resulting from both the manufacture and the disposal of PVC piping, we recommend seeking alternatives for waste lines as well.

Water Supply Pipe

Although we can choose the type of supply pipe we want in a new home, we have no control over how water is delivered to our property line. Well water is often delivered through PVC piping. Municipal water supply can be piped through a variety of unsavory piping, including PVC and asbestos cement. We recommend whole house water purification at the point where water enters the house. In Division 11 we outlined several whole-house water purification strategies. From the point at which water is purified, it makes sense to distribute it in piping that will not have an adverse affect on water quality. Your specifications could include one of the following acceptable alternatives for supply piping:

- **Type L or Type M copper: Solder shall be lead-free silver solder. The system shall be flushed prior to occupancy to eliminate any flux from the soldering operation.**
- **Wirsbo Aquapex: A crosslinked polyethylene that shall be installed by a certified installer.**

Waste Drain System

Waste drain systems do not have the same water quality concerns as supply piping does and are almost always plastic because it is most economical. We prefer to specify ABS piping because of the problems associated with the production and burning of PVC piping. Pipe assembly glues are highly volatile and toxic and their use onsite should be carefully managed to reduce pollution. You may wish to specify the following:

- **Assemble pipes with the longest pieces possible to minimize the amount of glue or solder required.**
- **When possible, glue waste pipe assembly outside the building envelope.**
- **Wipe up excessive glues and protect all surfaces from glue drips and spills.**
- **Whenever glue is being used inside the structure, provide adequate ventilation until all odors are dissipated.**

Floor Drains

Appliances containing water, such as water heaters and washing machines, can malfunction and leak. You can avoid the subsequent water damage and mold if you plan for this possibility. If floor drains or drain pans are strategically located, the water from accidental spills can be diverted to the sewer line or to the outdoors. Drains that lead to the sewer line should be installed with a trap to prevent unwanted sewer gases from entering the home. It is important that the traps be "primed," or kept filled with water, which creates a physical barrier against the entry of sewer gases. Self-priming drains can be installed so that the trap will remain filled with water without additional maintenance.

Plumbing Penetrations

Where plumbing penetrates walls and ceilings, the air space created around the opening must be completely sealed to prevent unwanted air infiltration. Consider specifying the following:

Wherever plumbing penetrates the wall, aquarium-grade 100 percent silicone caulking shall be applied to create an airtight seal.

Backflow Protection

In some communities, sewage systems periodically back up and flow into homes, leading to devastating contamination. Backflow prevention devices installed on the home waste line will usually prevent this. The local planning department may be able to help you determine if backflow prevention devices are advisable. In many communities, claims for sewage damage will not be paid unless such devices were in place prior to the incident.

Residential Heating and Cooling

Methods of heating, cooling, and ventilating homes have many important health ramifications that will affect us long after the initial building materials have outgassed and reached a neutral state. If we lived in a pristine natural environment with low humidity and mild temperatures, we would be able to condition our homes without mechanical assistance by means of solar gain, shading, and cross-ventilation. Residents throughout most of North America do not have this luxury. Cold and cloudy winters, hot and humid summers, and polluted or pollen-filled air are realities from which homes must shelter occupants.

We have come to expect a level of comfort and temperature control in our homes undreamed of by our not-too-distant ancestors. Along with the increased comfort level, we have unwittingly come to accept many health problems associated with heating and cooling

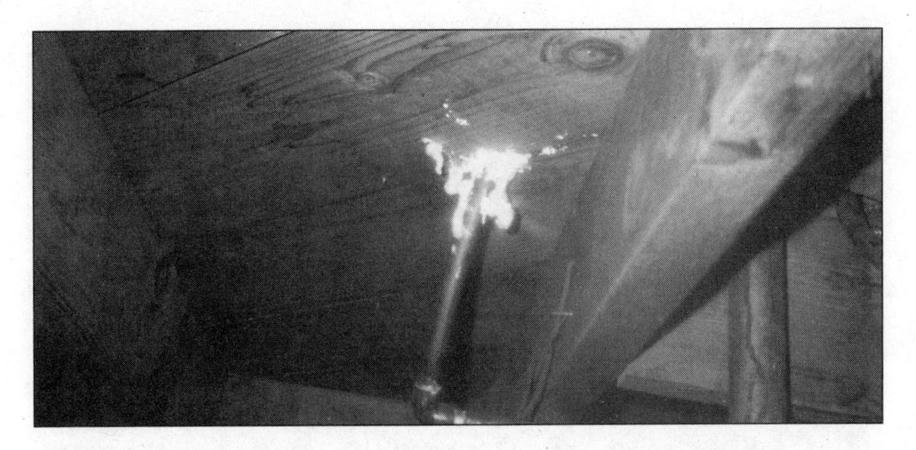

The Problem: Crawl space air was being drawn in to this home through plumbing penetrations before they were sealed Recommendation: Plumbing and other penetrations should be sealed to prevent infiltration. Photo: Restoration Consultants.

systems. In fact, more than any other building system or component, heating and cooling methods can be a major cause of sick building syndrome. Some of the problems include:

- toxic fumes from gas, oil, or propane fuels that work their way into the building envelope through leaky supply lines, from insufficiently ventilated or improperly sealed mechanical rooms, and from open combustion appliances
- backdrafting of hazardous and sometimes deadly gases into the living space from flues
- infiltration of pollutants from outside the building envelope resulting from depressurization
- fried dust resulting from hot surface temperatures on heating appliances
- circulation of dust through an unfiltered forced-air heating system
- contamination from mold growing in the ductwork and air conditioning equipment
- fiberglass fibers from ductwork insulation that circulate in the living space

In the following section we focus on ways of reducing the need for mechanical heating and cooling. Later in this chapter we present guidelines for healthier heating and cooling installations, language for specifications, and maintenance suggestions that will help eliminate some of the problems mentioned above.

Reducing Heating and Cooling Loads Through Design Strategies

The application of a few simple design and planning principles can greatly reduce the amount of mechanical heating and cooling required to live comfortably, thereby improving health and lowering energy consumption. In designing your home for energy efficiency, consider the following suggestions.

Create an Energy-Efficient Building Envelope

- Choose an exterior wall system with a high insulation value.
- Choose interior wall and floor systems with high levels of thermal mass to assist in

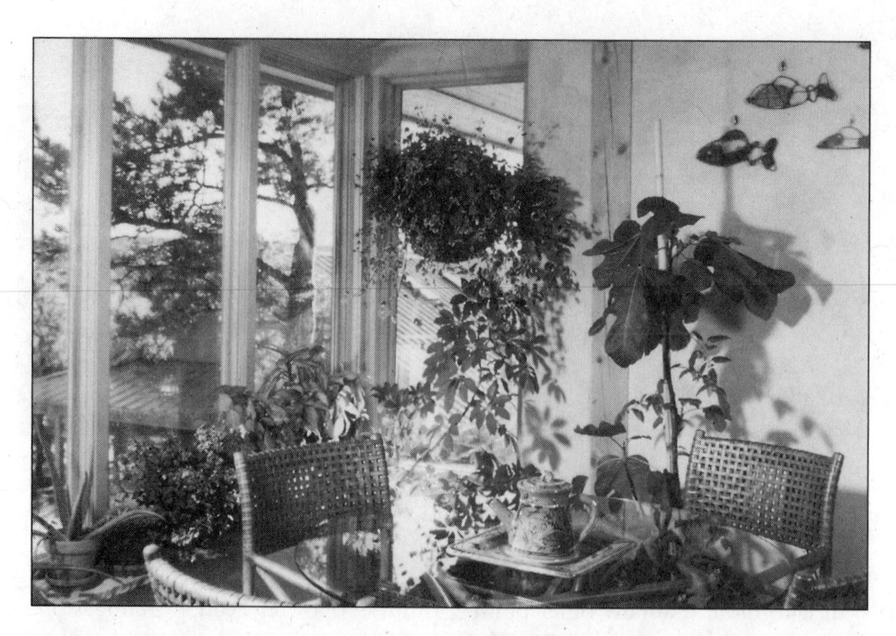

This winter garden located in New Mexico provides a large portion of the home's heat in the winter. A small overhang prevents excessive solar gain from the high summer sun. Architect: Paula Baker-Laporte; Builder: Econest Building Co.
Photo: Lisl Dennis.

keeping things cool in summer and retaining heat in winter.

- Seal cracks and joints to prevent unwanted infiltration and exfiltration.
- Choose a high insulation value for the ceiling. This measure will be especially cost effective because most heat escapes through the roof.

Consider the Surrounding Site as an Extension of Your Climate-Control Design

- Make use of deciduous trees to shade in summer and allow solar gain in winter.
- Observe prevailing wind patterns when planning for natural ventilation.
- Consider using trees as windbreaks to lower the heating load created by cold winter winds.
- Situate your home as far away from pollution sources as possible so that the site can provide a quality air supply for home ventilation.

Take Advantage of Solar Heat

- Orient the home to take advantage of solar gain.
- Plan fenestration (arrangement of doors and windows) for the desired amount of heat gain.
- Make use of overhangs and sun angle information to prevent overheating in summer.
- Use light colors to reflect heat and dark colors to absorb and store heat.
- Provide thermal mass for heat storage.
- Provide cross-ventilation to facilitate nat-

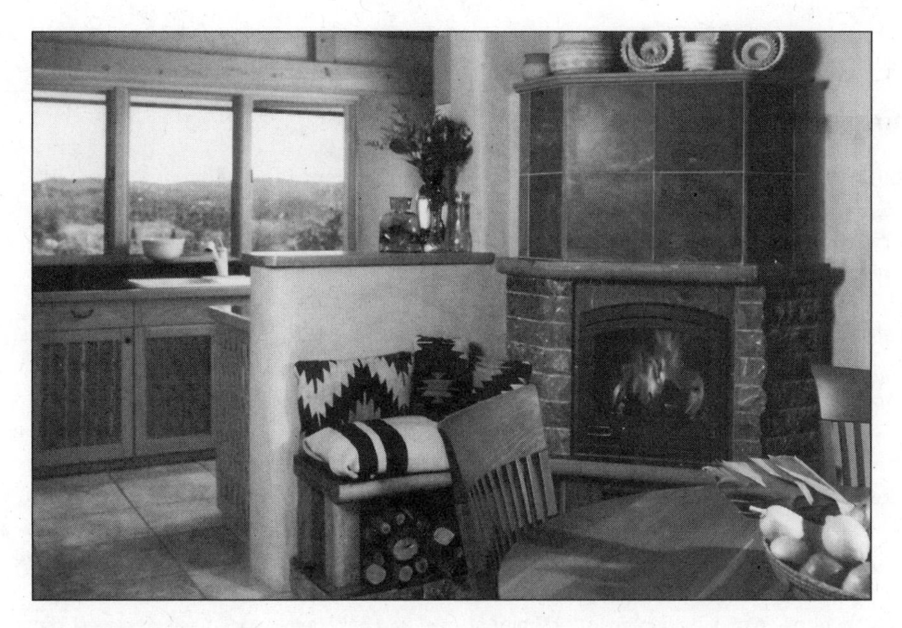

This "Tulikivi" brand masonry oven works on the principal of contra-flow design and mass storage capacity providing comfortable and energy efficient heat. Architect: Paula Baker-Laporte; Builder: Econest Building Co.
Photo: Lisl Dennis.

ural air exchange and to provide cooling in summer.
- Use thermal window-shading devices to control heat loss.
- Use specialized window coatings to enhance solar gain where desired and block unwanted heat gain.

Become a More Active Participant in Temperature Control
- Open and close windows to provide fresh air and control temperature.
- Open and close thermal shading devices to control heat gain and loss.
- Utilize automated thermostat controls to economize on heating and cooling when you are absent or asleep.
- Be willing to add and subtract layers of clothing to allow for a greater range of acceptable temperatures.
- Consciously acclimatize your body to a broader comfort range.

Healthier Heating and Cooling

Each heating and cooling system has advantages and disadvantages that you must weigh carefully when choosing a system that best fits your needs and budget. Once you have made a choice, there are several design, construction, and maintenance considerations that will optimize performance and minimize the health risks of the system. In the preliminary design phase, you and your architect must consider factors such as the location of the mechanical room. During the construction phase, the choice of materials and installation procedures

CASE STUDY 15.1

A Constant Supply of Warm Dust

A retired couple contacted John Banta because they were experiencing eye irritation and difficulty breathing caused by dust in their home. In spite of frequent vacuuming and dusting, an unusually heavy deposit of dust was noted on the furnishings during the house inspection. John suspected that the furnace system was the source of contamination because the heat registers in the home were lined with a fine dust and the clients' symptoms worsened when the furnace was on.

John was puzzled, though, by the lack of dirt on the cold air return filter and the absence of air movement. He opened the cold air return and examined the inside wall to see if there were any visible obstructions. To his surprise, he found no duct at all. The cold air return was a dummy and went nowhere.

Further investigation revealed that the furnace and duct system were located in the crawl space under the home. John inspected the crawl space, where he discovered that there was no connection between the cold air return port on the furnace and the rest of the house. In fact, the furnace was taking cold air from the crawl space and blowing the unfiltered, contaminated air directly into the house. Consultation with a heating and air conditioning company was recommended to correct this construction defect.

Discussion

HVAC duct systems should always be leak-tested to ensure that they meet specified standards. The stated industry standard for a sealed duct system is less than 3 percent leakage, which is rarely achieved. The furnace itself will account for much of the leakage since it is difficult to seal. The furnace should be mounted in a clean, easily accessible area such as a mechanical room and not in an attic or crawl space.

Leakage also occurs at unsealed joints where the metal ducts fit together. Since the return side of the furnace is sucking air back into the furnace, it will suck contaminants through leaks in the ductwork. If the unsealed ducts pass through walls or attics containing fiberglass, fiberglass particles are sucked into the ducts and blown into the house. If the unsealed ducts are in a crawl space under the home, then moldy, pesticide-laden or dusty air can be sucked into the furnace system and blown into the house.

can influence the ultimate outcome. For this reason we have provided specifications for the contractor where relevant. Finally, a regular cleaning and maintenance program is essential for optimal efficiency. This task will ultimately fall to the owner and may influence your choice of HVAC system.

Choice of Fuel Source

Gas and other sources of combustion fuels can pollute the airstream if you do not plan carefully. Electric heat is often considered "cleaner" heat because combustion does not occur in the home. However, environmental pollution from electricity generation plants must be acknowledged. Moreover, electric heating appliances generate electromagnetic fields, an invisible and often overlooked source of pollution. Whatever your choice of fuel source, there are several strategies that can be employed in the mechanical room that will make heating healthier.

Mechanical Room Design

- The mechanical room should be a dedicated room, insulated and isolated from the living space either in a separate building or in a well-sealed room that ventilates to the outside. It should be easily accessible for regular routine maintenance.
- The equipment in the mechanical room may produce elevated levels of electromagnetic fields and should not be located adjacent to heavily occupied living spaces.
- Ensure the supply of adequate combustion air to the mechanical room.
- We recommend that you locate a fire alarm in the mechanical room.
- If there is a water source in the mechanical room, there should also be a floor drain.

Heating and Cooling Appliances

We recommend the following guidelines for choosing, locating, and maintaining heating equipment:

- Purchase equipment designed for back-draft prevention.
- Use sealed combustion units to prevent transfer of combustion byproducts into the airstream. This is especially important where the mechanical room must be accessed directly from the living space.
- If you are using a forced-air system, we strongly recommend adding a good combination filtration system that will filter out both particulate matter and gas.
- If possible, choose a heating system that does not run hot enough to fry dust. Hydronic systems and heat pumps meet this requirement.
- Institute a regular maintenance program to clean components, change filters, and purge mold or mildew growth.

Hydronic Heating

Hydronic heating, delivered through hot water, is usually a wall-mounted baseboard or radiant floor system. Baseboard systems are usually made of copper tubes and aluminum radiating fins with painted steel covers. Baseboard radiators can be noisy if not maintained, and they can become traps for dust and dirt. Some baseboard units are subject to outgassing at first, when the factory-applied paint on them gets hot. Verify with the manufacturer if this will be a problem with the model you are considering.

Hydronic radiant floor systems are usually made of plastic, rubber, or copper tubing installed within or under the floor. Hot water circulating through the tubing heats the floor mass and the heat then rises through gentle convection. Radiant systems are silent and clean. Because this form of heating heats feet, occupants are comfortable at lower operating temperatures. The water running through the piping is not hot enough to fry dust. Note that hydronic radiant floor heating should not be confused with radiant electric heating, in which the heat source is heated electrical wiring. We do not recommend this type of heating because it will distribute a magnetic field throughout the home when in operation.

At one time, radiant floor heating used copper tubing almost exclusively but the rising price of copper, combined with the introduction of plastic and rubber tubing, made this a less common option. Metal tubing, such as copper, can conduct electromagnetic fields through the structure if it becomes charged at any point along its route and for this reason we do not recommend it. Some in-floor systems use very odorous rubber products. While this is not a problem where they are embedded in concrete, it can be a source of indoor pollution where the tubing is exposed at access points. **Wirsbo Hepex**, a crosslinked polyethylene tubing, or **Kitec**, a crosslinked polyethylene tubing with an aluminum core, are odorless products for radiant floor heating.

The advantages of a hydronic system include slightly lower operating costs, even heating, quieter operation, ease of zoning, and independent room-temperature control. Disadvantages of the hydronic system include slow response time and higher installation costs compared to forced air because of the number of mechanical components.

Forced-Air Heating

Throughout most of the country, forced air is the most common form of heating and cooling in new construction. Besides quick response time, the main advantage of forced-air heating lies in the opportunity it gives the homeowner to commission modifications and additions to standard equipment to create a healthy air-distribution system. A modified system can control humidity, filter air, and introduce fresh, conditioned air from the outside. Disadvantages of a forced-air system may include greater operating costs, noisy operation, larger space requirements for equipment installation and ductwork housing, depletion of negative ions, and the need for regular maintenance and cleaning of ductwork to prevent mold and dirt buildup.

Disadvantages of a standard forced-air system can also include distribution of odors and particulate matter, and unwanted dehumidification. Forced-air heating, which heats air, is considered to be far less comfortable than radiant heating, which heats objects. A forced-air system must be properly designed for appropriate balancing and distribution. Poor indoor air quality, energy inefficiency, and discomfort can result when system design is inadequate.

If forced air is your choice for heating and cooling (in much of the country this may be the only cost-effective choice), you can take advantage of the whole-house air distribution ducting that will already be in place to improve air quality by implementing the steps below:

- Use a fresh-air intake vent from the outside to the furnace to introduce and distribute fresh, tempered ventilation into your home. Locate the vent so that it receives "fresh" air; do not place the vent near trash storage areas or where auto exhaust and other pollutants could be brought inside the house.
- Install enhanced filtration in your forced-air stream. (See the Air Filtration section below.)
- Choose a furnace with sealed combustion to avoid the entry of combustion byproducts into the airstream.

Design of Healthier Forced-Air Ductwork

Care must be taken during the design, installation, and maintenance of forced-air ductwork because the means of air distribution is often the source of allergies and other health problems associated with forced-air heating and cooling.

Ductless air plenums are a common source of air contamination associated with HVAC systems. Joisted floors, and wall cavities without ductwork, act as pathways for contaminated attic or crawl space air to enter the building if air is forced through them. Fibers from wall and ceiling insulation are frequently sucked into the return side of the heating system and circulated throughout the building envelope. Furthermore, the plenums are inaccessible for cleaning and impossible to seal.

Floor registers should be avoided because debris will inevitably accumulate in them, not only during construction but also in the course of occupancy. For this reason, supply and return registers should ideally be located on walls or ceilings. Below-slab ductwork should be avoided because it can collect moisture and dirt, providing a breeding ground for microbes. Also avoid running ductwork through uninsulated spaces if at all possible. If this is unavoidable, the ductwork should be well insulated on its exterior.

Ductwork should be easily accessible for future inspection and maintenance. A good design should specify cleaning portals that will give access to all ductwork, especially points of probable condensation. Sheet metal is preferable to plastic flex ducts because the flex ducts are difficult to keep clean and are easily damaged. Ductwork may be coated with undesirable oils from the manufacturing process and should be cleaned of all oil prior to installation.

Installation of Forced-Air Ductwork

Quality control during the installation of a well-designed ductwork system will help ensure optimum efficiency and health. Ductwork should be well sealed with a nontoxic sealer. Ideally, an air distribution system should have a neutral effect on building pressurization.

A large amount of dust and debris is generated during the construction process, and it frequently finds its way into the ductwork, becoming a source of air contamination once the system is in operation unless measures are

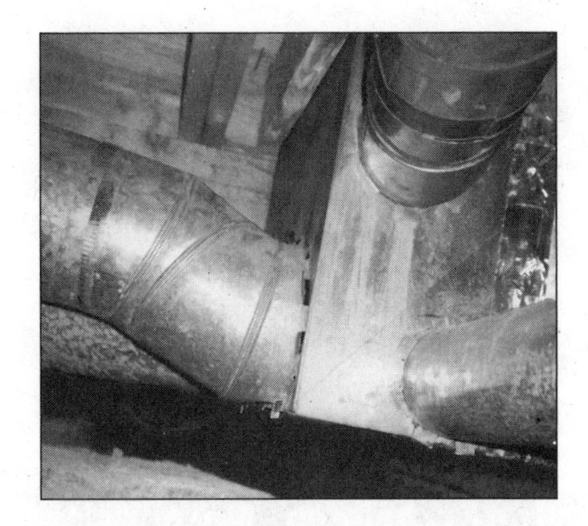

The Problem: Home investigation revealed that ductwork had not been sealed on the return side of this system causing contaminated air to be sucked in to the system and blown throughout the home. Recommendation: All ductwork should be throroughly sealed and tested for air leakage.
Photo: Restoration Consultants.

taken during construction to keep the ductwork clean.

In order to achieve an optimal ductwork system installation, we suggest the following specifications:

- **Metal ductwork shall be free of all oil residues prior to installation.**
- **Ductwork shall be well sealed with nontoxic compounds such as AFM Safecoat DynoFlex, RCD6, Uni-Flex Duct Sealer, Uni-Mastic 181 Duct Sealer, United Duct Sealer (Water Based), or approved equal. Mastics shall be water resistant and water-based, with a flame spread rating no higher than 25 and a maximum smoke developed rating of 50.**
- **During construction, the ends of any partially installed ductwork shall be sealed with plastic and duct tape to avoid the**

introduction of dust and debris from construction.

- All forced air must be ducted. The use of unducted plenum space for the transport of supply or conditioned air is prohibited.
- Cloth duct tape shall not be used. (It has a high failure rate that can result in undetected leakage.)
- All joints, including premanufactured joints and longitudinal seams, shall be sealed.
- Gaps greater than ⅛ inch shall be reinforced with fiber mesh.
- All ductwork running through uninsulated spaces shall be insulated to a minimum of R-10 to prevent condensation problems and to save energy.
- Any ductwork requiring insulation shall have the insulation located on the outside of the ducts.
- Ductwork must be professionally cleaned prior to occupancy. The duct-cleaning

The Kachelofen - Masonry Heater: The Ideal Heating for Room Climate and Health

ERNST KIESLING

Because humans do not have the ability to withstand the natural elements, we wear clothes and build shelters. In cold climates we heat those shelters. Many systems have been invented for heating the home, but not all systems are created equal. After examining the criteria that create health and a comfortable indoor climate, I chose to focus my career on the creation of Kachelofens, or masonry oven heating systems, because of their superior quality and performance. A Kachelofen-Masonry Heater is an individually designed, technically calculated, thermal mass wood-fired heating system.

From a Building Biology point of view, let us examine the criteria for creating a comfortable and healthy indoor environment and discover why the Masonry Heater is one of the best heating systems for meeting these criteria.

1. Type of Heat: A heating system should create radiant heat, like the heat from the sun. With a radiant heat source, the room air temperature can stay relatively low at 18 to 20 degrees Celsius (64 to 68 degrees Fahrenheit) and still be comfortably warm because, unlike the convection heat from a forced-air source, radiant heat warms walls, floors, and ceilings as well as furniture and bodies and not the room air. Therefore the room air is barely moving, or moving only at low speed, which means no electrostatic charge, no dust circulation, and no transfer of odors. Kachelofens–Masonry Heaters release about 60 to 70 percent radiant heat and only about 30 to 40 percent convection heat, an output not attainable with any other heating system.
2. Temperature: The quality of a heating system should not be measured by high room-air temperatures but rather by low differences between the room-air temperature and the temperatures of the walls, ceilings, and floors, as shown in the sketches.

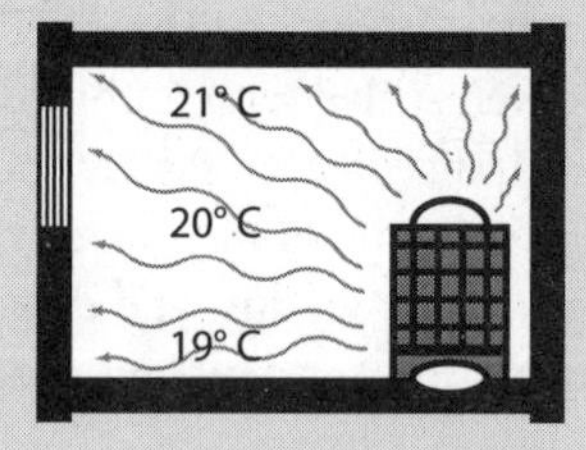

Kachelofen-Masonry Heater

vacuums should have true HEPA filtration or be exhausted to the outside. No chemicals shall be used in the process.

- **Prior to occupancy, the air distribution system shall be tested for leakage by a qualified third party or in the presence of the owner or architect. Any leakage greater than 3 percent shall be remedied by the contractor at no additional expense to the owner.**

Once the ducts are in place, a regular maintenance program is essential to maintaining a healthy system. Identify a professional maintenance company that uses high-powered duct cleaning equipment. Avoid the use of chemical cleaners.

Masonry Ovens

From a Building Biology perspective, the ideal heating system would have the following features:

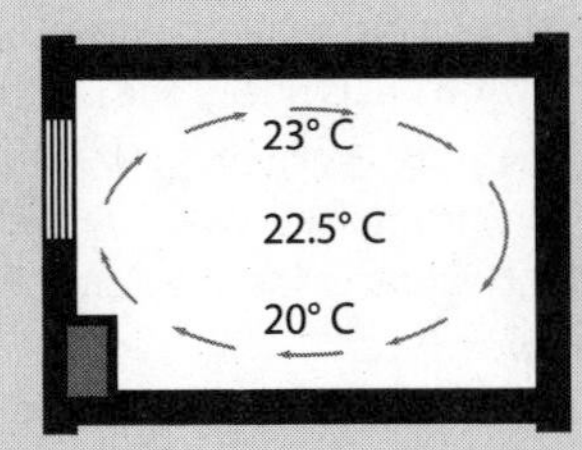

Electric Baseboard

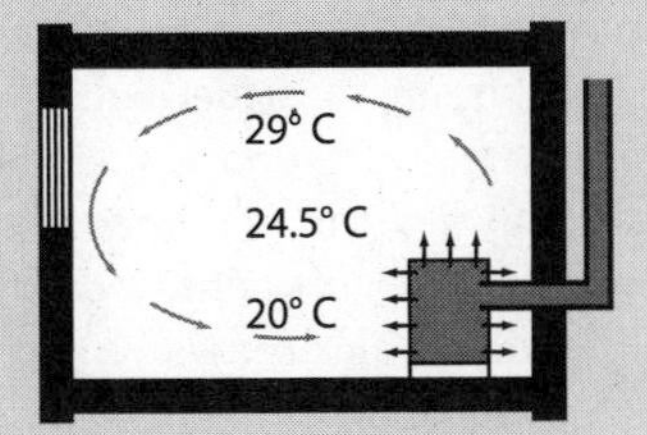

Iron Woodstove

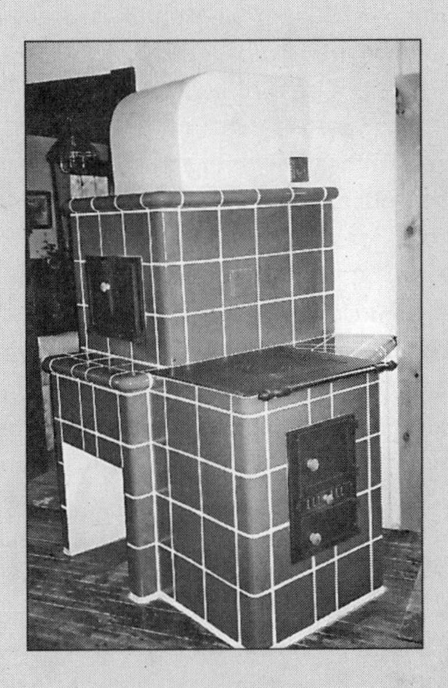

3. Heater surface temperature: A heater that has a high surface temperature, such as a radiator or woodstove, causes dust circulation, combustion of dust, and electric discharge of the room air. Electric discharge leads to "dead" air, or a predominance of positive ions. Air feels most vital when it has the same ion balance as is found in nature. Ideally this would be approximately five positive ions to four negative ions, but homes heated by forced-air or hot appliances create a predominance of positive ions. Dust circulation and electric

- It would be a radiant source.
- It would not rob the air of negative ions. (When air is forced through metal ductwork, negative ions will be attracted to the ductwork and room air ions will be depleted.)
- The appliance would not be hot enough to fry dust.
- It would not create "temperature monotony" (having all rooms the same temperature, which Building Biology considers unhealthy) or drafts.

discharge are major irritants to mucous membranes and cause many chronic illnesses and allergies. Since the surface temperatures of Kachelofens–Masonry Heaters are below 110 degrees Celsius, dust circulation, combustion of dust, and electric discharge of the room air do not occur.

4. Humidity: Room air should have a relative humidity of approximately 50 to 60 percent, which can be achieved only by radiant heat. Heating systems operating with mainly convection heat will bring the relative humidity in a room down to 30 percent. To compensate, some forced-air systems have built-in humidifiers, but these can cause condensation and mold buildup in the ductwork.
5. Temperature gradients: Convection heat creates horizontal layers of air in a room, with temperature differences up to 10 degrees Celsius from floor to ceiling, resulting in hot heads and cold feet. The temperature differences in rooms with radiant heat from Kachelofens–Masonry Heaters are only 1 to 2 degrees Celsius, meaning the room is evenly heated.
6. Electromagnetic fields: Heating systems with mainly convection heat (electric and hot-water baseboard heaters and hot-water radiators) create electromagnetic fields that cause electric stress. Permanent electric stress can be the cause of illnesses. Kachelofens–Masonry Heaters do not cause electromagnetic fields or electric stress.
7. Ionization of room air: Wood fire creates a negative ionization of the room air. Why is this important? An ion has either a positive or a negative charge. We have positive and negative ions in our body, but when we run, walk, work, or just generally move we lose negative ions. We are left with positive ions, or a positive charge in our body, and we need to find a source of negative ions to balance our positive charge. Wood fire is one of the best sources to recharge our body with negative ions.
8. Noise: The only noise created by Kachelofens–Masonry Heaters is the cozy crackling of the wood fire.
9. Environmental impact: Of all heating systems, the Kachelofen-Masonry Heater has the lowest overall impact on our environment, from production of the building materials to installation, to the amount of fuel required and pollution generated, to disposal after a lifetime of at least 80 years. Unlike a woodstove, which in cold climates must burn wood constantly to heat a home, a masonry oven is fired only for a short duration, fully burning the combustion gases and storing heat in its mass walls. It therefore uses far less wood than a woodstove and creates very little pollution in the form of smoke.

A study of Kachelofens–Masonry Heaters conducted by the Technical University of Vienna showed the following:

- There would be minimal byproducts of combustion.

Wood heat distributed through a masonry oven can fulfill these criteria. The masonry oven, not to be confused with other types of "fireplaces" or woodburning stoves, is designed to burn wood so that the gases are completely combusted. The generated heat circulates through multiple chambers within the oven and is distributed into the oven's massive walls before the relatively clean and cool

Criteria	Ideal	Kachelofen
Room Temperature	18 to 20° C	18 to 20° C
Temperature gradient	1 to 2° C	2 to 4° C
Wall temperature	20 to 22° C	18 to 20° C
Humidity	40 to 60 %	40 to 60 %
Air movement	<0.1 m/s	<0.1 m/s
Dust circulation	no	low
Odors	no	low and pleasant
Ionization	natural	natural
Noise	no/pleasant	no/pleasant
Design	individual	individual

The Baubiologische Institut Rosenheim (Germany) graded the various heating systems based on the criteria discussed above and came up with the following results:

Forced air/ fuel oil	7 points
Hot water in floor/ fuel oil	19 points
Wood-fired iron stove	21 points
Kachelofen–Masonry Heater	66 points

The masonry oven and its health, comfort, and ecological benefits are little known in North America, where forced-air heating is the norm. If you are interested in heating your home in this time-tested manner you will need to seek out a mason trained in the art of masonry oven building and installation. To find a certified mason in your vicinity you can refer to the member directory of The Masonry Heater Association of North America at mha-net.org.

Ernst Kiesling, an Austrian-educated structural engineer, has had a lifelong attraction to healthy living and green building methods. He has been involved with Kachelofens–Masonry Heaters for 31 years, starting out as a teacher for the profession at a vocational school in Austria and then going into business building individually designed Kachelofens–Masonry Heaters. After immigrating to Nova Scotia, Canada, he started Kiesling Construction Ltd. to bring the goodness of the Kachelofen – Masonry Heater to Canada. He can be contacted at Canadian Kachelofen, ermared@ns.sympatico.ca.

exhaust goes up the chimney. Most countries in northern Europe have developed this type of heating to perfection and masonry ovens are common there. There are many masons in the US trained in the art of masonry oven building. The **Masonry Heater Association of North America** has an informative website that lists trained and certified heater masons by location.

Combined Heating and Cooling Systems

Heat pumps are far more energy efficient than electric resistance heat and can be used for both heating and cooling. Heat pumps extract heat from outside air or, in some cases, from a water source. Air-source heat pumps are most common in areas where winter temperatures seldom fall below 30 degrees Fahrenheit and where summer cooling loads are high. As temperatures fall below 30 degrees, the heat pump must rely on electric resistance heating to make up the difference, at which point the system loses its economic advantage. The main advantages of a heat pump are that heating and cooling needs are met by a single unit, humidity is not added to the air, and operation is quiet.

Cooling Systems

Common types of air conditioners include condensing or refrigerated air conditioners, electric heat pumps as discussed above, and evaporative coolers.

Condensing air conditioners are available either as small units designed to cool one area of a home or as central air conditioners, which will cool an entire home via ductwork. Advantages of central air conditioners are their out-of-the-way location, quiet operation, integration with the forced-air heating system, and greater cooling capacity and efficiency than portable models. However, these central systems consume a lot of energy and cost up to seven times more to operate than evaporative cooling systems. It is important to choose an air conditioning unit that continues to blow air across the cooling coils for a time after the cooler is turned off. This allows any moisture remaining on the coils to be dried off, discouraging mold growth. Room air conditioners are less expensive to install than central air conditioners. Since they cool only designated areas, they save money and energy, but they do tend to be noisy.

Evaporative coolers are practical in very dry areas and are available either as a direct model, which adds humidity to the home, or an indirect model, which does not add humidity. The operating costs for evaporative coolers are significantly lower than those for condensing units, and evaporative units are fairly inexpensive to install. They bring fresh outdoor air into the living space and exhaust stale air. Evaporative coolers have a lower cooling capacity and work well only in low-humidity conditions, such as those found in the southwestern states. Another name for evaporative coolers is swamp coolers. They must be kept clean or they truly become swamps, filled with microorganisms.

When using mechanical air conditioning, you can save energy and money by keeping the windows closed. One exception to this rule is the case of evaporative coolers, which are more efficient when windows are left partially open. Air conditioners should be shut off and windows opened at night if it is cool outside. Do not cool unoccupied rooms or homes. Insulating all exterior ducting can save you at least 10 percent of the energy costs of

Chart 15.1: Heating and Cooling Systems

Type of system	How it works	Advantages	Disadvantages	Comments
Heating Systems				
Forced air heat	A fan pulls air through a heating unit and distributes the air throughout the house via ducts.	• Can be easily adapted for filtration, humidification, and dehumidification • Almost immediate response time • Inexpensive to operate	• Less comfortable than radiant heat • Stirs up and fries dust • Can exacerbate allergies • Ductwork is architecturally cumbersome • Leaky ducts can depressurize home • Noisy • Needs regular cleaning • Metal ductwork grounds negative ions • Fumes from gas or oil fuel can enter airstream • Insulation particles can enter airstream	• Many of the disadvantages of forced air can be rectified by adding filtration to the system at the furnace and where the air enters the room
Radiant hydronic floor heat	Hot water is run through tubing in or under the floor. Natural convection gently distributes heat.	• Even, comfortable heating • Comfortable at lower temperatures • Efficient • Not hot enough to fry dust • Silent • Low maintenance • Easy zonation • Invisible	• Slow response time • Initial installation costly • Does not filter air • Not practical for cooling	• Avoid metal tubing, which can transmit EMFs
Liquid-filled baseboard heaters	Hot liquid is circulated through fin tube baseboard units and radiates into the room.	• Heats quickly • Comfortable radiant heat • Not hot enough to fry dust • Less expensive than in-floor heating	• Baseboard units are dust traps • Limits furniture placement • Can be hot to touch	• Heated surfaces of baseboard units may outgas • Leaks (other than water) may be toxic
Electric radiant floor, wall, or ceiling heat	Electric current passes through resistant wiring embedded in walls, floors, or ceilings.	• Even heating • Comfortable radiant heat	• Expensive to run • Can create high levels of EMFs • Less expensive systems run hotter and fry dust	• Not recommended in a healthy home because of EMFs and high degree of energy consumption

Chart 15.1: Heating and Cooling Systems (cont'd.)

Type of system	How it works	Advantages	Disadvantages	Comments
Electric baseboard heating	Individual units are plugged in.	• Initial installation inexpensive and easy • Does not require centralized machinery • Puts heat only where required	• Expensive to run • Hot to touch • Traps and fries dust • Emits EMFs	• Heated surfaces may offgas
Woodburning stoves	Wood fire is contained in a noncombustible stove. Heat radiates into the room.	• Radiant heat source • No central equipment required • Inexpensive to install and operate	• Messy to run and requires high maintenance • Burn and fire hazard • Chimney can be subject to backdrafting • Burning wood produces more than 200 toxic byproducts of combustion and studies show higher rate of respiratory problems in children where woodstoves are the primary heat source • Most heat escapes up the chimney	• Not recommended in a healthy home • Choose the most efficient models available, burn hardwoods, and clean the flue often
Masonry heater (Kachelofen)	Heat from wood fire travels through a series of masonry chambers, is stored in the masonry mass, and slowly radiates into the room.	• Very efficient use of fuel • Requires less tending than conventional woodstoves • Burns cleaner • Produces comfortable radiant heat that does not fry dust or burn people • Inexpensive to operate, requires no further equipment • Can incorporate cookstove or oven • Can be an architectural feature • Short duration of fire time; full combustion of gases creates little pollution inside and outside the home	• Initial installation is costly • Generates a small amount of combustion byproducts	• Less convenient than central heating systems • Considered by Bau-Biologie as one of the most healthful ways to heat

Chart 15.1: Heating and Cooling Systems (cont'd.)

Type of system	How it works	Advantages	Disadvantages	Comments
Passive solar heating	Heat from the sun is captured through glazing and stored in building components with high thermal mass such as concrete and adobe walls and floors.	• No operation expenses • Does not consume fossil fuels • Does not fry or circulate dust	• Dependent on weather • Requires a relatively high degree of human interaction. • Must be incorporated into architecture	• For more information, refer to the Further Reading section
Heat pump	Heat or cold is extracted from outside air and transferred to inside air.	• Can be used for heating or cooling • Cost effective in mild climate • Quiet	• Not cost effective where temperatures are frequently below 30 degrees F. • Uses Freon (an atmospheric ozone depleter) as transfer medium	
Cooling Systems				
Central refrigerant coolers	Freon gas is passed through a condenser. Heat is transferred to the outdoors and the cool air is distributed throughout the house via ductwork.	• Can also dehumidify air • Will handle large cooling load • Can be quiet to operate if condenser is remote • Shares ductwork with central heating	• Expensive to operate • High energy consumption • Uses Freon (an atmospheric ozone depleter) • Requires maintenance to prevent mold	• Drip pan must be inspected and cleaned regularly for mold-free operation
Room refrigerant coolers	Freon gas is passed through a condenser. Heat is transferred to the outdoors and the cooled air is blown into the room.	• Inexpensive initial installation • Because it cools only designated areas, energy waste and expense are reduced	• High energy consumption • Uses Freon • Requires maintenance to prevent mold • Noisy	
Evaporative (swamp) coolers	Air is passed over a wet medium. As evaporation occurs, air is cooled and then blown into the home.	• Low cost initially and when in operation • Uses no CFCs or HCFCs • Requires 80% less energy than refrigerant coolers • Works well in hot, dry climates	• Subject to mold and other microorganism growth • Not suitable in humid conditions • Cannot take as large a load as refrigerant models • Can be noisy • Requires maintenance to keep mold-free and needs frost protection in cold winter climates	• Should be drained and cleaned monthly

cooling. Maintain systems regularly, keeping coils and filters clean. Locate the cooler in a shaded area.

Ventilation

Until the 1960s, ventilation in homes occurred naturally, obviating the need for intentional ventilation systems. Homes were loosely built, allowing enough outside air to make its way through the home to keep it fresh. By some accounts, this loose construction contributed to as many as three to four air exchanges per hour. Although there were ample air exchanges, there was also an unacceptable amount of energy required to run such a home, and uncontrolled ventilation through air leakage can cause serious harm to a building. Currently, with energy-efficient construction, much of the unintentional air exchange has been eliminated. However, while homes were built of more natural, nonpolluting materials in the past, in recent years indoor air has become at least five to ten times more polluted than outdoor air and it is often too polluted for optimal health. Although minimum air-exchange rates are enforced for commercial structures, this is generally not the case for residential construction, except where exhaust fans are mandated.

Like many other components essential to health, ventilation is considered an "extra" in standard construction. The American Society for Heating, Refrigeration, and Air Conditioning Engineers (ASHRAE) has set a standard of .35 air exchanges per hour, or 15 cubic feet per minute per resident, for residential ventilation. Although this may be sufficient to dispel pollutants created by human activity, it may not be enough to dispel the chemical pollution generated by standard construction or the thousands of other chemicals introduced into homes through furnishings, clothing, cleaning products, cosmetics, and other scented products. ASHRAE determines its requirements based on the level at which 80 percent of a test population feels comfortable. It should be noted that it is quite possible to feel comfortable in environments that are polluted enough to be detrimental to health. The human body has the ability to become accustomed to harmful chemicals, much as one might adapt over time to the toxic effects of tobacco smoke. Whether or not the ASHRAE standard is sufficient to meet health requirements is irrelevant because in fact most homes are not equipped with ventilation other than spot exhaust fans and do not meet the ASHRAE recommendations.

With tight construction, ventilation strategies are necessary in a healthy home to ensure fresh air and dispel odors from everyday living. Care should be taken to locate the fresh-air supply away from exhaust-air piping and in the best location for receiving an unpolluted airstream.

Air Filtration

The addition of filters to ventilation and forced-air heating and cooling systems allows for greater control of air quality. As discussed above, indoor air is often too polluted to properly nourish occupants. The first line of defense against such pollutants is to provide an ample supply of fresh outdoor air through ventilation. Unfortunately, "fresh" air, although considerably cleaner in most cases than indoor air, often contains allergens in the form of molds, pollens, and manufactured pollutants,

Chart 15.2: Ventilation Strategies

Type	Purpose	How it works	Advantages	Disadvantages	Comments
Natural ventilation	To bring fresh air into the home and exhaust stale air	Takes advantage of natural air patterns. Strategically placed openings encourage fresh air to move diagonally through the space, entering low and exiting high.	• Quiet • Free • Maintenance-free • Does not require energy to operate	• Can be drafty and create greater heating/cooling load • Air cannot be filtered • Allows for only minimal control • Requires high level of occupant participation • Suitable as sole means of ventilation throughout the year only in very temperate climates • Outdoor air must be clean	This strategy works best in mild climates and can be enhanced through various roof-ventilation techniques.
Exhaust fans	To remove localized pollution at the point of generation, primarily in kitchens and baths	Stale and moisture-laden air is sucked out of the house at the point of generation, using a powerful fan.	• Pollution is quickly removed before the rest of the home is affected	• Can depressurize home, causing infiltration and possible back-drafting	It is important to supply replacement air when fans are in operation. Exhaust fans are required by code in bathrooms and laundry rooms without operable windows.
Supply fans	To provide fresh air	A fan blows fresh outside air into the home, creating positive pressurization that forces stale air out.	• Inexpensive • Pressurization of home prevents contaminants from infiltrating from outdoors	• Cold drafts around fan in winter • Pressurization can cause hidden moisture problems as humid air is forced through wall openings and then condenses	Adequate and strategically placed vents are required to exhaust air. This is a good strategy for venting a basement. Supply fans are not suitable for dispelling kitchen- and bath-generated pollution.

Chart 15.2: Ventilation Strategies (cont'd.)

Type	Purpose	How it works	Advantages	Disadvantages	Comments
Balanced mechanical ventilation	To provide fresh air and exhaust stale air while controlling pressurization	A set of fans brings in fresh air through intake and distributes it, then exhausts stale air to the exterior.	• Provides balanced pressurization • Comes equipped with, or can be adapted for, various filtration strategies	• Does not moderate temperature or humidity of incoming air • Can be noisy • Relatively small fans are standard and are insufficient to handle large amounts of gas filtration	
Air-to-air heat exchange or HRV (heat recovery ventilator)	To supply fresh outdoor air into the home while exhausting stale air and maintaining indoor temperatures	Incoming fresh air passes through a series of chambers adjacent to outgoing exhaust air. Heat, but not air, is transferred.	• Reduces heating and cooling costs by recovering 60 to 80% of heat	• Chambers can be made of paper, which collects dirt, or plastic, which can outgas; choose one with metal chambers • More costly initially than other balanced ventilators • Causes condensation; must be maintained to remain mold-free	Most effective for tight homes in cold climates. Energy recovery ventilators (ERVs) also recover humidity VenMar Ventilation, Inc.
Fresh-air intake incorporated into forced-air system	To provide fresh air when the central forced-air system is operating	A 3" to 6" metal pipe with damper valve provides fresh air into the furnace supply stream.	• Inexpensive to retrofit • Ventilation supply air is preheated or precooled • Makes use of existing ductwork for distribution • Creates slight positive pressurization and can compensate for air lost through leaky ducts	• Operates only during heating or cooling season • Depends on a well-maintained heating and cooling system to deliver good-quality air	Screen all intake pipes to prevent rodent infestation.

including exhaust fumes, smoke, and pesticides. When your immediate surroundings are less than perfect, you may wish to incorporate some form of filtration into your home.

Home ventilation systems can easily be adapted to filter large particles like pollen and mold spores. However, most home ventilation systems are not equipped with very powerful fans and therefore cannot handle the air resistance created by some of the more efficient filtration methods, especially those designed to remove gases. Consequently, whole-house filtration is often more successfully combined with the forced-air distribution system. Standard filters used with most forced-air systems are designed primarily to prevent large particles from harming the motor, and are insufficient to effectively filter out small particles injurious to human health. Most forced-air equipment must be adapted to receive additional filtration systems. When equipped with good filters, a forced-air system will not only clean fresh intake air but also continue to clean air as it recirculates.

Filter efficiency rating systems such as the "dust spot" and "arrestance" systems have been developed by filter manufacturers to provide information about the ability of a filter to remove large particles from the airstream. This information is of limited use when evaluating filter effectiveness for removing small particles of less than 5 microns, which can be the most damaging to health. In 1999, the American Society of Heating, Refrigeration and Air Conditioning Engineers published a new filter rating system that goes by the acronym MERV. This stands for Minimum Efficiency Reporting Value and is a much better way of rating the ability of filters to remove small particles. The system currently rates filters on a scale of 1 to 16, with the higher number ratings representing filters that can remove smaller particles. Although they are currently not rated by the MERV system, a HEPA filter would likely rate a 17 or higher.

Adequate MERV filters are currently available that will fit into a standard furnace filter slot. For example, a MERV 8 filter is rated to remove greater than 70 percent of particles in the 3- to 10-micron range. This will remove most, but not all, mold spores and dust and should be considered as a much better alternative to the standard fibrous furnace filter. The **Filtrete Ultra Allergen Reduction Filter #1250** is a MERV 11 filter (removes 65 to 80 percent of 1- to 3-micron particles) manufactured by 3M. It is commonly available at Lowe's and Home Depot and will also fit in standard 1-inch furnace-filter slots.

While higher MERV-rated filters as well as HEPA systems are available, these more efficient filters tend to create more resistance, requiring a much larger filter to allow air to flow through them. They do not fit into or work well with standard HVAC systems. Note that when changing from a standard furnace filter to a more efficient filter it is important to replace it after one month's use before going to the regular three-month maintenance schedule recommended by the manufacturers because the filter will be overworked when first installed in a dirty environment. If the new type of filter continues to clog too quickly, there may be a larger than normal dust load in the building. John has observed this when an air path to the attic or crawlspace exists that pulls dirt or insulation fibers into the system.

Most mechanical filters that remove particles by filtration actually become more efficient as air flows through them. They remove particles as a sieve does. As the filter loads, the airflow slows and smaller particles can then be removed. The filter must be replaced before airflow is impeded. Electrostatic filters don't do as good a job of removing particles when they get dirty and must be cleaned often to achieve the manufacturer's stated MERV ratings.

Further Reading

Bower, John. *Understanding Ventilation: How to Design, Select and Install Residential Ventilation Systems.* The Healthy House Institute, 1995.

Mazria, Edward. *The Passive Solar Energy Book.* Rodale Press, 1979.

Chart 15.3: MERV Ratings Compared to Other Filter Ratings

	Particle size range			Test			
MERV	**3 to 10 µm**	**1 to 3 µm**	**.3 to 1 µm**	**Arrestance**	**Dust spot**	**Particle size range, µm**	**Applications**
1	<20%	—	—	<65%	<20%	>10	• Typical residential filters • Pollen, dust mites
2	<20%	—	—	65–70%	<20%		
3	<20%	—	—	70–75%	<20%		
4	<20%	—	—	>75%	<20%		
5	20–35%	—	—	80–85%	<20%	3.0–10	• 1" residential pleated filter • Pollen, dust, dust mites, most molds, most spores
6	35–50%	—	—	>90%	<20%		
7	50–70%	—	—	>90%	20–25%		
8	>70%	—	—	>95%	25–30%		
9	>85%	<50%	—	>95%	40–45%	1.0–3.0	• Moderate efficiency residential pleated filter (some may need furnace modification for installation) • All of above and *Legionella*
10	>85%	50–65%	—	>95%	50–55%		
11	>85%	65–80%	—	>98%	60–65%		
12	>90%	>80%	—	>98%	70–75%		
13	>90%	>90%	<75%	>98%	80–90%	0.3–1.0	• Specialty filter (usually need furnace modification for installation) • All of above and smoke, bacteria
14	>90%	>90%	75–85%	>98%	90–95%		
15	>90%	>90%	85–95%	>98%	~95%		
16	>95%	>95%	>95%	>98%	>95%		

Chart 15.4: Filtration Strategies

Filter type	Purpose	How it works	Efficiency	Advantages	Disadvantages	Comments
Standard furnace filter, MERV 1–4	Filters out large particulate matter to safeguard the motor, not the inhabitants	A coarse, 1"-thick filter traps large particles.	Removes less than 20% of particulate matter; does not significantly remove small particles	• Inexpensive • Easy to change	• Indoor air quality not significantly improved • Does not remove significant levels of mold spores	Can easily be replaced with 1" pleated panel filter, which will raise efficiency to MERV 6–11
Medium efficiency extended surface (pleated panel) filter, MERV 6–11	Particulate filter	Air is strained through a pleated (extended surface area) filter that maintains airflow.	Removes 20–70% of particulate matter	• Relatively inexpensive • Sufficient for most general filtration • Airflow resistance can be low enough to use with most HVAC ventilation systems • Removes many mold spores	• Filtration is inadequate for very polluted environments and/or very sensitive people • Does not filter out gaseous pollution	Many are now available that will work with standard HVAC systems. Media filters become more efficient with time as pores become smaller, but air resistance increases.
HEPA (high efficiency particulate air) filter	Particulate filter	Polyester or fiberglass fibers are bound with synthetic resins, creating a medium with extremely small pores.	Removes over 99.97% of particulate matter at 0.3 microns	• Can remove minute particles for extremely clean air • Can remove cigarette smoke and almost all mold spores	• High airflow resistance requires powerful fan • Expensive • May require custom design • Does not filter out gaseous pollution such as VOCs	Not commonly used in residential filtration. A carbon post-filter will help eliminate odor generated by the HEPA filter. An inexpensive, frequently changed prefilter will extend the life of the HEPA filter.

Chart 15.4: Filtration Strategies (cont'd.)

Filter type	Purpose	How it works	Efficiency	Advantages	Disadvantages	Comments
Electro-static precipitator (ionizer)	Particulate precipitator	Mechanism is mounted to ductwork, which statically charges dust. Dust is collected at oppositely charged plates in a filter.	Removes 90% of particulate matter when clean	• No resistance to airflow • Efficient when clean • Does not require replacement	• Must be adapted for residential use • Ozone is produced as byproduct of high voltage • Relatively expensive • Does not filter out gaseous pollution • Efficient only when clean • Generates EMFs	Plates must be cleaned frequently.
Electrostatic air filter (passive)	Particulate filter	Electrostatic charge is generated by friction as air moves through special media.	Removes 10 to 15% of particulate matter	• Good for large mold spores and pollen • No customization required on some filters used with HVAC • Inexpensive (washable/reusable)	• Not efficient for capturing small particles • Limited efficiency • Does not filter out gaseous pollution • Requires frequent cleaning to maintain filter efficiency	May be substituted for standard furnace filters. An inexpensive way to relieve pollen and mold allergies. Medium efficiency extended surface (pleated panel) filters are making these obsolete.
TFP (turbulent flow precipitator)	Particulate precipitator	Turbulent airstream "drops" particles into collection space, where there is no airflow.	Manufacturer claims 100% removal of particulate matter	• No resistance to airflow • Can be used with ventilator • Very low maintenance.	• Does not filter gaseous pollution	Actual performance varies widely.

Chart 15.4: Filtration Strategies (cont'd.)

Filter type	Purpose	How it works	Efficiency	Advantages	Disadvantages	Comments
Partial by-pass filter	Absorption of gaseous pollutants	Granules of absorptive material are held in place and separated by a metallic grid. Some air passes through the medium and some flows past unrestricted.	Efficiency varies widely based on amount of air that bypasses the filter	• Allows some air to flow through, thereby cutting down air resistance and requiring less powerful fan	• Not suitable where air is highly polluted • Not suitable in ventilator	Works in conjunction with HVAC, where the same air is repeatedly run through the filter.
Activated carbon filter	Adsorption of gaseous pollutants (not for particles)	Gases cling to many-faceted carbon granules.	Varies	• Effectively removes gases with high molecular weight • Offered in standard furnace sizes for low-pollution situations	• Does not remove certain lightweight pollutants such as formaldehyde or carbon monoxide • Filters become contaminated with use and can release pollutants if not changed	Can be treated to remove more gases. Must be changed regularly per manufacturer's recommendations.
Activated alumina	Adsorption and transformation of gaseous pollutants (not for particles)	Activated alumina is impregnated with potassium permanganate. It acts as a catalyst in changing the chemical composition of harmful gases and also acts through adsorption.	Varies	• Will remove gases not removed by carbon, including formaldehyde • Lasts longer than carbon	• Not as adsorptive as carbon • More expensive than carbon	Activated alumina changes color when depleted.

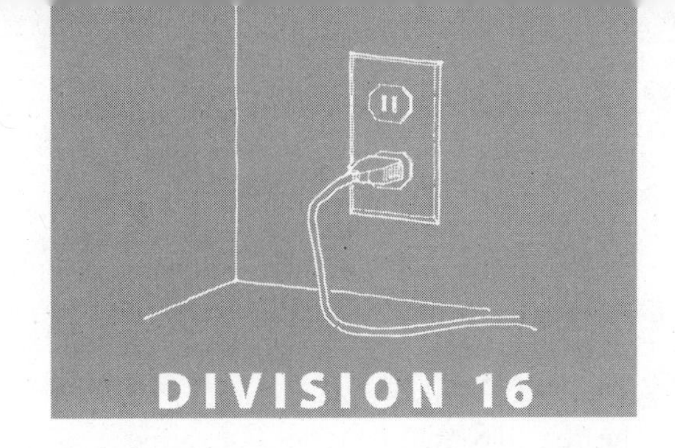

Electrical

Electromagnetic Fields

Electric and magnetic fields are commonly discussed as if they were a single entity termed electromagnetic fields or EMFs. In fact, the two phenomena, although interrelated, are distinctly different and they will be discussed separately in this chapter. Chart 16.1 presents a comparison of the two.

Magnetic Fields

Basic Home Wiring and Net Current

Although the relationship between human health and elevated fields remains controversial, there are definite safety concerns associated with wiring techniques that cause magnetic fields. In recognition of such hazards, the National Electrical Code has mandated safer wiring. Your electrician may be puzzled if you declare that you want a home free of all elevated magnetic fields, but if you say you want a home free of net current in compliance with the electrical code, you are saying the same thing in a language electricians understand.

Most household wiring consists of 110-volt lines. If you were to peel back the outer insulating plastic on a piece of Romex, the most common wiring used, three strands would be revealed — one black, one white, and a third either green or bare copper. The black strand is referred to as the hot wire because it draws electricity from the breaker box or panel and delivers it to light fixtures and appliances. The white wire, called the neutral, returns the electricity to the panel after it is used. The green or bare copper wire is the ground wire. Under normal conditions, it does not carry electricity. However, if a malfunction such as a short occurs, it serves as a fail-safe protective device, carrying power back to the ground until the breaker is tripped and the power to the faulty circuit is cut off, thereby helping to prevent shock and electrocution.

When the electrical system is functioning as it should, the amount of electricity flowing out to an appliance through the hot wire is equal to the amount of electricity flowing back through the neutral wire. This equal and opposite flow of current through the wires creates a net current that cancels to zero, which is the desired condition. When, for various reasons, unequal supply and return currents are unable to cancel each other out, a net current is present and a magnetic field is created.

A second condition that creates net current with associated magnetic fields occurs when the neutral and hot wires are separated by distance. When Romex wiring is used, the hot and neutral wires run adjacent to one another inside the plastic insulating sheathing, allowing them to cancel each other out. In an older wiring system known as knob and tube, the hot and neutral wires were run on separate studs. The distance between the wires resulted in an uncancelled magnetic field. There was also no grounding. Although now prohibited by code, this dangerous system of wiring, along with its associated elevated magnetic fields, is still found in many older homes.

The National Electrical Code prohibits the production of net current. This requirement should protect people from elevated magnetic fields as well. Unfortunately, subtle code violations resulting in the production of net current frequently occur, not only causing elevated magnetic fields but also increasing the risk of fire and electrocution.

We have identified several commonly used wiring techniques that create very high

Chart 16.1: Comparison of Electric and Magnetic Fields

Electric fields	Magnetic fields
Flow in straight lines in all directions from the source unless conductors attract them	Radiate out from the source, flowing in loops
Can be easily shielded	Difficult and expensive to shield (even lead is not effective)
Attracted by conductors such as metal, saltwater bodies, and people	Penetrate all normal building materials
Present when switches for machinery are off or on	Occur only when appliances are switched on and current is flowing
Not widely recognized presently in conventional circles as a health threat	Safe-exposure limits not regulated by the US government, though Sweden has set limits
Reportedly affect the nervous system and can cause insomnia, anxiety, depression, aggressive behavior, and a higher risk of leukemia[1]	Reportedly affect cellular function and have been statistically linked in some studies with increased cancer cell growth rate, Alzheimer's, miscarriage, and birth defects, while some sensitive individuals report physical reactions
Electrical code permits but does not mandate wiring for reduced electric fields	Electrical code offers protection against exposure to magnetic fields produced by wiring in the structure, with some exceptions
Proper use of electric field meters requires expertise	Easily measured with a gaussmeter

magnetic fields. Although these techniques are considered to be code violations by most code interpreters because they create net current, they often go unnoticed by building inspectors. Case studies 16.1 and 16.2 are accounts of such occurrences. Following are specifications for wiring techniques and inspections for preventing and detecting elevated magnetic fields in wiring:

- **All wiring shall be performed in strict accordance with the National Electrical Code.**
- **The ganging of neutral wires from different branch circuits is prohibited.**
- **Hot and neutral wires must be bundled together, as in Romex. Separate wires following separate paths are prohibited.**
- **Bonding screws shall be removed from the neutral bus of all subpanels per manufacturer's instructions.**
- **When wiring a half-switch outlet using two separate breakers for each half of the outlet, the two neutral wires must not make electrical contact. This is accomplished by breaking off the prescored conductive tabs between the two sections of the outlet per manufacturer's instructions.**
- **Neutral wires on half-switched outlets shall not be mixed. They shall remain paired with corresponding hot wires.**
- **When wiring enters an electrical box from more than one circuit, care must be taken to ensure that the wires from the different circuits are isolated from one another so that electricity return paths are not shared. This can be done by installing wiring so that all wiring entering an electrical box is from the same circuit.**
- **At the time of the final electrical installation, and in the presence of the general contractor, architect, or owner, the electrician shall apply a minimum load of three amps to the distal end of each electrical circuit. The home shall be inspected under load using a gaussmeter. Any elevated ambient magnetic fields greater than 0.5 milligauss will indicate the presence of net current. These measurements should be taken about a foot away from switches or outlets as the levels right at the switch or outlet will generally be greater than 0.5.**
- **It is the responsibility of the electrical contractor to locate and eliminate net current caused by the electrical installation.**
- **The home shall be reinspected for any net current resulting from the work of other trades in the completed building.**

An inspection should be performed after electrical installation but before wall surfacing is installed so that any net current resulting from errors in the electrical installation can be determined and easily remedied. The electrician should be responsible for correcting these errors. Reinspecting after the surfacing materials are installed will help determine if other trades have caused damage to the electrical system. For example, a nail might penetrate the wiring and cause electrical problems. This damage would not be the fault of the electrician, but the electrician would need to correct it.

Magnetic Fields from Three- and Four-Way Switches

Lights switched from two different locations are called three-way switches. When lights are switched from three or more locations, they

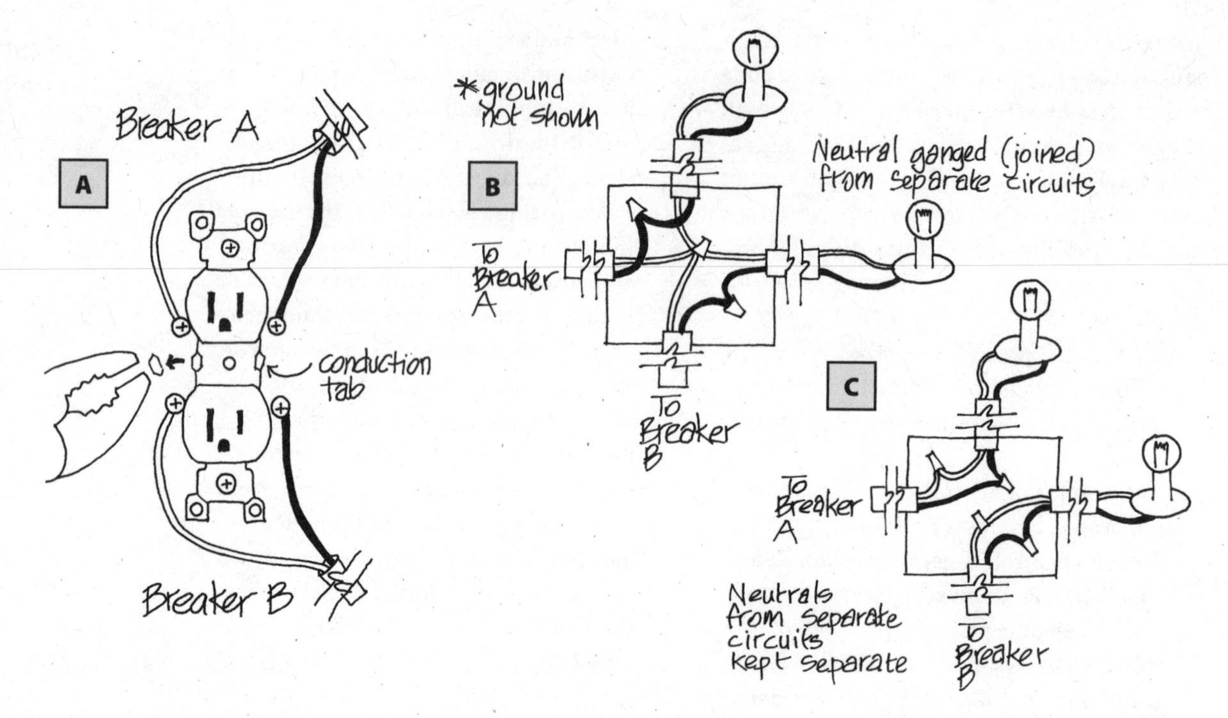

A: 1/2 switched outlet. Both hot and neutral pre-scored conduction tabs must be snapped off when the upper and lower outlets are supplied by separate breakers.

B: Ganging Neutrals.This wiring configuration is wrong and will create net current and magnetic fields.

C: This diagram shows the correct configuration, which will not generate magnetic fields.

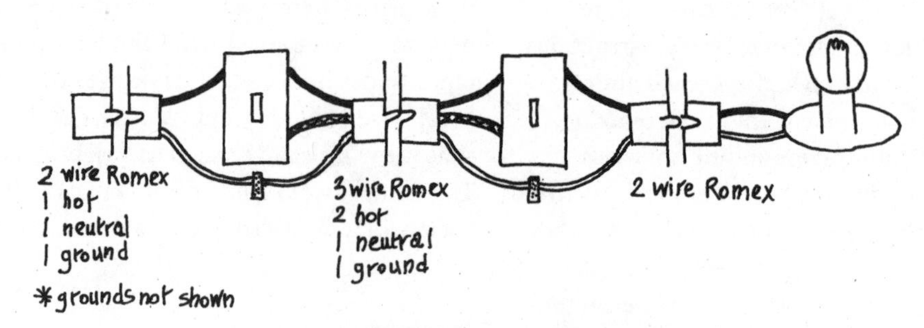

Properly wired 3-way switch.

are called four-way switches. A correctly wired three- or four-way switch will not emit magnetic fields. However, these switches are often wired incorrectly and thus become a source of magnetic fields that can radiate throughout the room. To avoid improperly wired three- or four-way switches, specify the following:

- **Three-wire Romex shall be used between the switches when wiring a three-way switch (see illustration). If alternate wire is used, it shall be twisted.**
- **Each three- or four-way switch must be controlled by a single breaker.**
- **All wiring for three- or four-way switches shall be contained in a single run of wire or a single metal conduit. All runs not in a conduit must be bundled.**

Fields from Dimmer Switches

Dimmer switches are a source of magnetic and radio frequency fields. If these switches are used, they should be located at a distance from seating and sleeping areas. The most expensive name-brand dimmers tend to emit smaller fields. Choose a model that emits no fields when all the way on or all the way off.

Magnetic Fields from Panels and Subpanels

Many electrical panels and subpanels emit substantially elevated magnetic fields. This problem arises because breaker and neutral bus bars are configured so that the neutral and hot wires are separated once fastened in place, causing magnetic fields as discussed earlier. Some electrical panels are configured with the neutral bus bar split to run alongside the breakers. To cancel the fields, the hot and neutral wires would be the same length and installed beside one another. We recommend that such reduced field configuration panels and wiring be specified as indicated below:

- **Panels and subpanels shall be configured so that hot and neutral field cancellation is possible.**
- **The following panels and subpanels are acceptable: Siemens EQIII, standard load center electrical panels, and subpanels with split neutral.**
- **Hot and neutral wires from the same run are to be installed adjacent to one another.**
- **Hot and neutral wire lengths shall be equal.**

Dielectric Unions

A dielectric union is a plastic joint that acts as an insulator, preventing the passage of electricity between conductive materials. In a typical home, conductive gas and water lines come into contact with appliances in several places. For example, water lines feed into refrigerators with icemakers, and gas lines feed into motorized furnaces. Should a fault occur in the appliance, wayward electricity will be distributed through the piping unless a dielectric union is used to isolate the appliance from the utility pipes. "Electrified" piping is undesirable for the reasons listed below:

- Magnetic fields will radiate out from the pipes.
- Net current in gas lines is an explosion hazard.
- Pipes carrying net current can become an electrocution hazard.
- Electric current flowing through pipes causes electrolysis, which results in decomposition of the pipes.

CASE STUDY 16.1

Magnetic Field Caused by Wiring Errors

John was called to the home of a client who was concerned about the high magnetic field in the apartment she was renting. The living room, dining room, and kitchen showed a reading of around 16 milligauss. After carefully tracing the wires, John discovered the problem. The apartment had two light switches by the front door. One switch controlled the outdoor lights and the other the living room lights. The two switches were controlled by different circuit breakers. When the switches were wired into the box, the neutral wires were joined with a single electrical connector nut, a situation known in the trade as "ganged neutrals." The problem was easily remedied with the addition of a 14-cent electrical nut to separate the two neutral wires. The magnetic fields throughout the house dropped to 0.5 milligauss, considered to be an acceptable level.

Discussion

This case study illustrates a simple code violation that went unnoticed by the electrical inspector. If the inspector had used a gaussmeter, the error would have been easily detected before final closeout. Surprisingly, such testing is not common practice. Had the tenant not used a gaussmeter, the code violation might never have been revealed.

The installation of dielectric unions is an inexpensive safeguard against a rarely occurring phenomenon but one with potentially devastating results. We recommend specifying dielectric unions in healthy homes as follows:

When permitted by code, metallic gas and water lines shall have dielectric unions installed wherever they enter into contact with any electrical appliance.

Bonding and Grounding

As discussed in Division 2, it is important to choose a site that is free from elevated magnetic fields generated from overhead power lines. Magnetic fields caused by faulty wiring in a neighbor's home also can be transferred into your home through utility service lines. Because electricity will follow all available paths, metal plumbing, gas lines, cable TV lines, and telephone lines can become pathways for uninvited net current. Consequently, taking simple precautions to prevent such an occurrence is prudent when site conditions allow. Although the National Electrical Code mandates grounding and bonding, it does not dictate the configuration of utilities entering residential structures. By grouping the entry points of all utilities and providing proper bonding, any net current traveling through public utility lines will be shunted back without ever entering the home. However, pathways of elevated magnetic fields may be created in your yard. These too can be blocked, but will require the expertise of a knowledgeable consultant.

If site conditions do not allow for the grouping of all utilities, then testing with a gaussmeter for unwanted fields with the house power turned off would be a prudent safety precaution, both during construction and periodically thereafter. If new magnetic fields are

CASE STUDY 16.2

Magnetic Fields

The importance of checking the electrical installation under load with a gaussmeter before occupancy is demonstrated in this case study. An electromagnetically sensitive client consulted with John by telephone throughout the construction of her home, which was built according to specifications similar to those outlined in this book. After the client moved into her new home, she began experiencing symptoms that occur when she is exposed to elevated magnetic fields, such as ringing in the ears and inability to concentrate. Using a gaussmeter, she discovered that about half of the home registered over 5 milligauss. She called John in a state of panic, convinced that her house was ruined and that she would never be able to live in it.

John contacted the client's electrician and offered to help him diagnose the problem over the telephone. Under John's guidance, the electrician conducted field testing with the client's gaussmeter. From the measurements, it became clear to John that the problem was located in the subpanel controlling a section of the house. At that point, the electrician immediately realized what he had forgotten to do. Some panels and subpanels are interchangeable except for a single screw that must be removed from the neutral bus bar to electrically isolate it from the ground wires in the panel. Called a bonding screw, it was causing net current in all circuits in the subpanel. The electrician simply removed the bonding screw and the magnetic fields dropped in an instant to less than 0.2 milligauss.

detected throughout the structure before it is energized, there is reasonable cause to suspect that fields are entering from an outside source. At this point, consult an expert who can properly block them. Because neighborhood conditions may change over time, fields should be checked regularly.

Along with proper bonding and grounding, grouping the entry points of all utilities will also provide more protection against lightning damage. However, this is not a substitute for lightning rods and lightning surge protection, which are designed to protect the home during a lightning storm.

The following are specifications for preventing the entry of magnetic fields through utility services:

- **All utilities, including telephone, cable TV, gas, and water, shall enter the building at approximately the same location, within a four-foot radius.**
- **All utilities entering the structure shall be properly bonded immediately prior to entry in accordance with the National Electrical Code (NEC).**
- **Bonds or grounds shall occur at only one point along each utility in accordance with the NEC.**
- **All utilities shall be tested with a gaussmeter when the house power is turned off. If magnetic fields are detected, inform the owner or architect immediately.**

Electromagnetic Fields: Challenging Unsafe Limits

ANDRÉ FAUTEUX

Take on the military, government, electric utilities, appliance and cell-phone manufacturers, and the owners of television, radio, and other high frequency antennas and you're in for a major fight. The stakes are huge because since 2003 insurance companies no longer cover eventual (because still unproven) damages caused by electromagnetic fields (EMFs). These are emitted by all from the smallest electrical devices and grounding circuits to high-tension power lines and radar systems.

"Scientists who have persisted in publicly raising the issue of harmful effects of any portion of the electromagnetic spectrum were discredited, and their research grants were taken away," says orthopedic surgeon Robert O. Becker.[a] In 2000, the double Nobel prize candidate stated,"I have no doubt in my mind that, at the present time, the greatest polluting element in the Earth's environment is the proliferation of electromagnetic fields."[b]

Power utilities and the communications industry are especially powerful, says David Carpenter, director of the Institute for Health and the Environment at the State University of New York (Albany). "They have infiltrated the world of science and become the dominant spokespersons to government and the public on this issue," he said in a telephone interview. "There's a huge amount of conflict of interest involved."[c]

Up to now, industry's public relations spin doctors have delivered. Most lay people, scientists, and journalists still scoff at the idea that EMFs could be dangerous. But the tide is turning. In recent years it seems not a month or season has gone by without another alarming study being published. PR spin is spinning out of control.

Since 1979, more than a dozen epidemiological studies have associated child leukemia with overexposure to residential magnetic fields. They found that the risk of leukemia doubled when the 24-hour average dose of EMFs measured as low as 1.4 milligauss in young boys. Some studies even found the risk quadrupled above 3 or 4 milligauss. Based on these studies, in 2001 the International Agency for Research on Cancer (IARC) classified residential — 60 hertz or Extremely Low Frequency (ELF) — magnetic fields as "possibly carcinogenic."[d] In Quebec, where 73 percent of homes are heated with cheap electricity, one out of five children receives a daily average dose of at least 2 milligauss, according to McGill University professor and Hydro-Québec researcher Jan Erik Deadman. Quebec also has the highest rate of child cancer in Canada (16.5 cases per 100,000 children), according to statistics obtained from the Public Health Agency of Canada. Besides ionizing radiation (X-rays), there are few proven causes of child cancer but many are suspected, including exposure to EMFs, says IARC, which is part of the World Health Organization (WHO).

Pressed by industry lobbyists, WHO has flip-flopped on whether to recommend countries take action to reduce public exposure. In the absence of direct proof of a biological mechanism by which EMFs damage genes, WHO still stands by the 1,000 milligauss daily public exposure limit recommended by the International Commission on Non-Ionizing Radiation Protection (ICNIRP).[e] But this limit only aims to avoid immediate effects of acute exposure, such as inducing current in the human body. It does not address cancer or other risks from long-term exposure.

Since magnetic fields are generated by the flow of electric current and since global power demand is always on the rise, public exposure has multiplied. Electric fields are generated when an appliance is plugged to receive voltage but not necessarily turned on to allow current flow. Few health studies have focused on electric fields. However, in 2007 British scientists discovered that electrically charged particles increase the risk of asthma because they stick to lung and respiratory tract tissue.[f]

In May 2007, the medical journal *The Lancet* criticized WHO for ignoring important evidence while developing international health guidelines.[g] WHO's EMF research project was also discredited for being 50 percent financed by industry. "Just months after leaving his post as the head of WHO's EMF project, Mike Repacholi is now in business as an industry consultant," reported *Microwave News*.[h] Repacholi denies ever putting industry's interests above the public's.

WHO responded by acknowledging that further EMF research is needed, that "the use of precautionary approaches is warranted" and that "exposure limits should be based on a thorough examination of all the relevant scientific evidence." However, it also stated that "assuming that the association is causal, the number of cases of childhood leukaemia worldwide that might be attributable to [EMF] exposure...represents 0.2 to 4.9 percent of the total annual incidence of leukaemia cases, estimated to be 49,000 worldwide in 2000. Thus, in a global context, the impact on public health, if any, would be limited and uncertain."[i]

This assertion is challenged by experts such as Carpenter. From 1980 to 1987, he coordinated EMF studies as head of the New York State Power Lines Project. "WHO is grossly underestimating the impact," he said in a telephone interview. "It is ignoring exposures from appliances, radio frequencies (from wireless appliances and antennas, etc.), as well as other exposures outside of homes, for example in school. In the mid-1980s, the Savitz study concluded 10–15 percent of all child cancers resulted from magnetic field exposure from powerlines. Nobody pointed out any errors in Savitz's logic. It is not unreasonable to say the total contribution of EMFs is 20 to 35 percent of child cancers. In my mind, the evidence is overwhelming."

Hundreds of medical studies have also linked various sources of EMFs to numerous ailments and diseases, ranging from depression to skin, eye, heart, reproductive, and neurological problems. That's why a number of public health experts have mandated or recommended stricter exposure guidelines and regulations to protect public health:

- Physicians Suzanne and Pierre Déoux,[j] French experts in healthy housing, recommend keeping these distances from transmission lines: 250 meters from 400 kilovolt lines, 150 meters from 225 kilovolt lines, 100 meters from 63 to 90 kilovolt lines, 40 meters from 20 kilovolt lines, and 5 to 10 meters from transformers. These are conservative by North American standards since magnetic fields are weaker in Europe, where 220-volt tension is used. (Electric fields are thus higher and more worrisome there.)
- In January 2007, the Connecticut Department of Public Health recommended imposing a 10 milligauss limit at the edge of rights-of-way

(land reserved for passing powerlines). Connecticut Light and Power's consultants (including Mike Repacholi) claim 100 milligauss is a safe limit.

- In 1996, Sweden recommended that new homes and schools be built at least 75 meters from powerlines and electrical equipment to avoid exposures above 2 milligauss.[l]
- Since 2000 in Switzerland, new electrical lines and equipment must emit below 10 milligauss in areas where people spend several hours a day.[m]
- Ontario and Wisconsin politicians have proposed legislation requiring that utilities stop using the ground as a return path for over 70 percent of electrical current. Ground currents often harm farm animals as well as humans worldwide.[n]
- Since 1999, several jurisdictions limit the power densities emitted by new or modified base cellular telephone antennas. In Switzerland and Toronto, for example, they must be 90 percent lower than the international standard of 1,000 microwatts per square centimeter.[o]
- In 2007, Carpenter led a group of experts who reviewed 2,000 scientific studies before declaring that current EMF public safety limits are inadequate to protect public health.[p] They recommended: a 1 milligauss limit for housing adjacent to all new or upgraded power lines and a 2 milligauss limit for all other new construction; a 1 milligauss limit for existing housing to protect children and pregnant women; and a limit of 0.1 microwatt per square centimeter (also 0.614 volts per meter) for outdoor cumulative exposure to radio frequencies.

While outdoor sources are not always the dominant source of electropollution, many countries and public utility commissions in California, Colorado, Connecticut, and Hawaii have adopted "prudent avoidance"[q] policies. These strike a balance between protecting public health from potential effects of EMFs and implementing reasonable- or modest-cost mitigation measures to lower public exposure. Such efforts send clear signals to building owners: they too should apply simple and affordable mitigation measures because in most cases the dominant sources of EMFs originate indoors.

a. Robert O. Becker. *Cross Currents*. Tarcher, 1990, page 300.
b. Linda Moulton Howe. *British Cell Phone Safety Alert and an Interview with Robert O. Becker, M.D* [online]. [Cited November 23, 2007.] Council on Wireless Technology Impacts, 2000. energy fields.org/science/becker.html
c. See Albany.edu.ihe.
d. International Agency for Research on Cancer. *IARC Finds Limited Evidence that Residential Magnetic Fields Increase Risk of Childhood Leukaemia* [online]. [Cited November 23, 2007.] Press Release No. 136, June 27, 2001. iarc.fr/ENG/Press_Releases/archives/pr136a.html
e. International Commission on Non-Ionizing Radiation Protection. *Guidelines for Limiting Exposure to Time-Varying Electric, Magnetic, and*

Electromagnetic Fields (Up to 300 GHz) [online]. [Cited December 10, 2007.] icnirp.org/documents/emfgdl.pdf

f. K.S. Jamieson et al. "The Effects of Electric Fields on Charged Molecules and Particles in Individual Microenvironments." *Atmospheric Environment*. Vol. 41, no. 25 (April 2007), pp. 5224–5235.

g. Maria Cheng. "WHO Criticized for Neglecting Evidence" [online]. [Cited November 27, 2007.] ABC News, May 7, 2007. abcnews.go.com/Health/wireStory?id=3149740 See also Andrew D. Oxman et al. "Use of Evidence in WHO Recommendations" [online]. [Cited December 10, 2007.] *The Lancet*. Vol. 369, no. 9576 (June 2, 2007), pp. 1883–1889. thelancet.com/journals/lancet/article/PIIS0140673607606758/abstract

h. "It's Official: Mike Repacholi is an Industry Consultant." *Microwave News*. Vol. 26, no. 8 (November 13, 2006), pp. 1–3.

i. World Health Organization. *Extremely Low Frequency Fields* [online]. [Cited December 10, 2007.] Environmental Health Criteria Monograph No. 238, 2007. who.int/peh-emf/publications/elf_ehc/en/index.html

j. See medieco.info.

k. "Public Health Officials Urge Precaution to Limit Cancer Risk" [online]. [Cited December 10, 2007.] *Microwave News*. Vol. 27, no. 1, pp. 1–3. microwavenews.com/docs/mwn.1-07.pdf

l. J. M. Danze et al. *L'habitat sain? L'électrosmog: le maîtriser, le connaître et s'en protéger*. Editions Marco Pietteur, 2002.

m. Swiss Agency for the Environment, Forests and Landscape. *Electrosmog in the Environment* [online]. [Cited December 10, 2007.] Swiss Federal Office for the Environment, 2005. bafu.admin.ch/php/modules/shop/files/pdf/phptbA19J.pdf

n. *Electrical Pollution Solutions* [online]. [Cited November 27, 2007.] electricalpollution.com

o. City of Toronto. *Reports and Publications: Radiation* [online]. [Cited December 10, 2007.] toronto.ca/health/hphe/radiation/radiofrequency.htm

p. David Carpenter and Cindy Sage, eds. *BioInitiative Report: A Rationale for a Biologically-Based Public Exposure Standard for Electromagnetic Fields (ELF and RF)* [online]. [Cited December 10, 2007.] BioInitiative Working Group, August 31, 2007. bioinitiative.org/report/docs/report.pdf

q. Leeka I. Kheifets. *The Precautionary Principle and EMF* [online]. [Cited December 10, 2007.] who.int/pehemf/meetings/southkorea/en/Leeka_Kheifets_principle_.pdf

Other excellent sources of information on EMFs are: powerwatch.org.uk/docs/emhealth.asp; next-up.org; and buildingbiology.net (to find an EMF inspector in the US and Canada).

André Fauteux, a journalist by training, has specialized in healthy housing since 1990. A former *Montreal Gazette* reporter, in 1994 he launched the newsletter *La Maison du 21e siècle* (21st-Century Housing), which in 1997 became Canada's first green-home magazine. See 21esiecle.qc.ca.

CASE STUDY 16.3

Net Current in Utilities

After purchasing a gaussmeter, an electrician was surprised to discover an elevated magnetic field throughout his entire driveway and a portion of his home. Upon learning that the field did not decline when he shut off the power to his home at the main breaker, he concluded that the source of the field was from net current in the gas line. A gas company technician visited the site and confirmed that the gas line was carrying electricity. There was no cause for concern, he said, because the amount of electricity was small.

The electrician was not comforted by such reassurances. As a specialist in complex wiring techniques for boats and marinas, he was familiar with the problems of electrolysis and galvanic action resulting from electricity straying from its intended path. He had even witnessed boats at the local marina whose metal had gradually dissolved from exposure to net current. Thus, the electrician reasoned, the net current in his plumbing and gas lines would cause the lines to deteriorate at an accelerated rate. After informing the gas company that the galvanic action in the pipes was a liability for the company because of the possibility of an explosion, the electrician was finally able to persuade the them to take his complaint seriously.

Measuring Magnetic Fields

Magnetic fields are measured with a gaussmeter. A homeowner might consider purchasing a gaussmeter for one or more of the following reasons:

- to determine safe distances from various household appliances
- to help detect wiring errors that not only produce magnetic fields but also may be fire and electrocution hazards
- as a periodic safety check to determine that no new problems have developed in household appliances
- as a periodic safety check to ensure that no new magnetic fields are entering the home through utility lines

There are two basic types of gaussmeters: single and triple axis. Single-axis meters tend to be less expensive and are slightly more difficult for a novice to use because they must be rotated to align with the flow of the magnetic field in order to detect it. Orienting a triple-axis meter with a field is not necessary because this meter requires positioning only within the range of the field. Less expensive gaussmeters will give false readings when measuring certain magnetic fields such as those generated by computers and electrically ballasted fluorescent lights. The following gaussmeters are widely available and are generally adequate for measuring household fields:

- **MSI EMF Meter** is a single-axis meter that is accurate for field frequencies between 60 and 180 hertz but does not measure higher frequency fields.
- **Tri-Field Meter** is a low-cost triple-axis meter for measuring magnetic and other fields. The meter may overestimate 60-hertz fields because of interference when higher frequency fields can also be detected.

Electric Fields

Wiring to Reduce Electric Fields

In Germany, Bau-Biologists have long been concerned about the negative health effects associated with exposure to electric fields. In the United States, mainstream science has given little credence to the notion that electric fields pose a health threat and remains skeptical in spite of continuing evidence of biological effects.

A 1996 study by the Ontario Hydroelectric Company indicated a greater than sevenfold increase in cancers among long-term workers exposed simultaneously to magnetic and high electric fields.[2] The study suggests that the presence of electric fields potentiates the health impact of magnetic fields. Additional data published in 2000 support the role of electric field exposure in leukemia.[3] These findings may shed light on why various studies of the impact of magnetic fields alone on humans have been inconclusive.

A proportion of the population appears to suffer from hypersensitivity to electric fields. These individuals may react to exposure with immediate neurological symptoms such as insomnia, depression, and anxiety. One frequently reported symptom is that of feeling physically exhausted but too jittery to sleep, or "wired and tired."

Wiring for reduced electric fields is not required by the electrical code and can be costly. Electric fields generated by wiring can be shielded in metal conduit. This practice is standard in commercial construction but rarely found in residential construction. Even if metal conduit is used, electric fields will still be emitted from appliances or fixtures once they are plugged in unless they have been specially wired or renovated. For people with hypersensitivity to electric fields, special wiring techniques similar to those used to block electrical interference in hospitals and sound studios may be a necessary expense. Techniques for this type of specialty wiring are beyond the scope of this book and will require consultation with an expert.

Wiring for Household Electric Field Reduction

The following instructions may be specified to reduce electric fields generated by household wiring:

- **All household wiring shall be placed in MX, MC, or rigid metal conduit.**
- **All electrical boxes and bushings shall be metal in order to provide shielding of electrical fields throughout the entire run to the panel.**
- **Avoid running wire behind or under bed placement locations.**

Wiring for Electric Field Reduction in the Bedroom with a Kill Switch

A less expensive approach is to reduce electric fields exclusively in the bedroom by employing a kill switch, which cuts the power to an individual circuit. You can turn off the power to the bedroom just before you retire at night, creating a field-free sanctuary. Because the presence of high electric fields is most commonly associated with sleep disturbances, we believe that such a device is an important feature in electric field reduction for the healthy bedroom.

Kill switches are most effectively used when wire runs are planned in advance. In brief, certain wiring, such as the wires leading

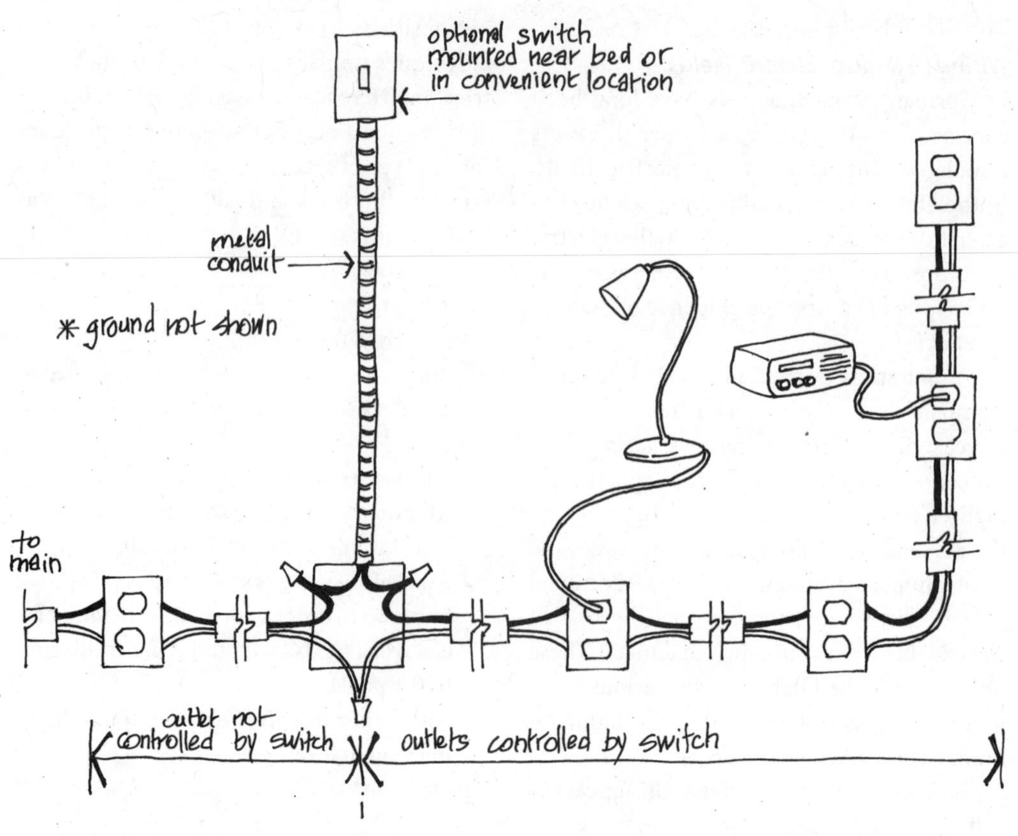

Kill Switch: The kill switch is used to eliminate electric and magnetic fields from plugged in appliances. When the kill switch is off the appliance is off and the fields are eliminated.

to smoke detectors or refrigerators, should not be included with bedroom runs. Typical electrical switches used for freestanding lamps and other electrical appliances turn that equipment off by cutting the power to the hot (black) wire of the equipment. This does not cut off the electrical field as long as the equipment is still plugged in. The entire run of wire up to the switch ends up radiating electric fields even when the switch is off. A kill switch is designed to cut off the fields in any given run of wiring. Using a kill switch is especially appropriate for bedrooms, where power isn't usually desired or necessary while the occupants are asleep.

The least expensive way to accomplish this is to install a double-pole switch in a convenient location along the run of electrical wire well before it enters the area of the home to be controlled. Heavy-duty switches have an increased amperage limit rating and can perform this task as long as the amperage on the circuit beyond the switch does not exceed the amperage limit rating of the switch. Combination electrical outlet and double-pole heavy-duty switch units are available. These contain

CASE STUDY 16.4

Electric Fields and Insomnia

Several years ago, John was asked to investigate the house of a woman who claimed she had not slept well since moving in. Upon inspection of the bedroom, John noted that the electric fields registered over 5,000 millivolts on the meter. He explained that the goal for a healthy house is 20 millivolts or less. (These measurements are relative, and are measured in the body using special equipment and techniques.)

The elevated electric fields were a result of the electrical wiring in and near the bedroom. The fields were being concentrated in the metallic bedsprings, which acted as an antenna, redirecting the electric field upward toward the client. John explained that the easiest way for an electrician to lower the electric fields in the bed would be to install a remote controlled switch on three of the circuit breakers in the basement that controlled the electrical wiring in and around the bedroom. The client's husband expressed his skepticism regarding the investigation and findings. He doubted that the electric fields could explain his wife's sleeplessness since he did not experience similar symptoms. He was reluctant to follow John's recommendations.

John then suggested that the couple try an experiment to ensure that a remote switch would indeed be money well spent. They were instructed to turn off the three breakers in the basement every night before they went to bed to determine if the woman slept better. John reminded them that since there would be no power in the bedroom they should have a battery operated alarm clock and flashlight available.

A few weeks later, the client contacted John to report that she was sleeping soundly for the first time in years and that both she and her husband were elated. She related to John what had transpired after he left their home. When the time came to turn off the breakers on the first night, she could hear her husband grumbling with resentment and stomping loudly down the steps to the basement to turn off the breakers. That night she slept so long and soundly that she barely made it to the bathroom in time the following morning. Her husband took note of her improvement and the second night went into the basement to shut off the breakers without saying a word. Again she slept soundly and awoke with the sun, feeling refreshed. By the third night she began to feel romantic, a feeling she had not experienced in a long time. By the fourth night her husband was whistling while he took the basement stairs two at a time. At this point the couple was eager to invest in a remote switching device.

Discussion

Because of standard wiring practices, readings of 1,000 millivolts or higher in a home are typical. Wiring homes for low electric fields is much easier and more cost effective when this consideration is part of the initial building plans. Wiring paths, for example, can be situated to limit the number of circuits involved, and high-field emitters can be placed at a safe distance from the sleeping area. Electric fields in existing homes cannot always be controlled by simply shutting off the breakers. Sometimes expensive shielding is needed. Sensitivity to electric fields varies from person to person. In the case described above, the client developed severe insomnia while her husband experienced no ill effects.

an outlet and a switch in the same unit and can be installed in a typical outlet box. The switch is designed to cut off power to the adjoining outlet and to all outlets downstream from it. When the switch is on, electricity flows through the hot wire and anything plugged into the controlled electrical line will function normally. When the switch is off, the electrical wiring from the switch and beyond is "dead" and no fields will be present in the rest of the circuit downstream from it.

This method of controlling fields may be inconvenient because the switch must be turned off at a distance from the items to be controlled and cannot be reached easily from the bedside. Kill switches can be wired into bedrooms and other chosen areas and placed more conveniently if the wires to the kill switch are run inside grounded metal conduit. When wired in this manner, the switch can be placed so that you can reach it without getting out of bed. The hot wire leading to the kill switch is still energized, but the field from it is shielded by the metal conduit. The room must be wired so that the kill switch is first on the circuit. When the switch is turned off, the fields are blocked and none of the electrical equipment plugged in along that run of wire will operate or produce fields.

Electrical runs from adjoining areas need to be carefully considered so that their fields do not enter areas designated to be free of fields. It is important that smoke detector and refrigerator/freezer circuits are never on a circuit with a kill switch that might turn them off. All equipment that must operate twenty-four hours a day should be specially shielded or positioned far enough away to prevent the fields from penetrating walls into the sleeping area. The electric fields generated by this type of household equipment generally do not extend more than 12 feet from the equipment.

A cut-off or demand switch can be installed as an alternative to a kill switch to eliminate unnecessary AC electric fields from dedicated rest and sleeping areas.

Cut-off or Demand Switches [4]

Automatic demand switches are readily available in German-speaking countries, and have been introduced into North America. These switches are a convenient solution because they do not require any lifestyle changes. The automatic demand switch cuts off power from selected circuits when there is no need for power consumption. The switch is installed next to the circuit breaker at the electric panel, making use of the existing wiring to control the circuit. When the power is cut off, a 3-volt DC control voltage monitors the circuit to ensure that it comes back on as soon as a switch is turned on demanding electricity.

For example, a demand switch can be installed for the bedroom circuit in the main panel. The bedside lamp is usually the last thing turned off at night. Once it is switched off, the bedroom circuit will go into sleep mode because the demand switch senses that no current is flowing and therefore cuts off the power. Since no more AC electric fields emanate from this particular circuit, no body voltages can be induced. (Only the very low DC control voltage is still present.) As soon as the bedside lamp or any other device in this circuit is turned on, the required power (and with it the undesired fields) will reappear.

This type of demand switch works only when a bedroom is serviced by a single electrical circuit. Unfortunately, it is common practice in the United States to connect the wall outlets of a given room to a different branch circuit than the ceiling light of the same room. Also the wiring for adjacent rooms with common walls may be on still another energized branch circuit.

The successful operation of an automatic demand switch depends on its proper installation. The selected electric circuit must not supply any electric appliances or electronic devices that draw power on a permanent basis, such as clock radios, video recorders, TV sets with stand-by mode, refrigerators, intercoms, antenna amplifiers, battery chargers, answering machines, and cordless phones. These devices need to be either disconnected or, better yet, kept out of the bedroom. If they must remain, they will need to be connected to other circuits not controlled by any demand switch. If one of these appliances were mistakenly connected to a protected circuit, it would render the demand switch inoperative.

Sources for automatic demand switches in North America are:

- **Breathing Easy**
- **Safe Living Technologies, Inc.**

In North America, switch modules are offered by home automation specialists. The modules require either an additional bell wire to transmit the control signal, which would be suitable only for new construction, or a dedicated regular circuit separate from the one you wish to control. There are also automatic wireless modules available, which we do not recommend because most of them emit radio frequency radiation while there is a load on the line.

Before you consider installing a cut-off or demand switch, you should have a Building Biology survey performed. A professional assessment will clarify whether a demand switch is necessary and, if so, on which circuit or circuits it should be installed. Often it is not sufficient to cut off power only to the circuit for the bedroom you are concerned about because AC electric fields emanating from wiring of adjoining rooms beside, below, or above the bedroom may affect the room in question. A mistake in the installation of a demand switch may also become the source of elevated AC electric fields caused by the loss of the electric field from the shut-off circuit. Sometimes the elimination of a field has the unintended consequence of no longer canceling electric fields from other circuits in the area of concern. For example, if you cut off the power from the bedroom wiring running through the wall behind your head, it is possible that the AC electric fields from the wiring of an adjoining room in the same wall will extend even more intensely into the head area of your bed.

It is important to note that cut-off or demand switches might be installed either in the wrong panel or on the wrong circuit. The electric field distribution of all circuits needs to be carefully surveyed by a qualified consultant in order to single out the circuits of concern and select the appropriate number of switch modules. A preventive installation without a professional survey is never a good idea.

Another caution is that most voltage testers will not detect all electric circuits governed by an automatic demand switch, which operates with a low control voltage. However, if a person touches one of the electrical conductors, the automatic demand switch might be initiated to turn the power back on, with the potential risk of an electric shock. To ensure safe usage, all electric circuits controlled by an automatic demand switch must be clearly labeled in the

Guidelines for Creating a Safe Electroclimate in the Bedroom

VICKI WARREN

The Standard of Building Biology Testing Methods (SBM) was pioneered by Bau-Biologist Wolfgang Maes in cooperation with the Institut für Baubiologie und Ökologie Neubeuern (IBN). The place where we spend most of our time should have the lowest electromagnetic readings possible. Based on the precautionary principle, the Building Biology Guidelines for Sleeping Areas are designed to provide optimal conditions for maintaining long-term health and apply mainly during sleep and regeneration, when humans are most vulnerable to electromagnetic influences. The recommendations are based on input from medical doctors and on decades of testing experience and thousands of sleeping-area surveys.[a]

A Building Biology survey will measure primarily six parameters of the electromagnetic spectrum: alternating current (AC) electric fields, AC magnetic fields, radio frequency radiation (RF), static fields, also known as direct current (DC) electric fields and DC magnetic fields, and radioactivity.

Sleeping Area Survey

AC Electric Fields

The human body is an amazing self-rejuvenating entity that can repair itself while it sleeps. This is accomplished with its own internal electrical system, which functions with very weak electrical impulses. Electrical impulses generated by the brain are used for intercellular communication. This is possible because the body is composed mainly of water with a high mineral content, making it highly electrically conductive.

Vibration tells cells when to divide. Brain cells, nerve cells, and bone cells all vibrate at different rates to communicate with one another. Unfortunately, our bodies act as tuning forks. When you vibrate a tuning fork (an external electrical influence), any other tuning fork in its vicinity (such as the body) will start vibrating at the same rate, or frequency, and cells will be confused about how fast to grow.[b]

In the typical sleeping area, electrical exposure from external sources (live electrical wiring in ceilings, walls, and floors) is thousands of times stronger than the body's own electrical system. Long-term exposure to these high-level electric fields can impact health by impairing the body's ability to communicate within itself. You spend about a third of your life sleeping. Doesn't it make sense to reduce exposure to electric fields in your sleeping area?

To test body voltage, the voltage, or electrical pressure, between a person and a dedicated rod driven into the Earth is measured. Tests are done with electrical appliances on and off, with circuits energized and de-energized, to determine what devices and circuits affect the electric field strength in the sleeping area. Goal: Body voltage should be less than 100 millivolts, and preferably less than 10 millivolts.

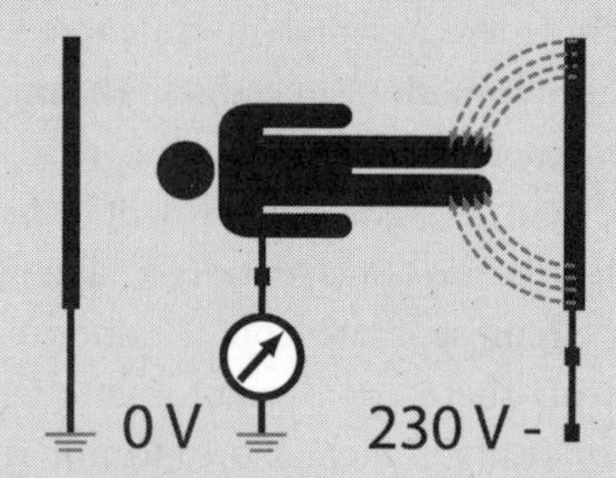

Electric field testing measures electric field strength using an electric field meter. The sleeping area is carefully surveyed until all sources are identified. Goal: Electric field strength should be less than 10 volts per meter and preferably less than 1 volt per meter.

AC Magnetic Fields

Magnetic fields travel unimpeded through almost any material. Alternating magnetic fields cause eddy currents (the induction effect) in the human body and can lead to abnormal nerve, bone, and muscle stimulation.[c,d] Therefore, appliances such as refrigerators, freezers, swimming pool pumps, and breaker boxes should be located far from sleeping areas. A survey will help establish safe distances from TV sets, electric baseboard heating elements, and clock radios. Additional problems of net currents on building wiring and plumbing systems are a reality, especially in urban areas. The resulting elevated magnetic fields need to be carefully traced and eliminated.

A gaussmeter or tesla meter is used to survey the sleeping area for elevated magnetic fields. These meters can be either a single-axis or triaxial instrument. Goal: Less than 200 nanoteslas (2 milligauss), and preferably less than 20 nanoteslas (0.2milligauss).

Since net current causes magnetic fields, the other main measuring instrument is the ammeter. Once the identified internal magnetic fields are removed by turning off the power, a clamp-on ammeter is used to measure current on the grounding system, especially the water service supply, TV cables, telephone lines, and even the air conditioning system's Freon lines. Typical values are less than 150 milliamperes.

Radio Frequency Radiation

The higher the frequency of the electromagnetic radiation, the more the electric and magnetic field components meld. The energy level of radio frequency (RF) radiation is billions of times stronger than the natural high-frequency energies from the cosmos that existed during our biological development. Research shows that cataracts, blood composition changes, hormone alterations, and chromosomal abnormalities are induced at high-frequency energies.[e] Sources of high RF radiation located outside a home require changing the location of the bed or shielding with RF-reflective paint and/or material.

Internal RF sources, such as cellular phones, wireless communications, and cordless phones, should not be in or near the bedroom, or at least not while you sleep. Cordless phones based on 2.4 or higher gigahertz technology emits pulsed RF energy 24 hours a day. Choose analog 900 megahertz models instead and use them sparingly. It is also important to consider avoiding light dimmer switches and fluorescent lighting of any type, as they can create RF signals that travel on the electric house installation, contaminating the entire living space.

The RF detector (50–3000 megahertz) and RF analyzer (800–3300 megahertz) are used to detect pulsed radio frequency signals, track down their sources, and test the effectiveness of mitigation. Goal: Exposure limits are: pulsed less than 0.1 microwatt per square meter and nonpulsed less than 1 microwatt per square meter.

Static Electric Fields or DC Electric Fields

Static electric and static magnetic fields (also called DC fields) occur in nature, where they can surprise us with enormous intensities. These fields do not vibrate at any frequency but are static — that is, independent of time and unchanging. Adverse health effects from static fields can occur when the fields deviate from the natural background even to a small degree. Thus, for a healthy environment, deviations from these natural static fields need to be eliminated. Unfortunately, this condition is often overlooked by indoor environmentalists who are not Bau-Biologists.

Static electricity is produced between electric charges at rest. At the right dose, air electricity is essential for sustaining life, but, when unbalanced, static electric fields can cause subtle health effects that are not as obvious as a shock. These effects result when static electricity generating materials upset the natural air ion balance and concentration. Synthetic carpeting, stuffed animals, upholstered furniture, and blended bed sheets are the major sources of static electricity in the bedroom. The cure is easy: use natural materials that cannot become so highly charged and that discharge quickly, such as cotton, hemp, silk, and wool. If replacement is not possible, cover the offending material.

Static Magnetic Fields or DC Magnetic Fields

Often while sleeping we are not in sync with the Earth's natural static magnetic field because of highly magnetic metal mattress springs. A DC gaussmeter or a liquid (oil) filled compass moved slowly across a bed can detect static magnetic field anomalies. A compass is sufficiently accurate for risk assessment of the innerspring mattress. Goal: Size changes under 1 milligauss (100 microteslas) when using a DC gaussmeter, or less than a 10-degree change in direction in 3 inches (7.5 centimeters) when using a compass.

Radioactivity

Building materials such as concrete, glazed tiles, and granite countertops may show radioactivity levels far above the ambient level. Select materials with lower radiation. All radiation exposures should be As Low As Reasonably Attainable (the ALARA principle). Even the smallest radiation exposure should be avoided. All homes and sites should be tested for radon following the EPA guidelines.

A Geiger counter compares the ionization effect of radioactive radiation to the natural background. To establish the natural background radiation, it is necessary to take several measurements at various spots, diligently avoiding potential sources of radioactivity. Goal: Less than a 70 percent increase and ideally less than 50 percent.

Prudent Avoidance Strategies

There are many simple and inexpensive ways to make the bedroom a sanctuary that is free from these stressful fields. Here are five suggestions:

1. Use battery-powered clocks near the bed. Research has shown that exposure to high magnetic fields during sleep can cause severe long-term illness. Many electric clocks produce high magnetic fields.
2. Turn off circuit breakers affecting the bedroom while you sleep. A restful sleep is necessary for health and a strong immune system. Electric fields affect the biocommunication system, keeping you from sleeping soundly.
3. Use beds without metal. Metal frames and metal box springs can amplify and distort the Earth's natural magnetic field, leading to a non-restful sleep.
4. Make sure there are no elevated magnetic fields. Magnetic fields from appliances and building wiring can penetrate walls into a bedroom and disrupt the body's communication system.
5. Eliminate or shield from RF. Radio frequency signals from portable phones, cell phones, and wireless devices have been shown to interfere with the body's immune system. External sources need to be shielded. In today's world of

ubiquitous cell phone towers and radio communications, there are many things you can do when building to block RF that will be bombarding your home. The first line of defense, of course, to measure the site before purchasing it and reject it if there are unacceptable levels of RF. If RFs cannot be avoided or are anticipated, the following should be considered:

- Use solid, dense building materials such as stucco, stone, brick, or concrete.
- Use low-emissive (Low-E) dual-pane windows with metal frames or frames painted with RF-reflective paint.
- Use foil or RF-reflective netting under the roofing or a grounded metal roof.

If you are not able to make major structural changes to the home, another option is to buy special shielding fabric that can be tented around you while you sleep. A source for this fabric is safe livingtechnologies.com. Beware of the multitude of devices on the market that claim to be effective against RF. The vast majority of these are gimmicks with limited or no measurable effect.

The Property Survey

Based on the findings of a property survey, it is possible to provide specific recommendations for any planned construction activity. Anticipated future developments in the neighborhood should also be taken into consideration.

First, map the naturally occurring terrestrial radiation pattern to detect anomalies in the Earth's magnetic field as well as radioactivity.

Second, assess the risk of power frequency fields. Be aware that on days with little moisture in the air the electric fields from high-tension power lines might be overestimated, although in many cases building materials will attenuate the external fields. In contrast, alternating magnetic fields are mostly independent of the weather. Because power consumption fluctuates over any given day, week, or even season, data logging is necessary for proper risk assessment.

Third, measure RF radiation. Radio waves, or microwaves, ride along the airwaves with an intensity that varies with the distance from the source of emission and the time of day. To accurately assess the highly complex web of electromagnetic waves, data logging is a must. The main direction and specific frequency bands of the major sources of RF radiation need to be carefully monitored so that appropriate shielding advice can be given.

Remember that in creating a safe electroclimate in your bedroom any attainable reduction is worthwhile and nature is the ultimate guide.

a. Baubiologie Maes/Standard of Baubiologie Methods of Testing (SBM-2008) is available from the International Institute for Bau-Biologie & Ecology, buildingbiology.net.
b. James Oschman. *Energy Medicine.* Churchill Livingstone, 2000.
c. Robert O.Becker. *Cross Currents.* Tarcher, 1990.
d. James Oschman. *Energy Medicine.* Churchill Livingstone, 2000.
e. Robert O. Becker. *Cross Currents.* Tarcher, 1990.

Vicki Warren, BSEE, is the program director for the International Institute for Bau-Biologie & Ecology (IBE). IBE is a leader in natural healthy-building education. Vicki has taught in public schools and has worked in the power industry and traversed the globe as a test engineer and trainer. She is a certified Bau-Biologist Environmental Consultant (BBEC), Indoor Environmentalist (CIE), and licensed educator. She can be reached at vwarren@buildingbiology.net.

main or subpanel as well as on all connected outlets. To maintain proper functioning of an automatic demand switch in the long run, you should test it by inserting a control lamp once a month, just as you would test a ground fault circuit interrupter (GFCI).

If elevated AC electric fields originate from neighboring apartments or adjoining houses, demand switches will not help and shielding strategies will have to be explored.

Shielding Electric Fields Emitted from Refrigerators

Because refrigerators generate large electric fields, they should be given a dedicated circuit and the wiring should be shielded with one of the recommended metal conduits in order to block the fields. In addition, the metal refrigerator cabinet should be bonded to the electrical ground. Since the compressor motor and defroster will still produce high magnetic fields, the home should be designed with the refrigerator at least 12 feet away from living and sleeping areas.

Gasketed Electrical Boxes

As discussed in the section on air barriers in Division 7, electrical boxes must be sealed in order to make an exterior wall airtight. You may have experienced the flow of air coming through an outlet on a cold day if the boxes are not installed in an airtight manner. It is necessary to prevent air from flowing into the living space from a wall cavity not only for the sake of energy efficiency but also to maintain optimal indoor air quality. The following gasketed electrical boxes are designed to create an airtight seal:

- **AirFoil**
- **Lessco Air Vapor Barrier Boxes**
- **Allied Moulded Vapor Seal Boxes**

Residential Lighting

Residential lighting can also be a source of electromagnetic fields. Here are some pointers on residential lighting and EMFs:

- Transformers of low-voltage lighting produce a magnetic field. If you use low voltage lighting, choose remote transformers and locate them in closets at a distance from where you spend a lot of time.
- Fluorescent lighting with ballasts emits magnetic fields that may not be detectable on an inexpensive gaussmeter. Avoid fluorescent lighting with ballasts in areas where you spend a lot of time, and never locate it on a ceiling below a bedroom. It should also be noted that fluorescent light tubes and compact fluorescent lights contain mercury and should be properly recycled. Breaking the tubes may release the mercury. (For more information about proper disposal, see earth911.org.)
- If you are using recessed can lighting, specify insulation contact airtight (ICAT) cans. These cans save energy and prevent dust and attic gases from filtering into the cans.
- If wiring is run through a metal conduit, the metal housing of the fixture must be in electrical contact with the metal conduit in order to shield the occupied space from electric fields.

Smoke Detectors

The two basic types of smoke detectors are ionizing and photoelectric. The ionizing type contains a radioactive substance called americium-241. Although the radioactive substance is shielded, we cannot recommend this type because there is no safe place for disposal once the smoke detector is discarded. Smoke detectors are available for use with 9-volt batteries or for hardwiring into the 110-volt household wiring, with or without battery backup. We recommend a hardwired photoelectric system with battery backup, which can be purchased through **BRK/First Alert** and **MCS Referral & Resources**. If you are wiring so that your bedroom circuitry can be shut off, it is important to put the smoke detector on a separate circuit so that it will always remain active. If this circuit is run through a metal conduit, the electric field will be minimal.

Carbon Monoxide Detectors

All gas-burning appliances to which occupants are exposed, such as gas ranges and dryers, should be tested for carbon monoxide emissions prior to building occupancy. The installation of a simple monitoring device ensures that you will be alerted if a problem with carbon monoxide develops. The device should have battery backup and a digital readout. The following CO monitors meet these criteria:

- **Aim S-450** is a portable pocket alarm CO detector unit with a digital readout.
- **BRK/First Alert**
- **NightHawk Carbon Monoxide Detector** contains a sensor that samples the air every 2½ minutes and updates the digital readout.

Further Reading

Becker, Robert O. *Cross Currents.* J.P. Tarcher, 1990. A timely and eloquent warning on the hazards of electronic pollution

Von Pohl, Gustav Freiherr. *Earth Currents: Causative Factor of Cancer and Other Diseases.* Frech-Verlag, 1987.

APPENDIX A

MCS: What is It?

Multiple Chemical Sensitivity

Multiple chemical sensitivity (MCS), often referred to as environmental illness, is an immune and nervous system disorder involving severe reactions to many everyday chemicals and products. For some people MCS occurs with dramatic onset, precipitated by a major chemical exposure or industrial accident. But for most people the condition develops gradually as the result of the cumulative exposures of daily life.

The symptoms of MCS are diverse and unique to each person and can involve any organ of the body. Symptoms range from mild to disabling and can sometimes be life threatening. They include headaches, fatigue, sleep disturbances, depression, panic attacks, emotional outbursts, difficulty concentrating, short-term memory loss, dizziness, heart palpitations, diarrhea, constipation, shortness of breath, asthma, rashes, flu-like symptoms, and seizures. Symptoms may be chronic or may occur only when a person is exposed to certain substances. The particular organs affected depend on the individual's genetic background and prior history as well as the specific chemicals involved in the exposure.

Symptoms are often triggered by very low levels of exposure, including levels lower than permissible by government standards and typically below the levels tolerated by most people. Triggers include a wide range of substances found in the workplace and at home. Solvents, paints, varnishes, adhesives, pesticides, and cleaning solutions are most frequently implicated. Other substances include new building materials and furnishings, formaldehyde in new clothes, artificial fragrances in cleaning and personal care products, detergents, car exhaust, and copy machine and laser printer toner. Symptoms can occur after inhaling chemical vapors, after chemicals touch the skin, or after ingestion. Sensitivity to a particular chemical can lead to sensitivity to an ever-widening range of other, often dissimilar, chemicals. This characteristic is known as the spreading phenomenon.

It may be useful to think of environmental illness as a spectrum that encompasses a wide range of chemical sensitivities. At one end are individuals who may suffer from mild symptoms, such as simple sinus congestion or headaches, which usually resolve when the triggering chemical is removed. At the other end of the spectrum are individuals with full-blown MCS, who suffer extremely debilitating symptoms that can last for months or years after exposure.

Why do some people develop MCS while others with the same level of exposure do not? Because of biochemical individuality, all humans manifest disease according to their genetic makeup, past chemical exposure, and overall general state of health, which includes total load. Total load refers to all the stressors in a person's life, including chemical exposure, poor nutrition, emotional tension, allergies, infections, trauma, and physical stress.

Although the exact mechanism whereby chemicals create this heightened sensitivity has not yet been clearly elucidated, theories are emerging that will hopefully lead to greater understanding and better treatment of MCS. Recent studies have demonstrated how toxins, having gained access to the brain through the olfactory nerve, can cause release of excitatory amino acids that result in swelling, dysregulation, and destruction of brain cells. The olfactory nerve is also the pathway to the limbic system, which is an area of the brain where the nervous, immune, and endocrine systems interact. The limbic system regulates an extremely wide variety of body functions. Many of the varied and seemingly bizarre symptoms reported by persons with MCS are consistent with symptoms known in the medical literature to occur when various parts of the limbic system are damaged by chemicals or physical injury.

Toxic chemicals can also cause direct damage to specific tissues of the body such as enzymes in the liver that are essential in the detoxification pathway. Because of inadequate amounts of detoxifying enzymes, a person with MCS is less able to handle chemical loads. Also, recent data indicate that certain toxins in the environment, especially chlorinated compounds, mimic natural hormones, causing disruption of endocrine systems such as the thyroid, adrenal, and reproductive systems.

The first documented cases of environmental illness resulted from widespread chemical poisoning during World War I. The exposure to mustard gas had long-term consequences for soldiers, many of whom developed chronic symptoms of chemical sensitivities. More recently, thousands of veterans who fought in the Gulf War returned with symptoms similar to those found in patients diagnosed with MCS.

Since World War II, the production of synthetic chemicals has increased significantly. In 1945, the estimated worldwide production of these chemicals was less than 10 million tons. Today it is over 110 million tons. As more and more synthetic chemicals are introduced into the environment, larger numbers of healthy people are becoming affected. Most people with MCS have not been through a war. They have become ill from ordinary day-to-day, low-level exposures to poor indoor air quality in their homes and workplaces. MCS sufferers often say that their role in society is like the canary in the coal mine. When the canary collapsed, the miners were warned that lethal gases were in the air.

Although MCS is a rapidly growing problem, sometimes called a silent epidemic, health care workers know little about the subject. Chemical sensitivity is a relatively new field of medicine, controversial in nature, and not recognized or understood by most physicians. The illness does not fit neatly into the current medical model and, unlike diabetes or hypertension, there is no simple medical test for making the diagnosis. There are remarkably few individuals in medicine who have toxicology training and who are sensitive to the possible neurological, behavioral, and psychiatric problems resulting from chemical exposures. In addition, the chemical and insurance industries have played a major role in influencing the average person's perceptions about chemicals and their impact on living organisms.

One of the most important steps in the treatment of the chemically sensitive person is to avoid or reduce toxic chemical exposures as much as possible in order to allow the body to heal. A healthy home is a prerequisite for those who wish to regain their health. The person with MCS needs a sanctuary of peace and well-being in a world saturated with toxic chemicals.

In spite of widespread ignorance and vested financial interests, MCS is gradually becoming known to the public as more and more people are becoming ill. For several years a small but growing number of physicians specializing in environmental medicine have been focusing on this serious problem. If you would like information about a physician in your area with expertise in the diagnosis and treatment of chemically related health problems, contact the American Academy of Environmental Medicine in Wichita, Kansas, at 316-684-5500 or aaemonline.org.

Author Testimonials

Paula Baker-Laporte

If someone had told me in the early years of my career that I would be writing a technical "how to" book about healthy homes, I would have looked at them with total incredulity! I would have explained that, as an architect, my main concerns were with the creation of beautiful and interactive spatial forms and that my aspirations were artistic rather than technical. It seems that fate had a different course for me. I joined the ranks of the chemically sensitive.

In retrospect, the roots of my illness can be traced back to formaldehyde overexposure that I suffered when for a short period I lived in a brand-new mobile home. Working in standard residential construction, I found that my symptoms became severely aggravated whenever I visited a jobsite because of the prevalence of this toxic chemical in conventional construction materials. Erica Elliott, my friend and physician, diagnosed my condition and helped me get back on my feet, and it was through her that I first heard of healthy building. She told me of the alarming number of chronically ill patients consulting with her who were diagnosed with MCS. For many, the primary cause of illness was exposure to multiple toxins in the home.

Even though I specialized in residential architecture, I had to admit I knew little about the health implications of standard home construction. While working with Erica to design her home, I began intensive research into this new frontier in architecture and building. It was then that my personal and professional life took a new direction.

Once I learned the facts, I could never again allow certain products, techniques, or equipment to be used in projects with which I became involved. I understood the health threats they posed to my clients, other inhabitants, construction workers, and the planet. In my efforts to learn everything I could about healthy building, I came across a body of information translated from the original German called Bau-Biologie. Bau-Biologie advocates an environmentally sustainable approach to healthy building, in part through the use of natural, unprocessed building materials.

I used these principles when designing a new home for my family. Our home has a timber frame and clay/straw wall system. My husband and builder, Robert Laporte, introduced this building system to me when I first met him at a natural building workshop he was leading. Our home has earth plasters and earth and stone floors, and is heated primarily by solar heat and a masonry oven. The electrical wiring is in metal conduit. My own health has improved steadily, partly as a result of the clean and vital environment afforded to me by our natural home and unpolluted surroundings. Although the bulk of my professional design work now incorporates alternative natural building systems, I realize that the majority of people planning a new home do not have access to alternative materials and methods of construction. I also realize that, for some chemically sensitive individuals, many natural materials can elicit symptoms as readily as synthetic ones do. For these reasons, much of the information in this book is geared toward making conventional building practices healthier.

A healthy home is far more than a home that is free of toxins. It must safeguard the residents on many other levels, described throughout this book. As a result of my research, my goals as an architect have grown. To truly nurture us, our buildings must not only be beautiful. They must also be healthful and conceived with mindfulness of our limited planetary resources. The same building design can destroy human health or enhance vitality. The difference lies in the materials and construction methods we choose.

Erica Elliott

My involvement with indoor air quality issues began in 1991, when I went to work for a large medical corporation as a family physician. The building housing the clinic was new and tightly sealed, with nonoperable windows and wall-to-wall carpeting. Previously in excellent health, a world-class mountaineer and marathon runner, I began to develop unexplainable fatigue. After several months, more symptoms developed, including rashes, burning eyes, chronic sore throat, and headaches. The symptoms subsided in the evenings after I left the workplace, only to return when I reentered the building.

By my second year of employment, I had developed persistent migraine headaches, muscle and joint pains, insomnia, confusion, lack of coordination, memory loss, and mood swings. By then the symptoms had become permanent, continuing when I was away from my workplace on weekends. My physician colleagues were puzzled by my symptoms. Some felt I was suffering an unusual manifestation of depression and would benefit from antidepressant medication. These medicines were not helpful and only masked the problem.

I finally had the good fortune to find a physician trained in environmental medicine who believed I had nervous and immune system damage related to chronic, low-level exposure to poorly ventilated toxins in the workplace.

By the time I resigned my position on the staff of the clinic and the local hospital, I had a full-blown case of multiple chemical sensitivity, also known as environmental illness. Most synthetic chemicals commonly found in the modern world, even in minute amounts, caused me to have adverse reactions to such a degree that life became a painful ordeal. With diligent avoidance of toxins, abundant rest, detoxification therapies, and other measures, my life began to stabilize.

Since very few physicians are trained in toxicology and environmental medicine, I immersed myself in this field of study, to help myself as well as others. It wasn't long before my practice consisted primarily of patients with immune dysfunction, including multiple chemical sensitivity, autoimmune disease, chronic fatigue syndrome, fibromyalgia, and severe allergies. I was struck by the number of patients who dated the onset of their symptoms to a move to a new home or to the remodeling of a school or office. They invariably had been to many doctors who treated them for conditions such as allergies, asthma, sinusitis, and depression. The underlying causes were not identified. By the time the correct diagnosis was made, the patients' immune systems were often severely, sometimes irreversibly, damaged.

It was during my own recovery that I decided to build a home using nontoxic building materials. Paula Baker-Laporte was my architect, patient, and neighbor. Together we began researching various available products and associated health effects. Shortly thereafter we had the pleasure of meeting John Banta, and a fruitful collaboration began.

John Banta

My introduction to the downside of indoor air quality occurred along with my introduction to fatherhood in 1980. Like many first-time parents, my wife and I wanted to welcome our newborn by decorating the nursery. We painted and carpeted the room in anticipation of our new arrival. The room smelled of chemicals and I noticed that I did not feel well in there. But it wasn't until our baby became ill that I realized what a serious problem we had created. By the time I made the connection between my daughter's medical condition and the toxins in the nursery, she had become sensitized to even minute amounts of toxic chemicals commonly found in the environment and was in severe distress. My wife and I decided to buy an old Victorian home that had not been remodeled in over 40 years. We proceeded to convert the building into a chemical-free sanctuary where our daughter could begin to heal from her devastating illness.

During that time I was working as a medical technician in a research lab, where I was exposed to numerous toxic chemicals, including formaldehyde, benzene, toluene, xylene, and several disinfectants. Over the next four years, I felt progressively worse while at work, yet I would feel better once I returned to our carefully remodeled home. My job-related health problems finally became so severe that I made the difficult decision to quit. Little did I know that a new and exciting career was awaiting me.

Because of my hands-on experience in renovating my own healthy home, people began to ask for my advice. My wife urged me to begin consulting professionally, which I have done full time since 1986. Over the years, thousands of people have consulted me about their homes. Typically, I am contacted in the middle of a disaster: the walls are moldy, the paint is causing headaches, or the landlord sprayed pesticides to control insects. I am hired to determine the cause and suggest a remedy for the problem. My job often includes educating a skeptical landlord or spouse about the causal relationship between the problem in the home and health of the occupant.

The most rewarding work for me is consulting during the planning phase of new construction, where I can help my clients prevent problems before they occur. Although I do not design or build homes, I can troubleshoot and monitor to help ensure a nontoxic, healthful, and nurturing abode. I have really enjoyed working with Paula and Erica in writing this book. For me, it offers a way to reach more people with the information they need to create a healthy home.

APPENDIX B

Resource List

9400 W Impregnant
Solvent-free, water-repellent coating that provides ultraviolet, mildew, and frost protection while allowing wood to breathe.
Palmer Industries, Inc.
10611 Old Annapolis Rd.
Frederick, MD 21701
800-545-7383, 301-898-7848
palmerindustriesinc.com

86001 Seal
Clear, water-reducible sealer and primer for gypsum board.

ACQ-Preserve
Pressure treatment for wood that uses alkaline copper quaternary, which contains no known carcinogens or EPA listed hazardous compounds.
Chemical manufactured by
Chemical Specialties Inc.
200 East Woodlawn Rd., Suite 350
Charlotte, NC 28217
800-421-8661
treatedwood.com
Treated wood manufactured by
J.H. Baxter
1700 S. El Camino Real, Suite 200
San Mateo, CA 94402
800-780-7073, 650-349-0201
jhbaxter.com

AdvanTech
A durable subflooring and wall and roof sheathing product that uses phenolic glues.
Huber Engineered Woods
One Resource Square
10925 David Taylor Drive, Suite 300
Charlotte, NC 28262
800-933-9220
huberwood.com

Aercon
Aerated autoclaved concrete block.
Aercon
3701 CR 544 E
Haines City, FL 33844
800-830-3171, 863-422-6360
aerconaac.com

AFM Coatings, Stains, and Sealers

Products developed specifically for chemically sensitive people in consultation with environmental medicine physicians.

AFM MetalCoat Acrylic Metal Primer
For use on metal, iron, steel, aluminum, and masonry.

AFM Naturals Clear Penetrating Oil
Plant-based sealer for interior and exterior wood applications and interior clay plaster.

AFM Naturals Oil Wax Finish
Plant-based hardener and sealer for unfinished wood, bamboo, and cork.

AFM Safecoat AcriGlaze
Clear-mixing medium and finish, ideal for restoring old finishes and sealing and preserving painted work.

AFM Safecoat Acrylacq
High-gloss, clear, water-based wood finishes replacing conventional lacquer.
SCS IndoorAdvantage Gold certified

AFM Safecoat All Purpose Exterior Satin
For use on exterior walls and trim, wood, stucco, masonry, and primed metal.

AFM Safecoat CemBond Masonry Paint
Water-resistant coating for cement, concrete block, and masonry.

AFM Safecoat DecKote
Waterborne coating for use on concrete, magnesite, walkways, breezeways, and patios.

AFM Safecoat DuroStain
7 different earth pigment semitransparent wood stains. Interior/exterior, water-based.
SCS IndoorAdvantage Gold certified

AFM Safecoat DynoFlex and DynoFlex Roofguard
Available in sprayable form to use as topcoat over DynoSeal. Also used as a joint sealant treatment for HVAC ducts to eliminate toxic outgassing from standard sealants. Useful as a low-toxic roof coating to replace tar and gravel. Can be walked on and remains flexible.

AFM Safecoat DynoSeal
A flexible, low-odor, dampproof, vaporproof barrier.

AFM Safecoat DynoSeal Driveway/Asphalt Sealer
Low-odor elastomeric sealer and topcoating for asphalt surfaces. Helps to reduce the outgassing and odors generated by new asphalt.

AFM Safecoat Enamel
Comes in flat, eggshell, semi-gloss, and cabinet and trim. Water-based paints without extenders, drying agents, or formaldehyde.

AFM Safecoat Grout Sealer
A clear, moisture-resistant sealer for porous tile grout to help prevent staining.

AFM Safecoat Hard Seal
Water-based, general purpose clear sealer for vinyl, porous tile, concrete, plastics, particleboard, and plywood. Not recommended where exposed to heavy moisture or standing water.

AFM Safecoat Lock-In New Wood Sealer
Sandable sealer that helps raise grain on new woods in preparation for sanding prior to finish coat.

AFM Safecoat MexeSeal
A satin finish top coat. Very durable sealer providing water and oil repellency for use on Mexican clay tile, stone, granite, concrete, and stone pavers. Glossy when multiple coats are applied.
SCS IndoorAdvantage Gold certified

AFM Safecoat New Wallboard Primecoat HPV
Water reducible, one-coat coverage primer for new gypboard/greenboard and high recycled content material.
SCS IndoorAdvantage Gold certified

AFM Safecoat Penetrating WaterStop
Sealer for use on Mexican clay tile, stone, granite, concrete, stone pavers, or wood.

AFM Safecoat Polyureseal BP
Clear-gloss wood finish replaces conventional solvent and water-based polyurethanes for interior wood floor and furniture applications. High durability and abrasion resistance.
SCS IndoorAdvantage Gold certified

AFM Safecoat Safe Seal
Clear sealer for porous surfaces. Effective in blocking outgassing from processed woods. Improves adhesion of finish coats.

AFM Safecoat Transitional Primer
Designed to transition from existing oil-based surfaces to water-based coatings.
SCS IndoorAdvantage Gold certified

AFM Safecoat WaterShield
Water-repelling sealer for masonry and painted surfaces.

AFM Safecoat Zero VOC Paint
Flat, eggshell, and semi-gloss paint. No VOCs, formaldehyde, ammonia, or masking agents.

AFM Cleaning and Maintenance

AFM SafeChoice Glass Cleaner
Virtually odorless glass, mirror, and hard surface cleaner.

AFM SafeChoice Safety Clean
Industrial strength biodegradable cleaner and degreaser for high-moisture areas.

AFM SafeChoice Super Clean
All-purpose biodegradable cleaner/degreaser.

AFM SafeChoice X158
Low-odor liquid surfactant coating for prophylactic use where mold and mildew are likely to appear.

AFM Carpet Maintenance System

AFM SafeChoice Carpet Seal
Sealer designed to help prevent outgassing of harmful chemicals from carpet backing and adhesives.

AFM SafeChoice Carpet Shampoo
An odorless carpet shampoo that helps remove chemicals such as pesticides and formaldehyde from new carpet.

AFM SafeChoice Lock Out
A final spray application that seals harmful chemicals in carpet and repels dirt and stains.

AFM Other Products

AFM Safecoat 3 in 1 Adhesive
Adhesive for ceramic, vinyl, parquet, Formica, slate, and carpet.

AFM Safecoat Caulking Compound
Water-based elastic emulsion caulking compound designed to replace traditional caulk and putty for windows, cracks, and maintenance. Limited distribution.
Safecoat Caulking Compound is available through:
The Living Source
PO Box 20155
Waco, TX 76702
254-776-4878
livingsource.com
AFM (American Formulating and Manufacturing)
3251 3rd Ave.
San Diego, CA 92103
800-239-0321
afmsafecoat.com

AGLAIA Aquasol
Line of solvent-free plant- and water-based natural oil finishes for wood. Can be thinned and cleaned up with water.

AGLAIA Natural Paints
Plant-based natural paint products, free of petrochemical products and artificial resins.
aglaiapaint.com
Available through:
Environmental Building Supplies
819 SE Taylor St.
Portland, OR 97214
503-222-3881
Ecohaus.com

Agriboard
An energy efficient, environmentally engineered structural panel made from compressed wheat straw.
Agriboard Industries
100 Industrial Drive
Electra, TX 76360
940-495-3590, 903-814-2716
agriboard.com

AgriStain
Bio-based interior and exterior stain for metal, wood, gypsum, and cement.

AgriStain for Concrete
Clear sealer and stain for plaster, tile, or concrete.
New Century Coatings
4320 San Remo Ave.
Higley, AZ 85236
602-625-8925
newcenturycoatings.com
agristain.com

Aim S-450
Portable carbon monoxide alarm detector unit with digital readout.
Available through:
Professional Equipment (see listing)

Air Care Odorless Paints
Acrylic paints that are zero- to low-VOC.
Coronado Paint Co.
308 Old County Rd.
Edgewater, FL 32132
800-883-4193
coronadopaint.com

AirChek Inc.
Manufactures and sells a variety of test kits for radon, formaldehyde, and microwaves.
AirChek Inc.
1936 Butler Bridge Rd.
Fletcher, NC 28732
800-247-2435
radon.com

AirFoil
Airtight electrical outlet and device boxes.
AirFoil, Inc.
8685 Black Maple Drive
Eden Prairie, MN 55344
612-280-8331
airfoilinc.com

Air Krete
Cementitious foam insulation made of magnesium oxide, calcium, and silicate. High R-value (3.9/inch).
Nordic Builders
162 N. Sierra Court
Gilbert, AZ 85234
480-892-0603
Palmer Industries, Inc.
10611 Old Annapolis Rd.
Frederick, MD 21701
800-545-7383
palmerindustriesinc.com

Air Quality Sciences, Inc.
Commercial building indoor air quality test kit and mold and allergen test kit.
Air Quality Sciences, Inc.
Laboratory Services
1337 Capital Circle
Marietta, GA 30067
770-933-0638
info@aqs.com
aqs.com

Allergy Relief Store
Mold and mildew test kit.
Allergy Relief Store
250 Watson Glen
Franklin, TN 37064
800-866-7464
allergyreliefstore.com

Allermed
Air filtration systems, both whole-house and stand-alone.
Allermed
31 Steel Rd.
Wylie, TX 75098
800-213-6191
allermedcleanair.com

Allied Moulded Vapor Seal Boxes
Allied Moulded Products, Inc.
222 N. Union St
PO Box 587
Bryan, OH 43506
419-636-4217
alliedmoulded.com
Available through:
Energy Federation Inc.
40 Washington St., Suite 2000
Westborough, MA 01581
800-876-0660
efi.org

Allowood
FSC certified hardwood lumber substitute made from softwoods thermally cured with agricultural-based additives.
GreenGuard certified
EverTech
4191 Grandview Rd.
PO Box 2339
Ferndale, WA 98248
360-366-9378, 360-366-3831
allowood.com

AlphaLab Inc.
Electromagnetic instruments; trifield meter, gaussmeters, and others.
AlphaLab, Inc.
1280 South 300 West
Salt Lake City, UT 84101
800-658-7030
trifield.com

Aluma-foil
Aluminum radiant/air barrier; two sheets of foil laminated to both sides of a natural kraft paper with a nontoxic adhesive.
Advanced Foil Systems
820 S. Rockefeller Ave., Suite A
Ontario, CA 91761
800-421-5947
afs-foil.com

American Clay Products

American Clay Black Soap Finish
A gelatinous castile soap infused with potash to enrich color and create a soft patina.

American Clay Earth Plaster
An environmentally friendly alternative to cement, gypsum, acrylic, and lime plasters, it is compatible with "breathable" construction for new and historic buildings.

American Clay Gloss Sealer
Low-VOC product used for high-traffic areas, providing water resistance to walls; easy to clean.

American Clay Penetrating Sealer
A low-VOC soy resin/acrylic spray-on sealer that increases durability and water resistance.

American Clay Sanded Primer
Provides a uniform surface that insures a proper bond for plaster applications.
American Clay Enterprises, LLC
2601 Karsten Court, SE
Albuquerque, NM 87102
866-404-1634
americanclay.com

American Pride 100 Line
Interior latex zero-VOC paint line: primer, flat, ceiling, and eggshell. Should not be used for individuals with latex chemical sensitivities. Contains acrylic polymer.
Green Seal certified
Southern Diversified Products
2714 Hardy Street
Hattiesburg, MS 39401
601-264-0442
americanpridepaint.com

Andersen
Window and door manufacturer.
Andersen Corporation
100 Fourth Avenue North
Bayport, MN 55003
800-426-4261
andersenwindows.com

Anhydrous Calcium Chloride Vapor Emissions Test
Test kit available through:
Plaza Hardwood, Inc.
219 W. Manhattan Ave.
Santa Fe, NM 87501
800-662-6306, 505-992-3260
plzfloor.com

Aprilaire
High-efficiency air cleaners.
Research Products Corporation
1015 East Washington Ave.
Madison, WI 53703
800-334-6011
aprilaire.com

Aquapex
A crosslinked polyethylene nontoxic plumbing system by Wirsbo. Refer to **Wirsbo Hepex** for product information.

AquaRite Saline Generator
Swimming pool purification that converts common salt to free chlorine, with none of the smell or skin irritation associated with standard chlorination.
Solar Unlimited
52 East Magnolia Blvd.
Burbank, CA 91502
818-843-1633
solarunlimited.com

Aqua-Zar
Water-based, nonyellowing polyurethane in gloss, satin, semi-gloss, and antique-flat finishes.
United Gilsonite Laboratories
PO Box 70
Scranton, PA 18501
800-272-3235, 570-344-1202
ugl.com

Armor-Guard
Borate-based wood preservative. Refer to **Shellguard** for product information.

Armstrong/DLW Linoleums
Full line of linoleum products made with natural materials.
Armstrong World Industries
PO Box 3001
Lancaster, PA 17604
717-397-0611
armstrong.com

Arreis
Formaldehyde-free, interior-grade MDF (medium density fiberboard). SCS certified no added formaldehyde and 100% pre-consumer recycled wood fiber. Refer to **Medex** for product information.

Auro Products

Note: These products are made with natural plant and mineral derivatives in a process called plant chemistry. Some sensitive individuals may have severe reactions to the natural terpenes, citrus derivatives, and oils.

Auro Awalan Line Cleaning and Care Products
Full line of natural plant-based cleaning and care products.

Auro Cleaning and Care Products
Full line of natural plant-based cleaning and care products.

Auro Natural Paints
Made exclusively from natural sources, with efforts made to support ecological diversity. Packaged in powder form.

Auro Oils, Waxes, and Impregnations
Full line of natural plant-based oils, waxes, and impregnation products.

Auro No. 123 Natural Finishing Oil
Oil primer, sealer, and protective treatment.

Auro No. 143 Organic Linseed Oil Finish
Interior and exterior penetrating, protective, and conditioning treatment for wood.

Auro No. 160 Natural Wood Stain
Weather resistant, water-dilutable, solvent-free stain.

Auro No. 171 Floor and Furniture Wax Finish
Wax paste for wood floors.

Auro No. 173 European Furniture Wax
Wax paste for wood.

Auro No. 251 Clear-Coat Paint Glossy
Oil-based transparent finishing lacquer for use on indoor surfaces. Can be tinted.

Auro No. 382 Floor Covering Adhesive

Auro No. 383 Natural Linoleum Glue
Auro USA
1340 G Industrial Ave
Petaluma, CA 94952
888-302-9352
aurousa.com

Austin Air Healthmate Air Filtration System
Stand-alone HEPA air filtration.
Austin Air Systems, Ltd.
500 Elk Street
Buffalo, NY 14210
800-724-8403
austinair.com
Available through:
Healthy Home
2894 22nd Ave. North
St. Petersburg, FL 33713
727-322-1058
healthyhome.com

Authentic Roof
Recycled material, thermo polyolefin roofing tile; alternative to slate roofing tiles.
Crowe Building Products
116 Burns Street
Hamilton, ON
Canada L8M 2J5
909-529-6818
authentic-roof.com

Bamboo Flooring Directory
Internet directory of bamboo flooring and accessories.
bamboo-flooring.com

Bamboo Hardwoods
Bamboo flooring and accessories.
6402 Roosevelt Way NE
Seattle, WA 98115
800-607-2414
bamboohardwoods.com

Bangor Cork Company
Natural cork "carpeting" and battleship linoleum flooring.
William and D Streets
Pen Argyl, PA 18072
610-863-9041
bangorcork.com

Begley's Best
Biodegradable all-purpose cleaner. Some chemically sensitive individuals may have severe reactions to terpenes and citrus-based components found in this formulation.
Cradle to Cradle certified
Can be ordered online at
begleysbest.com

BIN Primer Sealer
A white, alcohol-based primer sealer that locks in vapors.

BIN Shellac
White paint-on vapor barrier sealer for use as prime coat on gypboard and wherever an opaque sealer is desired.
Wm. Zinsser & Company
173 Belmont Drive
Somerset, NJ 08875
732-469-8100
zinsser.com
Available at:
Home Depot and Coronado

BioBased Systems
Soybean oil-based semi-open-cell spray foam.

BioBased 1701
Soybean polyurethane water-based closed-cell spray foam insulation.
GreenGuard certified
BioBased Systems
1315 N 13th St
Rogers, AR 72756
800-803-5189
biobased.net

Bioform
100% biodegradable form release agent. Environmentally safe, VOC-compliant, does not freeze.
Universal Building Products
4120 York Street
Denver, CO 80216
800-726-6710
universalformclamp.com

BioShield Products

A line of environmental oil finishes that are free of formaldehyde, lead, heavy metals, and fungicides. As with many natural products, some chemically sensitive individuals may not tolerate terpenes, oils, and citrus-based and other aromatic components found in these formulations. Also has a complete line of biodegradable, soap-based household cleaning products.

BioShield Aqua Resin Stain
Solvent-free, water-based, zero-VOC, low-drip, resilient wood stain finish for interior and exterior applications.

BioShield Casein Milk Paint
Dry powder, zero-VOC milk-based paint in pastel colors.

BioShield Clay Paint #12
Made from naturally occurring earthborne clays; earth tone colors.

BioShield Earth Pigments #88
Natural water- and oil-soluble powders made from rocks, minerals, and earth.

BioShield Hard Oil #9
Especially recommended for high-moisture and high-traffic areas. One of the most durable low-VOC oils suitable for hardwood and softwood floors.

BioShield Natural Cork Adhesive
Elastic, waterborne latex glue designed for cork, carpeting, and linoleum tile with jute backing on concrete surfaces, wood, and plywood.

BioShield Penetrating Sealer #5
Crafted from linseed oil, plants and other less hazardous materials, a high-solids primer that excels at sealing cork, dry and absorbent woods, slate, stone, and brick.

BioShield Primer Oil #1
An oil-based sealer that creates an elastic and breathable grain-enhancing prime coat. Equally functional in sealing and priming hardwoods and absorbent softwoods.

BioShield Resin Floor Finish #4
Suitable for use on floors of all types. The finish is breathable and elastic and will create depth and dimension in flooring substrates of all types.

BioShield Solvent Free Wall Paint
Matt and satin finish, zero-VOC wall paints in a variety of colors.
BioShield Paint Company
3215 Rufina Street
Santa Fe, NM 87507
800-621-2591 (US & Canada)
bioshieldpaint.com

Bio-Wash
Line of water-based, non-solvent wood coatings, wood and deck stain strippers, and household cleaners.
Napier Environmental Technologies
720 Eaton Way
Delta BC
Canada V3M 6J9
800-663-9274, 604-526-0802
napiere.com/products/Bio-Wash.php

Block Oil
Natural and nontoxic wood finish. Some chemically sensitive individuals may react severely to lemon oils contained in the product. Available at most woodworking supply and natural homecare stores and at woodworker.com and planetnatural.com.

Bonakemi Mega Polyurethane
Oxygen crosslinking waterborne polyurethane wood finish.
GreenGuard certified
Bonakemi USA, Inc.
2550 South Parker Road, Suite 600
Aurora, CO 80014
800-872-5515
bonakemi.com

Bon Ami Polishing Cleanser
Kitchen and bath scouring cleanser without perfumes, dyes, chlorines, or phosphates. Available in grocery and health food stores.
Faultless Starch/Bon Ami Company
1025 W. 8th St
Kansas City, MO 64101
bonami.com

Bora-Care
Designed to penetrate and protect all types of wood from wood-boring insects. Contains disodium octaborate tetrahydrate in an ethylene glycol carrier. Water-based solution requiring paint or sealer over it.
Nisus Corporation
100 Nisus Dr.
Rockford, TN 37853
800-264-0870
nisuscorp.com

Brai Roof
Modified bitumen roofing.
US Intec, Inc.
1361 Alps Rd.
Wayne, NJ 07470
800-624-6832
www.usintec.com

Breathing Easy
Automatic demand switches and other EMF safety equipment.
4 Louisa Street East
PO Box. 775
Thornbury, Ontario
Canada N0H 2P0
519-599-1111
breathing-easy.net

BRK/First Alert Products
Photoelectric smoke detectors.
BRK Brands, Inc.

3901 Liberty Street Rd.
Aurora, IL 60504
800-392-1395, 630-851-7330
brkelectronics.com
Available at:
Home Depot, Costco, True Value, Target, and many independent hardware stores.

Building for Health — Materials Center
PO Box 113
Carbondale, CO 81623
Orders: 800-292-4838
Information: 970-963-0437
buildingforhealth.com

Casa Natura
Furniture from recycled or sustainably harvested wood, organic upholstered chairs and sofas, and organic mattresses and bedding.
Casa Natura
328 Sandoval Street
Santa Fe, NM 87501
505-820-7634, 877-650-1600
casanaturainc.com

C-Cure Products

C-Cure AR Sanded Grout 922
Blend of Portland cement, silica sand, and colorfast pigments that forms a dense matrix,
free of any voids.

C-Cure FloorMix 900
Blend of Portland cement, sand, and additives producing an excellent dry-set mortar for floor tile.

C-Cure MultiCure 905
Dry-set mortar with additives for use over cementitious and plywood substrates.

C-Cure PermaBond 902
A dual purpose (floor and wall) premium dry-set mortar, particularly suited for tile installation in hot, dry areas.

C-Cure Supreme 925 Grout
Portland cement-based grout, nonshrinking, nontoxic, and odorless.

C-Cure ThinSet 911
Blend of Portland cement, sand, and special additives for the installation of ceramic tile.

C-Cure WallMix 901
Dry-set mortar used for the installation of absorptive tiles (more than 7%).
C-Cure Corporation
13001 Seal Beach Blvd.
Seal Beach, CA 90740
800-895-2874
c-cure.com

Celbar
Spray-in or loose-fill cellulose insulation from fibers, organic in nature, treated with adhesive and borate compound as a fire retardant.
International Cellulose Corporation
12315 Robin Blvd.
Houston, TX 77045
800-444-1252
celbar.com

CertainTeed
Manufacturer of undyed, unbacked fiberglass batt insulation products.
GreenGuard certified products
750 East Swedesford Road
Valley Forge, PA 19482
Consumer line: 800-782-8777
Building professional line: 800-233-8990
certainteed.com

Certified Forest Products Council
(now Metafore)
Nonprofit organization with a database called The Certification Resource Center (CRC), which can be used by consumers, retailers, manufacturers, and processors to find FSC certified products, locate FSC certified forests, and confirm certifications.
certifiedwood.org

Cervitor
High quality steel and thermofoil cabinetry and components that contribute to indoor air quality.
GreenGuard certified
Dwyer
1226 Michael Drive, Suite F
Wood Dale, IL 60191
800-822-0092
dwyerkitchens.com

CHAPCO Products

CHAPCO 244
Acrylic urethane latex wood floor adhesive. Designed to install laminated plank and wood parquet.

CHAPCO Safe-Set 3
Solvent-free, nonflammable, nearly odorless. Contains one or more microbiocides to inhibit mold and mildew.

CHAPCO Safe-Set 88
Ceramic tile adhesive, freeze/thaw stable. May be used where a short open time is desired.

CHAPCO Safe-Set 90
Ceramic tile adhesive type I & II acrylic-based mastic. For tile no larger than 8" × 8".
Chicago Adhesive Products Company
1165 Arbor Dr.
Romeoville, IL 60446
800-621-0220
chapco-adhesive.com

Chromix Admixture and Lithochrome Color Hardener
Mineral pigments containing no chromium or other heavy metals; for use in concrete.
L.M. Scofield Company
6533 Bandini Blvd.
Los Angeles, CA 90040
800-800-9900
scofield.com

Cisco Brothers
Upholstered furniture featuring FSC certified wood, formaldehyde-free glues and finishes, and environmentally friendly manufacturing processes. Their Basal Living Collection features 100% pure natural latex foam, wool matting, and latex/jute ticking. Organic fabrics are available.
Corporate Headquarters
1933 W. 60th St.
Los Angeles, CA 90047
323-778-8612
ciscobrothers.com

Classic Gutter Systems
Distinctive copper gutters and downspouts.
PO Box 2319
Kalamazoo, MI 49003
269-665-2700
classicgutters.com

Clear Coat
Waterborne acrylic topcoat for use with Milk Paint. Protects against dirt abrasion and water spotting. Environmentally safe, nontoxic, odorless when dry. May be used as a clear seal over wood.
Refer to **Milk Paint** for more information.

ClearWater Tech, Inc.
Ozone generators for water and air purification.
ClearWater Tech, Inc.
850 Capitolio Way
San Luis Obispo, CA 93401
800-262-0203
cwtozone.com
Available through:
Healthy Home
2894 22nd Ave. N.
St Petersburg, FL 33713
800-583-9523
HealthyHome.com

Climate Pro
Formaldehyde-free blown-in loose-fill fiberglass insulation.
SCS recycled content certified
Johns Manville Insulation Group
PO Box 5108
Denver, CO 80217
800-654-3103
jm.com

ComfortTherm
A white fiberglass batt insulation with a polyethylene wrap.
SCS recycled content certified
Johns Manville Insulation Group
PO Box 5108
Denver, CO 80217
800-654-3103
jm.com

Contec
Aerated autoclaved concrete block.
Texas Contec, Inc.
1535 Brady Blvd, Suite 2
San Antonio, TX 78237
210-402-3223

Core Home
Cabinet manufacturer that meets European E1 emissions standards and uses FSC certified cabinetry products.
Core Home LLC
PO Box 8200
Santa Fe, NM 87504
505-988-3435
corehome.net

Coyuchi
Organic cotton bedding.
Coyuchi
PO Box 845
Point Reyes Station, CA 94956
888-418-8847
coyuchiorganic.com

Cradle to Cradle
Cradle to Cradle Certification provides a company with a means to tangibly, credibly measure achievement in environmentally intelligent design and helps customers purchase and specify products that are pursuing a broader definition of quality.
c2ccertified.html

Crate and Barrel
Solid wood, glass, and metal furnishings and accessories.
Crate and Barrel
1250 Techny Rd
Northbrook, IL 60062
800-967-6696, 847-272-2888
crateandbarrel.com

Crete-Lease
Very low-odor, nontoxic, nonflammable, biodegradable spray-on concrete form release agent.
Cresset Chemical Company
One Cresset Center, PO Box 367
Weston, OH 43569
800-367-2020 (USA & Canada)
cresset.com

Cross Tuff
Cross-laminated polyethylene air barrier and under-slab radon barrier.
Manufactured Plastics and Distribution Inc.
PO Box 488
Palmer Lake, CO 80133
800-FLEX-FILMS
mpdplastics.com

Custom Woolen Mills
Manufacturers of wool insulation products.
RR #1
Carstairs, AB
Canada T0N 0N0
403-337-2221
customwoolenmills.com

The Cutting Edge Catalog
Moldcheck test kit.
Watercheck test kit for pesticides in water.
The Cutting Edge Catalog
PO Box 4158
Santa Fe, NM 87502
800-497-9516, 505-982-2688
cutcat@cutcat.com
cutcat.com

DAP
Building Green/Living Green sealants and adhesives for residential and commercial use.

Silicone Sealant and Silicone Plus.
2400 Boston Street, Suite 200
Baltimore, MD 21224
800-543-3840
dap.com
Available at many hardware chains including:
Home Depot, Ace Hardware, Hacienda Homecenters, Builders Square

Davis Colors
Mineral-based pigments for concrete.
3700 E. Olympic Blvd.
Los Angeles, CA 90023
800-356-4848
daviscolors.com

DCAT (Development Center for Appropriate Technology)
Nonprofit organization that works to enhance the health of the planet and our communities by promoting a shift to sustainable construction and development through leadership, strategic relationships, and education.
DCAT
PO Box 27513

Tucson, AZ 85726
520-624-6628
dcat.net

Dekswood
Cleaner and brightener for exterior wood.
The Flood Company
PO Box 2535
Hudson, OH 44236
800-321-3444
floodco.com

DEL Industries
Water ozonation systems for residential applications.
DEL Industries
3428 Bullock Lane
San Luis Obispo, CA 93401
800-676-1335
delozone.com

Dennyfoil
Two-sided foil-laminated virgin kraft paper bonded with sodium silicate adhesive.
Denny Wholesale Services, Inc.
141 NW 20th St., Suite B9
Boca Raton, FL 33431
800-327-6616
Distributed by:
E.L. Foust Company
754 Industrial Drive
Elmhurst, IL 60126
800-353-6878
foustco.com

DensArmor Plus
Paperless interior drywall gypsum panel that is highly mold-resistant.
Georgia-Pacific Building Products
55 Park Place
Atlanta, GA 30303
800-284-5347, 404-652-4000
gp.com

Dodge-Regupol, Inc.
Manufacturers of high-quality cork and recycled rubber products for flooring in 18 colors.
Dodge-Regupol, Inc.
715 Fountain Avenue
PO Box 989
Lancaster, PA 17601
866-883-7780
regupol.com

Dragonboard
Multipurpose construction panel made of MgO that can replace gypsum board, OSB, and plywood.
866-447-3232
dragonboard.com

DriTac 7500
Solvent-free, zero-VOC urethane wood flooring adhesive.
DriTac Adhesives Group
59 Ingraham Street
Brooklyn, NY 11237
800-394-9310
dritac.com

Durisol
Wood insulated concrete forms made of recycled clean waste softwood lumber. Special "thermal" units incorporate mineral fiber (rockwool) insulation.
Durisol USA, Inc.
8270 Greensboro Drive, Suite 810
McLean, VA 22102
866-801-0999
inquiries@durisol.com
durisol.com

Durock
Cementitious substrate board for glass/ceramic mosaics, ceramic/quarry tile, thin stone, and brick.
United States Gypsum Company
125 S Franklin St., # 2
Chicago, IL 60606
800-874-4968, 312-606-4000
usg.com

Duro Design
Low-VOC, renewable, and sustainable bamboo, cork, and wood flooring materials.
Duro Design
2866 Daniel Johnson Blvd.
Laval, QC
Canada H7P 5Z7
888-528-8518
durodesign.com

Eagle System 3
Tilt-and-raise blind system. Blinds are sandwiched between insulating glass for dust-free and odorless window dressing; 4 blind colors, 6 shade styles.
Eagle Window and Door
2045 Kerper Blvd.
Dubuque, IA 52001
800-324-5354
eaglewindow.com

Earth Friendly Products
A complete line of environmentally safe domestic cleaning products derived from renewable resources.
Earth Friendly Products
44 Green Bay Rd.
Winnetka, IL 60093
800-335-3267
ecos.com

Earthweave Bio-Floor
Nontoxic natural wool carpeting without dyes, pesticides, or stain protections.
Earth Weave Carpet Mills, Inc.
PO Box 6120
Dalton, GA 30722
706-278-8200
earthweave.com

ECO 2000
Manufacturers and suppliers of environmentally aware, nonhazardous products.
Greencross Certified
KC Products
707 N.E. Broadway, Suite 210
Portland, OR 97232
800-927-9442
kcproductsinc.com

Eco Design/Natural Choice
Cork floor tiles, adhesives, and nontoxic wood floor finishes.
1365 Rufina Court
Santa Fe, NM 87501
800-621-2591

Ecological Paint
Water-based acrylic urethane paints, zero-VOC, formaldehyde-free, formulated especially for chemically sensitive people.
Innovative Formulations
1810 South 6th Avenue
Tucson, AZ 85713
520-628-1553
innovativeformulations.com

Eco-terric
Green and healthy furnishings for the home. Healthy-home consultation and interior design.
Eco-terric
866-582-7547
716 E Mendenhall St.
Bozeman, MT 59715
406-582-7643
Eco-terric
1812 Polk St.
San Francisco, CA 94109
415-558-8700
eco-terric.com

EcoTimber
Supplier of bamboo and sustainably harvested wood floorings produced without harmful chemicals.
EcoTimber
1611 Fourth Street
San Rafael, CA 94901
415-258-8454
ecotimber.com

Eco Wool
Premium-quality wool batting products.
Woolgatherer Carding Mill
610 S. 11th St.
Montague, CA 96064
530-459-5900

ELM Concrete Form Release WS
Low-odor, nontoxic biodegradable concrete form release agent.
Environmental Lubricants Manufacturing, Inc.
1307 Badger Ave.
Plainfield, IA 50666
319-276-4801
elmusa.com

Elmer's Carpenter's Glue
Solvent-free glue.
Borden, Inc.
180 Broad Street

Columbus, OH 43215
800-435-6377, 800-848-9400
elmers.com
Available in many retail outlets.

El Rey Stucco
Manufacturers of exterior wall coatings and stucco products.
3830 Singer Blvd. NE, Suite 2020
Albuquerque, NM 87109
505-873-1180
elrey.com
Available in many retail outlets.

Endurance II
Odorless, hypoallergenic synthetic jute pad.
Shaw Contract Group
380 S. Industrial Blvd.
Calhoun, GA 30701
800-257-7429
shawcontract.com

Enertia Padding
Wool-based carpet padding without dyes, fire retardant, mothproofing, or adhesives.
Earth Weave Carpet Mills, Inc.
PO Box 6120
Dalton, GA 30722
706-278-8200
earthweave.com

Enviro Care
Environmentally preferred green cleaning products, some Green Seal certified.
Available through:
Liberty Enterprises
43 Liberty Drive
Amsterdam, NY
518-842-5080
info@libertychoices.com
libertyarc.org

Enviro-Cote Paint
Acrylic, low-odor, low-VOC interior and exterior paints in flat, satin, and semi-gloss finishes.

E coat Paint
Recycled post-consumer paint line containing 0.8% ethylene glycol by weight and some solvents from recycled paints.
Kelly-Moore Paint Co.
987 Commercial St.
San Carlos, CA 94070
888-677-2468
kellymoore.com

Environ Biocomposites Products

Formaldehyde-free, agribased sustainable panel products for interior finishes and cabinetry.

Environ Biocomposite
Recycled newsprint, soy-based resin interior decorative panel product.

Environ Biofiber Wheat
Wheat straw panel alternative to traditional hardwood or panel products.

Environ Dakota Burl
Burled sunflower hull panel product for interior applications.

Environ Microstrand
Line of industrial-grade panel products as replacement for standard particleboard and/or plywood products.
Environ Biocomposites
221 Mahr Dr.
Mankato MN 5601
800-324-8187
environbiocomposites.com

Environmental Health Center
Home mold test kit.
Environmental Health Center
8345 Walnut Hill Lane, Suite 220
Dallas, TX 75231
214-368-4132
ehcd.com

Environmental Home Center (ecohaus)
Natural and organic wool and cotton bedding, natural mattresses and box springs.
Environmental Home Center
4121 1st Avenue South
Seattle, WA 98134
800-281-9785, 206-682-7332
environmentalhomecenter.com

Environmental Testing and Technology
Wide variety of indoor air-quality testing services

and consultation.
Environmental Testing and Technology
Peter H. Sierck
5431 Avenidas Encinas, Suite F
Carlsbad, CA 92008
760-804-9400
PSierck@baubiology.com

Enviro-Pure
Interior latex zero-VOC paint line in flat, eggshell, and semi-gloss. Should not be used for individuals with latex sensitivities. Contains acrylic polymer.
Green Seal certified
M.A. Bruder & Sons, Inc.
600 Reeder Rd.
Broomall, PA, 19008
800-MAB-1899
customer_service@mabpaints.com
mabpaints.com

Enviro Safe Paints
No-fungicide, low-biocide paints mixed to order.
Chem Safe
PO Box 33023
San Antonio, TX 78265
210-657-5321

Envirotec Health Guard Adhesives
A line of zero-VOC, solvent-free adhesives without alcohol, glycol, ammonia, or carcinogens. Call distributor to find best product for a particular installation.

Envirotec Health Guard Seaming Tapes
For carpeting.
Refer to **Taylor Adhesives** for product information

Extra-Bond
A concentrated acrylic, nontoxic bond that can be mixed with a first coat of Milk Paint to promote adhesion on surfaces other than bare wood.
Refer to **Milk Paint** for more information.

Faswall
Wood insulated concrete form made of softwood lumber.
K-X FASWALL International Corporation
PO Box 328
Montmorenci, SC 29839
800-491-7891
faswall@faswall.com
faswall.com
Available in the Western US through:
Shelter Works Ltd.
PO Box 832
Corvallis, OR 97339
541-760-3644

Fibermesh 650
Macro synthetic fiber alternative for secondary concrete reinforcement.
PROPEX (formally known as SI Corp)
800-621-1273
siconcretesystems.com

Filtrete Ultra Allergen Reduction Filter #1250
3M Corporate Headquarters
3M Center
St. Paul, MN 55144
1-888-364-3577
3m.com
Available through:
Home Depot and Lowe's

FloodStop
Automatic shut-off equipment for hot and cold water supply valves serving washing machines.
Water Alarm
1424 South 700 West
Salt Lake City, UT 84104
801-501-7952
thewateralarm.com

Florapan
Hempwool building-insulation mats.
Moy Isover Ltd.
Ardfinnan, Clonmel,
Co. Tipperary
Ireland
353-52-66100
info@moyisover.ie
moyisover.ie/index.htm

FoamSealR
Polyethylene sill-plate gasket.
GreenGuard certified
1 Owens Corning Pkwy
Toledo, OH 43659
419- 248-8000, 800-766-3464
owenscorning.com

Forbo
Linoleum floor coverings with natural adhesives and antibacterial properties.
2 Maplewood Drive,
PO Box 667
Humboldt Industrial Park
Hazelton, PA 18201
Commercial: 800-842-7839
Residential: 866-Marmoleum
forboflooringna.com

Forest Stewardship Council
International organization that sets standards for sustainability and accredits independent third-party certifiers.
fscus.org

Formula G-510
Nontoxic concentrated multipurpose colloidal industrial cleaner.
Air Control Technologies, Inc.
14120 W. August Zupec Dr.
Wadsworth, IL 60083
847-623-2903, 877-272-4510
www.gaylordg510.com

Furnature
Manufacturer of a natural, organic furniture line and mattresses and bedding for people with multiple chemical sensitivities.
Furnature
86 Coolidge Ave.
Watertown, MA 02472
800-326-4895
info@furnature.com
furnature.com

Gaiam
Organic bedding, towels, and shower curtains.
Gaiam, Inc.
360 Interlocken Boulevard, Suite 300
Broomfield, CO 80021
877-989-6321
customerservice@gaiam.com
gaiam.com

Genesis Odor Free Paint
Interior paints without intrusive paint fumes.
Duron Paints
10406 Tucker St.
Beltsville, MD 20705
800-723-8766
duron.com

GE Silicone II
Clear silicone sealant.

GE Silicone II Household Glue
Use as a glue, sealant, or caulk for many repair applications.
General Electric Company
9930 Kincey Avenue
Huntersville, NC 28078
24-hour hotline: 800-ASK-GESA
Customer Service: 877-943-7325
gesealants.com
Available at: True Value, Ace Hardware, Home Base

Glacier Clear
MDF (medium density fiberboard) with no added urea-formaldehyde.
Plum Creek Timber Company, Inc.
999 Third Ave., Suite 4300
Seattle, WA 98104
800-858-5347, 206-467-3600
plumcreek.com

Good Shepherd Wool Insulation
Natural wool batt and wool rope insulation for log buildings.
Good Shepherd Wool Insulation
RR #3
Rocky Mountain House, AB
Canada T4T 2A3
403-845-6705
goodshepherdwool.com

Good Water Company
Water filtration and consultation.
Stephen Wiman
2778 Agua Fria, Bldg. C, Suite B
Santa Fe, NM 87501
505-471-9036, 800-471-9036
goodwaterglobal.com.

Great Stuff
Expanding foam sealant that is free of CFCs, HCFCs, and formaldehyde.
Insta Foam, Division of Dow Chemical Co.

1881 W. Oak Pkwy
Marietta, GA 30062
800-800-3626
dow.com/greatstuff
Available at: Ace Hardware, Home Depot

Green
Personal care soap; contains fragrance.
GNLD
3500 Gateway Blvd.
Fremont, CA 94538
800-227-2926
gnld.net (search for Green)

GreenGuard
GreenGuard Environmental Institute
Industry-independent, nonprofit organization that oversees the GreenGuard Certification Program.
greenguard.org

Green Planet Paints
Zero-VOC clay-based paints utilizing soy resin and mineral pigments.
PO Box 13
Patagonia, AZ 85624
520-394-2571
greenplanetpaints.com

Green Seal
Organization that offers third-party certification of environmental claims made by a wide variety of products and services in the marketplace.
greenseal.org

Green Unikleen
Water-based emulsion multipurpose cleaner, nontoxic, no VOCs, biodegradable.
Green Seal certified
IPAX Cleanogel, Inc.
8301 Lyndon Avenue
Detroit, MI 48238
313-933-4211
info@ipax.com
ipax.com

Guardian Plus
HEPA filtration, fresh air ventilation and heat recovery systems.
Broan-NuTone LLC
PO Box 140
Hartford, WI 53027
800-558-1711
GuardianPlusAirSystems.com

H3Environmental
Healthy home products and services.
H3Environmental
12439 Magnolia Blvd., PO Box 263
Valley Village, CA 91607
480-946-9600
h3environmental.com

Hardibacker Board
Cementitious tile backerboard for use in moist/wet applications.
James Hardie Building Company
26300 La Alameda, Suite 250
Mission Viejo, CA 92691
888-542-7343
jameshardie.com

Harmony
Low-odor vinyl acrylic interior latex paint. It is more durable than some of the other commercially available low/no-odor paints but also has more odor.
The Sherwin Williams Company
101 Prospect Avenue NW
Cleveland, OH 44115
800-524-5979
sherwin-williams.com

Hartex Carpet Cushion
Odorless synthetic jute underpadding for carpet.
Leggett & Platt
1100 S. McKinney Street
Mexia, TX 76667
800-880-6092
leggettandplatt.com

Healthy Buildings Made Easy
Manufacturer of wood insulated concrete forms.
1621 Villa Strada
Santa Fe, NM 87506
505-466-2012
healthybuildingsmadeeasy.com

Healthy Home
Retail and online store for a variety of products for a healthy home, including mattresses and bedding.

2894 22nd Ave. North
St Petersburg, FL 33713
727-322-1058
healthyhome.com

Heart of Vermont
Organic futons, mattresses, and bedding.
Heart of Vermont
131 South Main Street
PO Box 612
Barre, VT 05641
800-639-4123
heartofvermont.com

Heavenly Heat Saunas
Environmentally safe saunas.
PO Box 2892
Crested Butte, CO 81224
800-697-2862
heavenlyheatsaunas.com

Hendricksen Naturlich
Natural organic fiber carpeting, felt underpads, adhesives, wood, cork, linoleum, and bamboo flooring.
7120 Keating Ave.
Sebastopol, CA 95472
707-829-3959
info@naturalfloors.net
naturalfloors.net

Hepex
A crosslinked polyethylene nontoxic tubing system for radiant floors by Wirsbo. Refer to **Wirsbo Hepex** for product information.

Homespun Fabrics and Draperies
Natural, woven 100% cotton nontoxic fabrics.
Homespun Fabrics and Draperies
PO Box 7287
Chandler, AZ 85246
480-699-9376
homespunfabrics.com

Honeywell
Air purifiers and filters that help reduce contaminants.
877-633-9464
honeywellpurifiers.com

Humabuilt Products

Company specializing in the marketing and sale of healthy, sustainable building solutions.

Humabuilt HumaBlock
Autoclaved aerated interlocking concrete block.

Humabuilt WheatCore Cabinets
Cabinets manufactured from rapidly renewable resource cores and premium-grade woods and veneers, assembled with ultra-low-VOC adhesives and finishes. No added formaldehyde.

Humabuilt WheatCore Doors
Solid core doors made from rapidly renewable resource cores and quality veneers. No added formaldehyde.
Humabuilt
2305-C Ashland Street, #511
Ashland, OR 97520
541-488-0931
info@humabuilt.com
humabuilt.com

Hydrocote Products

Manufacturers and distributors of environmentally safe, virtually odorless, nonflammable, and nontoxic wood finishing products.

Hydrocote Danish Oil Finish
A nontoxic penetrating oil. One-step stain and seal in 9 wood tones.

Hydrocote Hydroshield Plus
Clear coat available in gloss or satin sheen. Water-based polyurethane, giving impact- and weather-resistance for interior or exterior.

Hydrocote Polyshield
A tough, super-hard, nonyellowing polyurethane that is UV stable. Use with Hydrocote stains. Can be used with Hydrocote Ultraviolet Light Absorber Blocker to increase UV resistance.
Hydrocote Company.
1000 Somerset St., Bldg 3B
New Brunswick, NJ 08901
800-229-4937
hydrocote.com

Hydroment
Ceramic tile grout (sanded) and dry tile grout (unsanded). Blend of quartz aggregates, specialty cements, and colorfast pigments. Available in 46 colors.
Bostik, Inc.
211 Boston St
Middleton, MA 01949
978-777-0100
bostik-us.com

IBP Glass Block Grid System
Extruded aluminum glass block grid system for floors.
Innovative Building Products, Inc.
PO Box 425
Fort Worth, TX 76101
800-932-2263
ibpglassblock.com

Icynene Insulation System
A modified, low-density urethane sprayed-foam insulation. Good performance and extremely low outgassing make this product acceptable for those with chemical sensitivities.
Icynene
6747 Campobello Rd.
Mississauga, ON
Canada L5N 2L7
800-758-7325 (US & Canada)
icynene.com

Ikea
Swedish-based company offering solid-wood and veneered furnishings sourced from sustainably managed forest resources and meeting E-1 emissions standards.
For nearest location see ikea.com/us.

Indoor Environmental Technologies, Inc.
Wide variety of indoor air-quality testing services and consultation.
Indoor Environmental Technologies Inc.
William H. Spates
1384 Pierce St.
Clearwater, FL 33756
866-446-7717
inevtec.com

Institute of Inspection, Cleaning and Restoration Certification
Provides certification and referrals for water damage and fire/smoke damage restorers.
IICRC Administrative Office
2715 E Mill Plain Blvd.
Vancouver, WA 98661
800-835-4624
iicrc.org

InsulSafe 4 Premium Blowing Wool
Odor-free, non-corrosive, formaldehyde-, asbestos-, and chemical-free insulation used for thermal and acoustical applications.
CertainTeed Corporation
PO Box 860
Valley Forge, PA 19482
800-233-8990
certainteed.com

International Institute for Bau-Biologie & Ecology (IBE)
A nonprofit educational institute disseminating information and offering courses and seminars on natural, healthy buildings, indoor environmental quality, and electromagnetic radiation. Referrals to certified Bau-Biologie environmental inspectors and consultants.
IBE
1401 A Cleveland St.
Clearwater, FL 33755
727-461-4371
buildingbiology.net

IQAir HealthPro
Stand-alone HEPA air filtration.
Sylvane, Inc.
1495 Hembree Road, Suite 400
Roswell, GA
800-934-9194
sylvane.com
Available through:
Healthy Home
2894 22nd Ave. North
St. Petersburg, FL 33713
727-322-1058
healthyhome.com

Iron sulfate
An iron-based agricultural fertilizer that can be used in a water solution to stain concrete slabs. Some testing samples may be required; staining hues vary. Available at garden centers.

Jandy 3-way diversion valves
For gray-water systems.
1 Valves
PO Box 910996
San Jose, CA 95355
800-688-1233
1valves.com/jandyvalve.html

Janice's
Natural and organic bedding.
30 Arbor Street South
Hartford, CT 06106
Orders: 800-526-4237
Inquiries: 860-523-4479
janices.com

Japanese Wall
Natural clay-based plasters for interior and exterior from Japan.
North American Headquarters
110 E Remington Dr., Suite #30
Sunnyvale CA 94081
626-278-9998
japanesewall.com

Johns Manville
A line of formaldehyde-free fiberglass products.
SCS certified
Johns Manville Insulation Group
PO Box 5108
Denver CO 80217
800-654-3103
jm.com

Junckers
Dust-free wood flooring systems produced without insecticides or laminating adhesives.
Junckers Hardwood, Inc.
95 Grand Street, Unit 3
New York, NY 10013
800-878-9663
junckershardwood.com

Kahrs
A solid wood prefinished engineered floor system.
Kahrs International, Inc.
Oasis Office Center
940 Centre Circle, Suite 1000
Altamonte Springs, FL 32714
800-800-5247
kahrs.com

KD Gold
All-purpose natural, nontoxic, biodegradable soap cleaner/degreaser.
Natural Soap Formulas
Fort Lauderdale, FL
888-759-7256 (US & Canada)
kdgold.com

Kitec
A composite pipe made with an aluminum core bonded to interior and exterior crosslinked polyethylene. Used for radiant in-floor heating.
American Radiant Technologies and Supplies
67 Industrial Park Access Road
Middlefield, CT 06455
860-349-3555
americanradiant.com

Knauf Fiber Glass
Fiberglass insulation products.
GreenGuard certified
Knauf Insulation
One Knauf Drive
Shelbyville, IN 46176
800-825-4434, ext. 8300
knaufusa.com

Laticrete 254 Platinum Thinset mortar
Polymer-fortified thinset mortar.
GreenGuard certified
Laticrete Additive Free Thinset
For use over concrete, cement backerboard, or wire-reinforced mud. Contains Portland cement and sand.
Laticrete International, Inc.
1 Laticrete Park N.
Bethany, CT 06524
800-243-4788
laticrete.com

LESSCO Air Vapor Barrier Boxes
Airtight electrical boxes.
LESSCO Low Energy Systems Supply Co., Inc.
W1330 Happy Hollow Rd.
Campbellsport, WI 53010
920-533-8690
lessco-airtight.com
Available through:
Shelter Supply Inc.
151 East Cliff Rd.
Burnsville, MN 55337
800-762-8399
sheltersupply.com

Less EMF Inc.
EMF-reduction supplies.
LessEMF Inc.
809 Madison Ave.
Albany, NY 12208
888-537-7363
lessemf.com

Lifebreath
Air filtration systems.
Nutech Brands, Inc.
511 McCormick Blvd.
London, ON
Canada N5W 4C8
519-457-1904
lifebreath.com

Lifekind Products
Full line of organic mattresses, linens, bedding, and furniture. Chemically sensitive individuals may react severely to natural rubber compounds found in these products.
Specific products GreenGuard certified
PO Box 1774
Grass Valley, CA 95945
800-284-4983
lifekind.com

Lifemaster 2000
Commercially available paint without petroleum-based solvents. Zero-VOC.
ICI Dulux Paints
925 Euclid Avenue
Cleveland, OH 44115
800-984-5444
iciduluxpaints.com

LifeTime Wood Treatment
Wood preservative, wood stain, wood treatment.
Cedar Mountain Wood Products
143A Great Northern Rd.
Sault Ste. Marie, ON
Canada P6B 4Y9
888-874-7717, 705-941-9945
valhalco.com

Lithochrome Color Hardener
Refer to **Chromix Admixture**.

Lithofin
Stone sealers.
US distributor:
GranQuartz Stone Care Systems
4963 Royal South Atlanta Dr.
Tucker, GA 30084
866-639-0960
lithofin.de

Lithoseal Building Caulk
High quality urethane modified polymer. Inert once cured.
LM Scofield Company
6533 Bandini Blvd.
Los Angeles, CA 90040
800-800-9900, 323-720-3000
scofield.com
Available in the Southwest through:
Lofland
2300 1st Street NW
Albuquerque NM 87124
800-737-1891, 505-247-4344

The Living Source
Source of nontoxic carpets and adhesives.
PO Box 20155
Waco, Texas 76702
Voice mail orders: 800-662-8787
Customer service/orders: 254-776-4878
livingsource.com

Livos Products

A line of plant chemistry products made from plant and mineral derivatives. As with many natural products, some chemically sensitive individuals may not tolerate terpenes, oils, and citrus-based and other aromatic components found in these formulations.

Livos Ardvos Wood Oil
Penetrating oil primer and finish for interior hardwoods. May be topcoated with Livos Bilo Floor Wax.

Livos Bilo Floor Wax
A clear, mar-resistant finish for wood, stone, terra cotta, and linoleum.

Livos Donnos Wood Pitch Impregnation
A penetrating preservative for exterior woodwork that is in contact with moisture. It is made of natural ingredients using plant chemistry.

Livos Dubno Primer Oil
A penetrating oil primer for use as an undercoat on exterior wood.

Livos Glievo Liquid Wax
Clear, apply-and-buff furniture and floor wax. We have also applied this product to plastered walls.

Livos Kaldet Stain, Resin & Oil Finish
A stain and finish oil for interior and exterior surfaces made of wood, clay, or stone. 12 colors.

Livos Meldos Hard Oil
A penetrating oil sealer and finish for interior absorbent surfaces of wood, cork, porous stone, terra cotta tiles, and brick.

Livos Naturals
Low-toxic paints. All ingredients listed on label, many organically grown. Water- and oil-based products available.

Livos Vindo Enamel Paint
Available in the Southwest through:
Building for Health — Materials Center
PO Box 113
Carbondale, Colorado 81623
Orders only: 800-292-4838
Information: 970-963-0437
buildingforhealth.com

Log Home Wool
Sheep wool insulation in batts or rope configuration.
Schroeder Log Home Supply, Inc.
Western Office
3919 Stevensville River Rd
Stevensville MT 59870
800-359-6614, 406-777-2999

MagBoard
Mineral-based nontoxic sheathing product that resists fire, moisture, mold, fungus, and impact.
775-338-2252
mag-board.com

Magnetic Sciences
Magnetometers, gaussmeters, and sensors.
Magnetic Sciences
367 Arlington Street,
Acton, MA 01720
800-749-9873
magneticsciences.com

Mapei 2½ to 1
An additive-free grout for joints larger than ⅜".
Mapei Ultramastic ECO
For ceramic tile installation on light-duty floors, walls, and countertops.
Mapei
1501 Wall Street
Garland, TX 75041
Technical Support: 800-992-6273
Customer Service: 800-455-1210
Customer Service in the Southwest: 480-968-7722
mapei.com

Marvin
Window and door manufacturer.
Marvin Windows and Doors
PO Box 100
Warroad, MN 56763
888-537-7828, 218-3861430
marvin.com

Mary Cordaro Collection
Natural, healthy beds and bedding.
H3Environmental
12439 Magnolia Blvd
PO Box 263
Valley Village, CA 91607
818-766-1787
h3environmental.com

Masonry Heater Association of North America
Membership directory and information source for masonry ovens.

Richard Smith, Administrator
rsmith@boreal.org
mha-net.org

MCS Referral and Resources
Professional outreach, patient support, and public advocacy devoted to the diagnosis, treatment, accommodation, and prevention of multiple chemical sensitivity (MCS) and multisensory sensitivity.
MCS Referral and Resources
10145 Falls Rd.
Lutherville MD 21093
410-889-6666
adonnay@mcsrr.org
mcsrr.org/whoweare.html

Medex
Formaldehyde-free medium density fiberboard for interior high-moisture areas.
No added formaldehyde. 100% preconsumer recycled wood fiber.
SCS certified

Medite ll
Formaldehyde-free, interior-grade medium density fiberboard.
No added formaldehyde. 100% preconsumer recycled wood fiber.
SCS certified
Medite Corporation
PO Box 4040
Medford, OR 97501
800-676-3339
sierrapine.com

Milk Paint
Made from milk protein, lime, earth pigments, and clay; petrochemical-free, biodegradable, nontoxic paint, odorless when dry. Comes in 16 colors. Sold in powder form.
Old-Fashioned Milk Paint Company
436 Main Street
Groton, MA 01450
978-448-6336, 866-350-6455
milkpaint.com

Miller Acro
Acro line has low biocide content and no fungicides. Solvent-free. Flat, satin, semi-gloss.
Miller Paint Company
12812 Northeast Whitaker Way
Portland, OR 97230
800-424-9300, 503-2255-0190
millerpaint.com

Minerva Finishes
Full line of natural interior and exterior lime-based primers, paints, and plasters. Refer to product literature for specific applications and use.
Minerva Finishes
54 White Horse Pike
Waterford, NJ 08089
888-768-3665
minervafinishes.com

Mirrorseal
A non-petroleum-based, polymer, fluid-applied roofing system. Can be applied and repaired by unskilled labor without specialized tools.
Innovative Formulations
1810 S. 6th Ave
Tuscon, AZ 85713
520-628-1553
mirrorseal.com

MSI EMF Meter
A single-axis meter that comes with a Magcheck sensor module.
Available through:
The Cutting Edge Catalog
PO Box 4158
Santa Fe, NM 87502
800-497-9516, 505-982-2688
cutcat.com

Multi-core
Hardwood veneered plywood panels with low formaldehyde emissions, suitable for cabinetry.
Longlac Wood Industries
2311 Royal Windsor Dr., Unit 1
Mississauga, ON
Canada L5Y 1K5
905-403-0425, 888-566-4522
kruger.com
Available in the Central West through:
Frank Paxton Lumber Company
4837 Jackson St,

Denver, CO 80216
303-399-6810
paxtonwood.com

Murco Products

Murco GF1000
Flat wall paint. Odorless when dry. In-can preservatives are entombed in dry paint. No slow-releasing compounds or airborne fungicides.

Murco LE1000
Higher gloss paint formulated as above for use where latex enamels are recommended.

Murco M-100 HiPo
Powdered all-purpose joint cement, a texture compound formulated with inert fillers and natural binders only. No preservatives.
Murco Wall Products
2032 N. Commerce
Fort Worth, TX 76106
800-446-7124, 817-626-1987
murcowall.com

Mystical
Odorless cleaner and deodorizer.
The Non Toxic Hotline
3441 Golden Rain Rd., #3
Walnut Creek, CA 94595
800-968-9355, 888-267-4600
nontoxic.com

National Electromagnetic Field Testing Association
Referrals to independent EMF consultants.
National Electromagnetic Field Testing Association
714 Laramie
Glenview, IL 60025
847-729-1532

The Natural
A complete line of cleaning and homecare products. Degreaser, Bath Tub & Tile Cleaner, and All Purpose products meet Green Seal standards.
The Clean Environment Co., Inc.
8609 I St.
Omaha, NE 68127
800-266-2353, 402-537-0011
cleanenvironmentco.com

Natural Cork Co
Natural cork flooring in a variety of colors and finishes.
Natural Cork Co., Ltd.
1710 N. Leg Ct.
Augusta, GA 30909
800-404-2675
naturalcork.com
Available in the Southwest through:
EcoBuild
PO Box 4655
Boulder, CO 80306
303-545-6255
eco-build.com

Natural Home
Natural beds and bedding.
Natural Home Design Center
461 Sebastopol Ave.
Santa Rosa, CA 95401
800-373-4548, 402-571-1229
naturalhomeproducts.com

Naturally Yours
A complete line of household cleaning products derived from pure, natural ingredients.
Naturally Yours
1926 S. Glenstone Ave., Suite 406
Springfield, MO 65804
888-801-7347
naturallyyoursclean.com

NaturalPAVE XL Resin Pavement
A combination of nontoxic, environmentally friendly organic and inorganic resin materials that creates a high-strength pavement.
Soil Stabilization Products Company, Inc.
PO Box 2779
Merced, CA 95344
800-523-9992
sspco.com

Naturel Cleaner and Sealer
Nontoxic, biodegradable, water-soluble flakes that clean, protect, and finish stone surfaces.
www.naturelsolution.com
Available through:
Building for Health — Materials Center
PO Box 113

Carbondale, CO 81623
Orders: 800-292-4838
Information: 970-963-0437
buildingforhealth.com

NatureWood
Alkaline copper quaternary preservative system developed to provide long-term protection of wood exposed in exterior applications.
Osmose
980 Ellicott Street
Buffalo, NY 14209
716-882-5905
osmose.com

Neff Cabinets
High-quality manufactured cabinets with low formaldehyde emissions. Boxes are made of phenolic glued plywoods. Solid wood doors can be ordered unfinished.
Neff Kitchen Manufacturers
6 Melanie Drive
Brampton, ON
Canada L6T 4K9
800-268-4527, 905-791-7770
neffweb.com

Neil Kelly Cabinets
Cabinetry system designed to meet the needs of the chemically sensitive.
Neil Kelly Cabinets
2636 NW 26th Ave., Suite 200
Portland, OR 97210
503-335-9207
centralpointsystems.com

Neogen Corporation Agri-Screen Ticket
Do-it-yourself pesticide testing kit.
Neogen Corporation
620 Lesher Place
Lansing, MI 48912
800-234-5333
neogen-info@neogen.com
neogen.com

next-ScaleStop
Water-scale control equipment that converts dissolved hardness into microscopic crystals. Does not require potassium or sodium. Not suitable for all water chemistries.
next filtration technologies inc.
PO Box 4010
Incline Village, NV 89450
800-783-0310
info@nextfiltration.com
nextfiltration.com

Nighthawk Carbon Monoxide Detector
A portable unit with battery backup and digital readout.
Positive Energy Conservation Products
PO Box 7568
Boulder, CO 80306
800-488-4340
positive-energy.com
Available at:
Ace, True Value, Home Depot

Nirvana Safe Haven
Organic futons; cotton and wool mattresses and bedding.
3441 Golden Rain Rd., Suite 3
Walnut Creek, CA 94595
800-968-9355, 888-267-4600
nontoxic.com

Novomesh
Synthetic fiber reinforcement for concrete.
SI Corp.
PO Box 22788
Chattanooga, TN 37416
800-635-2308, 423-892-8080
siconcretesystems.com

Obasan
Organic bedding products.
Obasan
50 Colonnade Rd.
Ottawa, ON
Canada K2E 7J6
800-313-3799 (US), 888-413-4442 (Canada)
obasan.ca

Okon Seal and Finish
Satin or gloss. Clear sealer that can be used to seal plaster.
Okon
800-237-0565
okoninc.com

Division of Zinsser Co., Inc
173 Belmont Drive
Somerset, NJ 08875
Zinsser.com

Optima
Blown-in blanket system fiberglass insulation without chemicals and with inert binders.
CertainTeed Corporation
750 East Swedesford
Valley Forge, PA 19482
800-274-8530
certainteed.com
For closest distributor, call 800-441-9850.

Organic Mattresses Inc.
Full line of organic mattresses, linens, and bedding. Chemically sensitive individuals may react severely to natural rubber compounds found in these products.
Organic Mattresses Inc.
sales@organicmattresses.com
omifactory.com

OS Products

OS Color Hard Wax/Oil
A satin matt oil/wax finish for interior wood floor and cork. Water repellent, easy to refinish.

OS Color One Coat Only
12 different stain colors in base of vegetable oils. Interior/exterior use. No preservatives or biocides.

OS Wood Protector
A natural oil-based penetrating wood preservative with zinc oxide. Use to prevent mold and mildew on wood exposed to high humidity and moisture. Does not prevent insect infestation.
Available from:
Environmental Home Center.
4121 1st Ave. South
Seattle, WA 98134
800-281-9785, 206-682-7332
environmentalhomecenter.com
Available in the Southwest and Central West through:
Planetary Solutions
2030 17th St.
Boulder, CO 80302
303-442-6228
planetearth.com
Building for Health — Materials Center
PO Box 113
Carbondale, CO 81623
800-292-4838, 970-963-0437
buildingforhealth.com

Ozark Water Service and Air Services
Air and water testing and consultation services for gases, molds, asbestos, VOCs, pesticides, and EMFs.
Ozark Water Service and Air Services
Warren Clough
114 Spring Street
Sulphur Springs, AR 72768
800-835-8908
ozarkwaterandair.org

Pacific Rim
Hand-crafted, solid western maple furniture grown in managed forests in Washington and Oregon.
Pacific Rim Woodworking.
1030 Tyinn St., # 12
Eugene, OR 97402
541-342-4508
pacificrimwoodworking.com

Pella Corporation
Windows come with optional Slimshade blinds between the two layers of glass, the blinds never requiring cleaning.
Pella Corporaton
102 Main Street
Pella, IA 50219
800-547-3552, 641-628-1000
pella.com

PermaBase
A rigid cementitious substrate suitable for use in wet areas.
Unifix Inc.
National Gypsum Co./Gold Bond
2001 Rexford Road
Charlotte, NC 28211
800-628-4662, 704-365-7300
nationalgypsum.com

Perma-Zyme
A biodegradable and environmentally safe road stabilization enzyme that can be used in place of asphalt paving.

Idaho Enzymes, Inc.
1010 West Main
Jerome, ID 83338
208-324-3642

Phenoseal Products

Water-based nontoxic, nonflammable caulks and sealants available in translucent and 15 colors.

Phenoseal Surpass Caulk and Sealant

Phenoseal Valve Seal

Phenoseal Vinyl Adhesive Caulk
Phenoseal
2400 Boston Street, Suite 200
Baltimore, MD 21224
800-543-3840, 410-675-2100
phenoseal.com

Plaza Hardwood, Inc.
Source for sustainably harvested and recycled wood and anhydrous calcium chloride vapor emissions test.
219 W. Manhattan Ave.
Santa Fe, NM 87501
800-662-6306, 505-992-3260
plzfloor.com

Plyboo
Bamboo flooring and accessories.
Smith & Fong Company
475 6th Street
San Francisco, CA 94103
866-835-9859
plyboo.com

Polyken Tape 337
Aluminum tape that forms an effective air barrier.
Covalence Adhesives (formerly Tyco Adhesives)
25 Forge Parkway
Franklin, MA 02038
800-248-7659
covalenceadhesives.com
Available in the Southwest through:
Perry Supply Company
Albuquerque: 505-884-6972
Santa Fe: 505-473-5177
perrysupply.net

Pottery Barn
Solid wood, glass, and metal furniture and accessories and cotton window dressings.
Pottery Barn
PO Box 7044
San Francisco, CA 75491
800-922-5507
potterybarn.com

Premium Interior Paint Zero-VOC (Olympic Paints)
Zero-VOC paint line; flat, eggshell, satin, and semi-gloss, kitchen and bath. Contains acrylic polymer.
Green Seal certified
Olympic Headquarters
PPG Industries
One PPG Place
Pittsburgh, PA, 15272
800-441-9695
tchsrvaf@ppg.com
olympic.com
Available at: Lowe's

Prestige Publishing
Mold plate test kit for home use. Does not identify mold types.
Prestige Publishing
PO Box 3068
Syracuse, NY 13220
800-846-6687
prestigepublishing.com

Prestowall Interior Wall System
Interior wall panel made of compressed wheat straw.
Available through:
Affordable Building Systems
2747 State Hwy 160
Whitewright, TX 75491
866-364-1198, 903-364-1198

Pristine Eco-Spec
Commercially available acrylic latex paint without VOCs. Available in several finishes.
GreenGuard certified
Benjamin Moore & Company
101 Paragon Drive
Montvale, NJ 07645
800-344-0400
benjaminmoore.com

Professional Discount Supply
Radon mitigation supplies and technical support. Test kits for radon in water and long-term and short-term test kits for radon in air.
Professional Discount Supply
19 W. Las Vegas Street
Colorado Springs, CO 80903
800-688-5776
info@radonpds.com
radonpds.com

Professional Equipment
Lead-check swabs #K910
Turns pink if lead is present; can be used on ceramics, paint, soil, and solder.
Mold test kit #K2400
AccuStar radon test kit #K550K
Professional Equipment
PO Box 5197
Janesville, WI 53547
800-334-9291
professionalequipment.com

Pro-Series H2U
A low-VOC exterior/interior urethane acrylic sealant.
OSI Sealants
Henkel Corporation
32150 Just Imagine Drive
Avon, OH 44011
Technical support: 800-624-7767
Customer Service: 800-999-8920
osisealants.com, henkel.com
Available at: Ace, Home Depot, Lowe's, True Value

PureBond
Formaldehyde-free hardwood plywood.
Columbia Forest Products
100 Paul Road
Chatham, VA 24531
800-237-2428 (East), 800-438-6069 (West)
ColumbiaForestProducts.com

PureColor (formerly Old Growth Aging and Staining)
Two-stage stain formulation of pure mineral ions and oxygen catalyst for wood and concrete surfaces. No solvents, oils, VOCs, odors, acids, or bleaches.
PureColor, Inc.
3900 Paseo del Sol
Santa Fe, NM 87507
505-438-4200
purecolorinc.com

PureKor
"Environmentally preferable panels," one FSC certified, one formaldehyde-free.
Manufactured by and shipped from:
Panel Source International, Inc.
23 Rayborn Crescent, 2nd Floor
St. Albert, AB
Canada T8N 5C1
780-458-1007
panelsource.net

PuriTec
Advanced air purifier and water filter systems, including ESF Enviro Scale-Free.
PuriTec
8879 West Flamingo Road,
Suite 203
Las Vegas, NV 89147
888-491-4100
puritec.com

Radalert 100
Geiger counter radioactivity measuring device.
International Medcom
6871 Abbott Ave.
Sebastopol, CA 95472
707-823-0336
medcom.com

Radon Mitigators, Inc.
Installation of Soil Gas Collector Matting.
505-986-8395
Services@RadonNewMexico.com
radonnewmexico.com

Rappgo
Prefinished engineered wood flooring system from Sweden with very low emissions.
Distributed in the US by:
Plaza Hardwood, Inc.
219 W Manhattan Ave.
Santa Fe, NM 87501
800-662-6303, 505-992-3260
plzfloor.com

Rate It Green
An online community committed to growing the green building market through shared resources and information.
216 Westerly Road
Weston, MA 02493
617-686-8977
rateitgreen.com

RCD6
Nontoxic water-based mastic for sealing ductwork and metal joints.
Positive Energy
PO Box 7568
Boulder, CO 80306
800-488-4340, 303-444-4340
positive-energy.com

Real Goods
Source of Floatron, a solar-powered pool purifier combining solar electric power with mineral ionization. Reduces chlorine usage up to 80%. Catalog sales for natural organic bedding, shower curtains, and towels.
Real Goods
360 Interlocken Blvd., Suite 300
Broomfield, CO 80021
888-212-5643
gaiam.com/realgoods

Reflectix Insulation
Foil faced and backed over plastic bubbles, especially designed to reflect heat.
Reflectix, Inc.
#1 School Street
PO Box 108
Markleville, IN 46056
800-879-3645, 765-533-4332
reflectixinc.com

Resource Conservation Technologies, Inc.
Acrylic polymer roll-on paint roofing without toxic dispersants or tints.
2633 N. Calvert Street
Baltimore, MD 21218
410-366-1146
Conservationtechnology.com

Restoration Consultants Inc.
Consultation and training in thermal imaging, mold investigation, and indoor environmental quality.
3284 Ramos Circle
Sacramento, CA 95827
888-617-3266, 916-736-1100
restcon.com

Restoration Industry Association (RIA)
Formerly ASCR
Certified Mold Professional Program
Mold professional certification program and referrals.
Water Loss Institute
Water-loss specialist technician certification and referrals.
Restoration Industry Association
9819 Patuxent Woods Dr., Suite K
Columbia, MD 21046
800-272-7012, 443-878-1000
ascr.org

rFOIL
Reflective foil insulation product.
WE International, Inc.
PO Box 97
Syracuse, IN 46567
574-457-3066
877-777-3645
we-intl.com, rfoil.com
Available in Santa Fe through:
Dahl Plumbing
1000 Siler Park Lane
Santa Fe, NM 87507
505-471-1811
dahlplumbing.com

Rocky Mountain Hardware
72% recycled content, 50% post-consumer architectural hardware.
SCS recycled content certified
Rocky Mountain Hardware
PO Box 4108
1030 Airport Way
Hadley, ID 83333
888-788-2013

RoofShield
Roofing underlayment.
Refer to VaproShield for product information.

RooftopGuard
Roofing underlayment.
Drexel Metals Corp.
204 Railroad Drive
Ivyland, PA 18974
888-321-9630
rooftopguard.com
drexmet.com

Roo Glue
Adhesives for most construction materials.
PO Box 299
Woodburn, OR 97071
877-766-4583, 503-981-5640
rooglue.com

Roseburg Plywood
Plywood product with no added urea-formaldehyde.
Roseburg SkyBlend Particleboard
Particleboard that has no urea-formaldehyde added during the manufacturing process.
SCS 100% pre-consumer recycled fiber certified
Roseburg Forest Products
PO Box 1088
Roseburg, OR 97470
10599 Old Hwy 99 S.
Dillard, OR 97432
800-245-1115, 541-679-3311
rfpco.com

Rub-R-Wall
Rubber polymer moisture-resistant foundation membrane containing no asphalt. Spray-on application. Manufacturer claims product is nontoxic once dry.
Rubber Polymer Corporation
1135 W. Portage Trail Extension
Akron, OH 44313
800-860-7721
rpcinfo.com

Sachi Organics
Manufacturers of organic cotton beds and futons and retailers of organic bedding and linens.
Sachi Organics
523 West Cordova Rd.
Santa Fe, NM 87505
877-997-2244
services@sachiorganics.com
sachiorganics.com

Safe Living Technologies, Inc.
Automatic demand switch.
Safe Living Technologies, Inc.
34 Queen St.
PO Box 72
Morriston, ON
Canada N0B 2C0
519-240-8735
safelivingtechnologies.ca

Samina
Manufacturers of organic cotton, wool, and latex mattress systems.
Samina USA
1530 Northern Blvd.
Manhasset, NY 11303
516-869-6004
samina.com

Scientific Certification Systems (SCS)
Scientific Certification Systems is a leading third-party provider of certification, auditing and testing services, and standards.
scscertified.com

Seagull IV Water Purification System
Chemical-free water purifier.
General Ecology, Inc.
151 Sheree Blvd.
Exton, PA 19341
800-441-8166
generalecology.com
Available through:
Nirvana Safe Haven
3441 Golden Rain Rd., Suite 3
Walnut Creek, CA 94595
800-968-9355, 888-267-4600
nontoxic.com

Shellguard
Borate-based wood preservative.
Perma-Chink Systems, Inc.
1605 Prosser Road
Knoxville, TN 37914

800-548-3554
permachink.com

Shepherd's Dream
Custom-made wool beds and bedding, solid wood bed frames, and organic linens.
140 S. 11th St.
Montague, CA 96064
800-966-5540
Also:
361 3rd St.
Steinbach, MB
Canada R5G 1P9
866-552-0167
shepherdsdream.com

Siemens EQ111
Standard-load center electrical panels and subpanels with split neutral.
Siemens
1 Internet Plaza
Johnson City, TN 37604
800-964-4114
usa.siemens.com

Sinak Corporation
pH test pencil for concrete slab alkalinity test. Reusable calcium chloride moisture and pH dome test kit for concrete slabs.
Sinak Corp.
1949 Walnut Ave.
San Diego, CA 92101
800-523-3147
sinakcorp.com

Sinan Company Products

Natural building materials company with wood finishes, wall paints, glues, cleansers, and polishes.

Sinan Company No. 143 Linseed Oil
Organically grown for plain oiled-rubbed finish.

Sinan Company No. 251 Natural Clear Varnish, Clear, Glossy and No. 261 Clear Satin
Varnish with good covering qualities for indoor wood use only.

Sinan Company No. 253 Natural Undercoat Enamel, White, Water-Based
Suitable for priming or intermediate coats for interior and exterior use on woods.

Sinan Company No. 260 Natural Enamel, White, Water-Based, Interior Satin
Low-gloss lacquer for interior use only. For use over No.153. Can be tinted.

Sinan Company No. 301 Natural Wall Paint Primer
Water-based paint for priming interior wall surfaces that are absorbent, such as Sheetrock and plaster.

Sinan Company No. 321 Emulsion Wall Paint, White
For application over No.301. Can be tinted.

Sinan Company No. 322 Professional Wall Paint, White
Water-based paint for indoor use over primer. Satin flat; can be tinted.

Sinan Company No. 380 Natural All-Purpose Floor Adhesive
Water emulsion organic binders for cork, tile, linoleum, carpeting, small parquet floors, etc., for use over cement-based substrates.

Sinan Company No. 390 Natural Contact Glue
Water emulsion organic binders for cork, paper, metal, plastic, and glass.

Sinan Company No. 751 Powder Chalk-Casein Wall Paint
Powdered paint for interior Sheetrock and woodwork.
Sinan Company
PO Box 857
Davis, CA 95617
530-753-3104
sinanco.com

SlabShield
Foam/foil sandwich slab insulation.
Environmentally Safe Products, Inc.
313 W. Golden Lane.
New Oxford, PA 17350
800-289-5693, 717-624-3581
low-e.com

Sleeptek
Oasis Collection
Custom-made organic mattresses and bedding sets distributed by Furnature. Refer to **Furnature** for information.

SmartWood Certification Program
Independent auditing, certification, and promotion of FSC certified forest products to improve forest management by providing economic incentives to businesses practicing responsible forestry.
rainforest-alliance.org/programs/forestry/smartwood

Smith and Hawken
Variety of sustainably harvested teak and cedar solid wood furniture.
Smith and Hawken
PO Box 8690
Pueblo, CO 81008
800-940-1170
smithandhawken.com

Soft Heat Infrared Sauna
Uses radiant (infrared) energy, unlike the more common hot-air saunas.
Available through:
The Cutting Edge Catalog
PO Box 4158
Santa Fe, NM 87502
800-497-9516, 505-982-2688
cutcat@cutcat.com
cutcat.com

Soil Gas Collector Matting
Used alongside perimeter at top of stem wall with "T" risers and piping. Effectively removes radon gas before it enters building.
Professional Discount Supply
19 W. Las Vegas St
Colorado Springs, CO 80903
800-688-5776, 719-444-0646
radonpds.com

Sound Deadening Board (Natural Panels)
Rigid 4' × 8' building panel with excellent noise control properties made from nontoxic, paraffin-impregnated organic materials and natural wood fibers.
Building Products of Canada Corp.
9510 St. Patrick Street
LaSalle, QC
Canada H8R 1R9
800-567-2726
service@bpcan.com
bpcan.com

SOYsolv
Very low-odor, water-based, nontoxic, nonflammable, biodegradable spray-on concrete form release agent.
SOYsolv
6154 N CR 33
Tiffin, OH 44883
800-231-4274
soysolv.com

Spectracidal Disinfectant Agent
Nontoxic germicide, EPA approved.
Apothecure, Inc.
4001 McEwen Rd., Suite 100
Dallas, Texas 75244
800-969-6601
apothecure.com

Spectra-Tone Paints
Zero-VOC, solvent-free latex paint; cost competitive with standard quality latex.
Spectra-Tone Paint Corporation
1595 E. San Bernardino Ave.
San Bernardino, CA 92408
800-272-4687, 909-478-3485
spectra-tone.com

Stabilizer
A colorless, odorless psyllium-based additive for pathways, trails, and driveways.
Stabilizer Solutions, Inc.
33 S. 28th Street
Phoenix, Arizona 85034
800-336-2468, 602-225-5900
info@stabilizersolutions.com
stabilizersolutions.com

Stevens EP
Low-odor, heat weldable ethylene propylene roofing membrane.
Stevens Roofing Products
9 Sullivan Road
Holyoke, MA 01040
800-621-7663, 413-552-1000
stevensroofing.com

Stratica
Resilient flooring that is PVC-free, very low-odor, and durable.
Amtico International, Inc.

Amtico Studio
6480 Roswell Road
Atlanta, GA 30328
800-268-4260, 404-267-1900
amtico.com
stratica.com

Strong-Enviro Board
Multiuse mineral and fiber board.
2323 S. Shepherd Dr., Suite 810
Houston, TX 77019
866-640-7895
strongenviroboard.com

StrongSeal Roofing Underlayment
Contains no asphalt; both nail-down and premium self-adhering membranes.
Cetco-StrongSeal Roofing Materials
1500 West Shure Dr.
Arlington Heights, IL 60004
800-527-9948
strongsealroofing.com

Styrofoam Weathermate Plus Housewrap
Nonwoven nonperforated polyolefin-based wrap.
Dow Building Solutions
200 Larkin
Midland, MI 48674
Call 866-583-2583 for distributors
dow.com/Styrofoam/na/weather

Summitville-700 SummitChromes
Sanded grout without polymer additives; available in 32 colors.
Summitville Tiles, Inc.
Summitville, Ohio 43962
330-223-1511
summitville.com

Super R and Tempshield
Radiant barriers and reflective insulation.
Innovative Insulation, Inc.
6200 W. Pioneer Parkway
Arlington, TX 76013
800-825-0123
radiantbarrier.com

Sure Seal Foam Tape
An adhesive-backed gasket that is extremely compressible and creates a tight seal. Must be mail ordered.
Denarco Inc
301 Industrial Drive
Constantine, MI 49042
269-435-8404

Sustainable Flooring
Supplier of Jelenik cork flooring and Hanlite bamboo flooring and millwork.
Sustainable Flooring
1336 Mountain Pine Rd.
Boulder, CO 80301
303-544-6076
sustainableflooring.com

Taylor Adhesives Products

Taylor Envirotec 901 Odyssey
Smooth-spreading mastic for interior ceramic wall and floor tile.

Taylor Meta-Tec 2084 Tuff Lok X Link
Solvent-free, low-odor linoleum adhesive.
GreenGuard certified

Taylor Meta-Tec 2086 Tuff Lok-Link
Solvent-free low-odor cork flooring, cork tile, and cork underlayment adhesive.
GreenGuard certified

Taylor MS Plus
Negligible-VOC, low-odor polymer-based wood flooring adhesive.
GreenGuard certified
WF Taylor Company
11545 Pacific Ave.
Fontana, CA 92337
800-397-4583 (CA office), 800-868-4583 (GA office)
wftaylor.com

Taylor Tools
Calcium chloride moisture and alkali test kit for concrete slabs.
Taylor Tools
303-371-7667
kpapulski@taylortools.com
sinakcorp.com

TC&I
Foam-in-place urethane insulation.
Thermal Coatings & Insulation Construction, Inc.
I-25 and Cerrillos Road Exit

Santa Fe, NM 87508
505-471-9230
tcandifoamroofing.com

Tectum
Acoustical ceiling tiles.
Tectum, Inc.
PO Box 3002
Newark, OH 43058
888-977-9691
tectum.com

Temstock-Free
Recycled and/or recovered fiber particleboard, manufactured with no added urea-formaldehyde.
Temple-Inland
1300 S. Mopac Expressway
Austin, TX 78746
512-434-5800
information@templeinland.com
templeinland.com

Teragren
Bamboo flooring and accessories (previously called Timbergrass).
Teragren LLC
12715 Miller Rd. NE, Suite 301
Bainbridge Island, WA 98110
800-929-6333, 206-842-9477
teragren.com

Terramica
Industrial-grade particleboard and particleboard underlayment with no added urea-formaldehyde.
SCS certified no added formaldehyde
Potlatch Forest Products Corp.
601 West Riverside Ave., Suite 1100
Spokane, WA 99201
505-835-1500
potlatchcorp.com

Therma-Stor Filter-Vent
Air purifying ventilator.
Therma-Stor LLC
4201 Lien Rd.
Madison, WI 53704
800-533-7533
sales@thermastor.com
thermastor.com

Thoroseal Foundation Coating
Cementitious waterproofing for concrete surfaces.
BASF Building Systems
889 Valley Park Dr.
Shakopee, MN 55379
800-433-9517, 952-496-6000
www.basfbuildingsystems.com

Tiger Foam
Low-VOC, formaldehyde-free spray-foam insulation.
Commercial Thermal Solutions, Inc.
6 Worthington Avenue
Spring Lake NJ 07762
800-664-0063
tigerfoam.com

Tillco Plastic Rebar
Fiberglass-reinforced plastic rebar alternative to metal rebar.
Tillco Company
PO Box 1127
Greenbrier, AR 72058
870-404-1922
tillco.com

Timberline 2051 Wood Flooring Adhesive
Refer to **Envirotec Health Guard Adhesives** for product information.

Timber Pro UV
Natural plant-based, oil-based, waterborne breathable stain that seals and protects. Available in 5 standard and 40 custom colors. Optional low-toxicity fungicide/algaecide (1% solution) provides mildew and algae resistance.
Timber Pro UV (USA)
2232 E. Burnside Avenue
Portland, OR 97214
888-888-6095, 503-232-1705
usainfo@timberprocoatings.com
timberprocoatings.com

TimberSIL
Nontoxic, arsenic-free wood treatment process that uses sodium silicate technology (SST).
Cradle to Cradle certified
TimberSIL
7481 Huntsman Blvd., Suite 520

Springfield, VA 22153
800-385-0450, 866-318-9432
timbersil.net

Tim-bor
Disodium octaborate tetrahydrate wood preservative that protects against termites, fungus, and wood-boring beetles.
Nisus Corporation
100 Nisus Dr.
Rockford, TN 37853
800-264-0870
nisuscorp.com

Titanium UDL
Non-asphaltic underlayment for sloped roofs.
InterWrap, Inc.
32923 Mission Way
Mission, BC
Canada V2V 6E4
800-567-9727
To find a distributor, see interwrap.com/titanium.

Titebond Solvent Free Construction Adhesive
Titebond Solvent Free Subfloor Adhesive
Multipurpose adhesives for a variety of porous surfaces, including plywood and wood paneling.
Franklin International
2020 Bruck Street
Columbus, OH 43207
800-877-4583
titebond.com

TransMineral USA, Inc.
St. Astier Natural Hydraulic Lime exterior plaster.
201 Purrington Rd.
Petaluma, CA 94952
707-769-0661
limes.us

Trewax Nature's Orange
Biodegradable cleaner, degreaser, deodorizer.
SCS biodegradable certified
Some chemically sensitive individuals may have severe reactions to citrus-based components in this formulation.
Trewax Neutral Cleaner
Biodegradable all-purpose cleaner (except unfinished wood) for no-wax floors, marble, terrazzo, pavers, etc.
SCS biodegradable certified
Beaumont Products, Inc.
1560 Big Shanty Dr.
Kennesaw, GA 30144
800-451-7096, 859-514-7400
trewax.com

Trip Trap Oils
A complete line of wood surface flooring treatment oils using only natural ingredients, imported from Denmark and designed to maintain and clean hardwood or engineered wood flooring.
Trip Trap USA
Special Hardwood Products Inc.
6728 Tribble St.
Lithonia, GA 30058
877-928-9663
specialhardwood.com

Tru-Spec
Urea-formaldehyde-free, low-VOC millwork-quality engineered wood product made with a water-resistant adhesive.
GreenGuard certified
Refer to **AdvanTech** for more information.

TruStone America
Autoclaved aerated concrete blocks.
2151 E. Broadway Rd., #115
Tempe, AZ 85282
877-351-4448
e-crete.com

Tulikivi U.S., Inc.
Scandinavian manufacturer of high-efficiency masonry and metal fireplaces and ovens.
PO Box 7547
Charlottesville, VA 22906
800-843-3473
tulikivi.com

Tu Tuf 4 or XF
4 mil thick, high-density, cross-laminated, puncture-resistant polyethylene air barrier. Can be effectively used under concrete.
Sto-Cote Products, Inc.
PO Box 310
Genoa City, WI 53128
800-435-2621, 262-279-6000

Available through:
Energy Federation Inc.
800-379-4121
energyfederation.org

Tyvek Products

Tyvek FlexWrap
Polyolefin-based flexible flashing.

Tyvek HomeWrap
Air and weather barrier.

Tyvek StraightFlash (new)
Polyolefin-based flexible flashing.

Tyvek StuccoWrap
Stucco weather barrier underlayment.
DuPont Co.
1007 Market St.
Wilmington, DE 19898
800-441-7515
dupont.com

UltraTouch
29 oz. carpet cushion, R-19 batts, and R-13 batts made of recycled cotton and other fibers.
Bonded Logic
411 East Ray Road,
Chandler, AZ 85225
480-812-9114
bondedlogic.com

Uni-Flex Duct Sealer
Uni-Mastic 181 Duct Sealer
United Duct Sealer (Water Based)
Low-VOC water-based duct mastics for residential use.
McGill AirSeal Corporation
2400 Fairwood Avenue
Columbus, OH 43207
800-624-5535
mcgillairseal.com

Vaprecision, Inc.
Anhydrous calcium chloride moisture vapor test kit and surface pH test kit for concrete slabs.
Vaprecision, Inc.
3211 W. MacArthur Blvd.
Santa Ana, CA 92704
800-449-6194
kits@vaportest.com
vaportest.com

VaproShield
Manufacturer of moisture-control products.
VaproFlashing
Bonded polypropylene fabric flexible flashing.
VaproShield
915 26th Ave. NW, Suite C5
Gig Harbor, WA 98335
866-731-7663
lees@vaproshield.com
vaproshield.com

Venmar Ventilation, Inc.
Heat/energy recovery ventilation.
550 Lemire Blvd.
Drummondville, QC
Canada I2C 7W9
800-567-3855
venmar-ventilation.com

Vocomp-25
Water-based acrylic concrete sealer.
W. R. Meadows
PO Box 338
Hampshire, IL 60140
800-342-5976, 847-214-2100
wrmeadows.com

Volclay
4' × 4' corrugted kraft panels filled with Bentonite clay that expands when wet to form a dampproof barrier.
Cetco
1500 West Shure Drive
Arlington Heights, IL 60004
800-527-9948, 847-392-5800
cetco.com/bmg

V-rod
Fiber reinforced polymer rebar for reinforcing concrete.
Trancels Construction Technologies
33 Pennsylvania Ave., Unit 5
Concord, ON
Canada L4K 4A5
888-726-2357, 416-410-2564
trancels.com

Warm Board
Structural subfloor and radiant heat system.
Warm Board
8035 Soquel Dr.
Aptos, CA 95003
831-685-9276, 877-338-5493
warmboard.com

Water Factory Systems
SQC Series: Reverse osmosis combined with premium activated carbon.
Available through:
Good Water Company
2778 Agua Fria, Bldg. C, Ste. B,
Santa Fe, NM 87501
800-471-9036, 505-471-9036
goodwaterglobal.com.

Weatherall Products

Sealings, coatings, and adhesives.

Weatherall UV Guard
Exterior acrylic wood finish that penetrates and seals, forming a protective shield against UV, rot, and decay. Comes in clear and semi-transparent finishes.
Weatherall UV Guard Premium Caulking
A professional strength acrylic-based sealant designed for use in a wide variety of construction applications.
Weatherall Co., Inc.
106 Industrial Way
Charlestown, IN 47111
800-367-7068
weatherall.com

Weather-Bos Products

Stains and finishes for durable, high performance protection.

The Boss
Four different formulas for protection of exterior wood surfaces.
Masonry Boss
Water-reducible sealer for all above-grade concrete and masonry surfaces. Helps reduce dusting, powdering, efflorescence, spalling, cracking, and freeze-thaw damage.

Distributed and drop shipped same day by:
Weather-Bos International
316 California Avenue, Suite 1082
Reno, NV 89509
800-664-3978
info@weatherbos.com
weatherbos.com

Weather Pro
A water-based, water-repellent wood stain for interior/exterior. VOC-compliant.
Okon
4725 Leyden St., Unit A
Denver, CO 80216
800-237-0565, 303-377-7800
okoninc.com

Wheatboard or Wheatstraw
Medium density fiberboard made from recycled wheatstraw, formaldehyde-free.
Eco-Products, Inc.
3655 Frontier Ave.
Boulder, CO 80301
303-449-1876

WindowWrap-Butyl
Self-adhering flexible flashing polyethylene film.
MFM Building Products
PO Box 340
Coshocton, OH 43812
800-882-7663, 740-622-2645
mfmbp.com

Wirsbo Hepex
Crosslinked polyethylene tubing for radiant floor heating.
Wirsbo
5925 148th Street W.
Apple Valley MN 55124
800-321-4739
wirsbo.com

Wood Flooring International
A source for engineered and solid FSC certified flooring. Their American Woods, Monteverde, Pacific Northwest, and Orchard Collections all meet E1 emissions standards.
Wood Flooring International
122 Kissel Road

Burlington, NJ 08016
866-764-2601
wflooring.com

Wood Pro UV (formerly Timber Tek UV)
A resin-based waterborne penetrating oil.
Timber-Pro UV Wood Finishes
2232 E. Burnside
Portland, OR 97214
888-888-6095
timberprocoatings.com
Distributed by:
Planetary Solutions
2030 17th St.
Boulder, CO 80302
303-442-6228
planetearth.com

Wow!
Stainless steel cleaner and protectant, biodegradable, no petroleum distillates.
SCS biodegradable certified
EZ Finishes, Inc.
78 Aurora St.
Hudson, Ohio 44236
866-969-3279
wowezfinish.com

Xypex
Concrete dampproofing by crystallization. EPA approved for potable water. Protects concrete against spalling, efflorescence, and other damage.
Xypex Chemical Corporation
13731 Mayfield Place
Richmond, BC
Canada V6V 2G9
800-961-4477, 604-273-5265
www.xypex.com

Yolo Colorhouse
Zero-VOC interior paints: primer, flat, satin, and semi-gloss. Contain acrylic emulsion.
Green Seal certified
Yolo Colorhouse LLC
1001 SE Water Avenue, Suite 140
Portland, OR 97214
877-493-8276
info@colorhouse.com
yolocolorhouse.com

Z-coat (59-Line)
Zero-VOC interior paint line (sealer, flat, eggshell, and semi-gloss) containing acrylic polymer.
Green Seal certified
General Paint
950 Raymur Ave
Vancouver, BC
Canada V6A 3L5
604-253-3131
generalpaint.com

Zip-Guard Environmental Wood Finish
Clear, water-based, low-VOC urethane finish for interior woodwork.
Star Bronze Co., Inc.
PO Box 2206
Alliance, OH 44601
800-321-9870, 330-823-1550
starbronze.com

Notes

Preface

1. David E. Jacobs et al. "Linking Public Health, Housing, and Indoor Environmental Policy: Successes and Challenges at Local and Federal Agencies in the United States." *Environmental Health Perspectives.* Vol. 115, no. 6 (June 2007), pp. 976–982.
2. Ibid.
3. US Environmental Protection Agency. *Identification of Non-Target List Analytes in Complex Environmental Samples* [online]. [Cited November 8, 2007.] epa.gov/ppcp/projects/non-target.html
4. Environmental Working Group. *Chemical Industry Archives* [online]. [Cited November 8, 2007.] chemicalindustryarchives.org/factfiction/facts/1.asp
5. Nicholas Ashford and Claudia Miller. *Chemical Exposures: Low Levels and High Stakes.* 2nd ed., John Wiley and Sons, 1998, p. 26.

Overview

1. "Environment 1992." Science News. Vol. 142, nos. 25–26 (December 17 and 26, 1992), p. 436.
2. William J. Rea. *Chemical Sensitivity, Volume 2.* Lewis Publishers, 1994, p. 706.
3. Marion Moses. *Designer Poisons: How to Protect Your Health and Home from Toxic Pesticides.* Pesticide Education Center, 1995, p. 309.
4. US General Accounting Office. *Lawn Care Pesticides: Risks Remain Uncertain While Prohibited Safety Claims Continue.* US Government Printing Office, March 1990, pp. 4–5.
5. Jay Feldman. "Press Release." Beyond Pesticides/National Coalition Against the Misuse of Pesticides, June 8, 2000.
6. Michael H. Surgan. "EPA Pesticide Registration: Our Safety in the Balance?" *NCAP News.* Vol. 4, no.3 (Fall 1993), pp. 21–23.
7. Steven Arnold et al. "Synergistic Activation of Estrogen Receptor with Combinations of Environmental Chemicals." *Science.* Vol. 272 (June 7, 1996), pp.1489–1492.
8. Marcia Nishioka et al. "Measuring Transport of Lawn-applied Herbicides from Turf to Home: Correlation of Dislodgeable 2,4-D Turf Residues with Carpet Dust and Carpet Surfaces Residues." *Environmental Science Technology.* Vol. 30, no.1, pp. 3313–3320.
9. Jack Leiss and David Savitz. "Home Pesticide Use and Childhood Cancer: A Case-control Study." *American Journal of Public Health.* February 1995, pp. 249–252.
10. E. Gold et al. "Risk Factors for Brain Tumors in Children." *American Journal of Epidemiology.* Vol.109 (1979), pp. 309–319.
11. American Cancer Society. "Drug-free Lawns." Pamphlet, 1993.
12. William J. Rea. *Chemical Sensitivity, Volume 2.* Lewis Publishers, 1994, p. 880.
13. D.J. Hunter and K.T. Kelsey. "Pesticide Residues and Breast Cancer: The Harvest of a Silent Spring?" *Journal of the National Cancer Institute.* Vol. 85 (April 21, 1993), pp. 598–599.
14. Robert Becker. *Body Electric.* Tarcher Press, 1985.

15. Research conducted by Anthony Coehlo and Steve Easley of Southwest Research Institute, San Antonio, TX. Cited in *The Sacramento Bee*, July 14, 1990.
16. "Leading Epidemiologists See Childhood Leukemia Risk at 4 mG." *Microwave News*. Vol. 20, no. 5 (September/October 2000), pp. 1, 11–13.
17. See, for example: US Environmental Protection Agency. *The Total Exposure Assessment Methodology (TEAM) Study: Summary and Analysis, Volume 1*. EPA Office of Research and Development, June 1987, and Nicholas A. Ashford and Claudia S. Miller. *Chemical Sensitivity*. The New Jersey State Department of Health, December 1989.
18. Committee on Science and Technology, US House of Representatives. Report 98-821, September 16, 1986. Cited in Cindy Duehring and Cynthia Wilson. *The Human Consequences of the Chemical Problem*. TT Publishing, 1994, p. 5.
19. "Neurotoxins: At Home and in the Workplace." Committee on Science and Technology, US House of Representatives. Report 99-827, September 16, 1986. Cited in Cindy Duehring and Cynthia Wilson. *The Human Consequences of the Chemical Problem*. TT Publishing, 1994.
20. Ibid.
21. Ibid.

Division 1

1. California Environmental Protection Agency, Office of Environmental Health Hazard Assessment. *Proposition 65* [online]. [Cited November 16, 2007.] oehha.ca.gov/prop65.html
2. Elizabeth Kersten and Bruce Jennings. *Pesticides and Regulation: The Myth of Safety*. California Senate Office of Research, Senate Reprographics, 1991.
3. Robert Abrams. *The Secret Hazards of Pesticides: Inert Ingredients*. New York State Department of Law, 1991.
4. B. I. Castleman and G.E. Ziem. "Corporate Influence on Threshold Limit Values." *American Journal of Industrial Medicine*. Vol. 13 (1988), pp. 531–559.
5. See hpd.nlm.nih.gov.
6. US Environmental Protection Agency. *EPA Releases RCRA Waste Minimization PBT Chemical List* [online]. [Cited November 9, 2007.] EPA Environmental Fact Sheet 530-F-98-028, November 1998. p2pays.org/ref%5C02/01851.pdf
7. California Environmental Protection Agency, Office of Environmental Health Hazard Assessment. "All Chronic Reference Exposure Levels as of February 2005" [online]. [Cited December 20, 2007.] oehha.ca.gov/air/chronic_rels/AllChrels.html
8. Green Seal. *Green Seal's Choose Green Report: Industrial and Institutional Cleaners* [online]. [Cited December 20, 2007.] September/October 1999. resourcesaver.org/file/toolmanager/O16F1993.pdf. For 2006 list, see greenseal.org/certification/standards/gs37.pdf.
9. Available through Green Seal, 1001 Connecticut Ave.; NW, Suite 827, Washington, DC 20036, 202-872-6400, greenseal.org.

Division 4

1. Gernot Minke. Earth Construction Handbook: The Building Material Earth in Modern Architecture. WIT Press, 2000, p.17. Test results show that a surface 1.5-centimeter-thick layer of mud brick is able to absorb 300 grams of water per square meter and that when ambient humidity levels drop, this moisture is released back into the room, causing a stability in ambient humidity levels.
2. David Malin Roodman and Nicholas K. Lenssen. *A Building Revolution: How Ecology and Health Concerns are Transforming Construction*. Worldwatch Paper 124, 1995.
3. Gernot Minke. *Earth Construction Handbook: The Building Material Earth in Modern Architecture*. WIT Press, 2000, p. 35.
4. R-value, a measurement of thermal insulation, indicates resistance to heat flow. The US Department of Energy has recommended R-values for every area of the United States, with higher values recommended for colder climates. See Zip Code Insulation Calculator at www1.eere.energy.gov/consumer/tips/insulation.html.

5. Lynne Elizabeth and Cassandra Adams, eds. *Alternative Construction: Contemporary Natural Building Methods.* John Wiley and Sons, 2000, p. 126.
6 Gernot Minke. *Earth Construction Handbook: The Building Material Earth in Modern Architecture.* WIT Press, 2000, p. 67.
7. J. Thornton. "Initial Material Characterization of Straw Light Clay." Research paper funded by Canada Mortgage and Housing Corporation under the terms of the External Research Program, 2004, p. 40. Can be ordered through cmhc-schl.gc.ca.

Division 7

1. Peter F. Infante et al. "Fibrous Glass and Cancer." American Journal of Industrial Medicine. Vol. 26 (1994), pp. 559–584.
2. P. Boffetta et al. "Lung Cancer Mortality Among Workers in the European Production of Man-Made Mineral Fibers: A Poison Regression Analysis." *Scandinavian Journal of Work, Environment, and Health.* Vol. 18 (1992), pp. 279–286.
3. US Environmental Protection Agency. *The Phaseout of Ozone-Depleting Substances* [online]. [Cited November 19, 2007.] epa.gov/ozone/title6/phaseout

Division 9

1. Monona Rossol. Acts Facts. Vol. 4, no.7 (July 1990, updated November 18, 1994).

Division 11

1. Environmental Working Group. A National Assessment of Tap Water Quality [online]. [Cited November 21, 2007.] ewg.org/tapwater/findings.php
2. See epa.gov/safewater.contaminants.
3. See ewg.org/tapwater/findings.php
4. Alfred Zamm. *Why Your House May Endanger Your Health.* Simon and Schuster, 1980.

Division 13

1. US Department of Energy, Office of Energy Efficiency and Renewable Energy. A Consumer's Guide to Energy Efficiency and Renewable Energy: Thermographic Inspections [online]. [Cited October 8, 2007.] eere.energy.gov/consumer/your_home/energy_audits/index.cfm/mytopic=11200

Division 16

1. "Strong Electric Fields Implicated in Major Leukemia Risk for Workers." Microwave News. Vol. 20, no. 3 (May/June 2000), pp. 1–3.
2. "Both Electric and Magnetic Fields Seen as Critical to Cancer Risk." *Microwave News.* Vol. 16, no. 1 (July/August 1996), pp.1, 5–6.
3. "Strong Electric Fields Implicated in Major Leukemia Risk for Workers." *Microwave News.* Vol. 20, no. 3 (May/June 2000), pp. 1–3.
4. This section on cut-off or demand switches has been based on the online Building Biology Correspondence Course: Electrical Home Wiring, International Institute for Bau-Biologie & Ecology (IBE), 2003, with permission from Katharina Gustavs, translator. See buildingbiology.net/elhowie.html.

Index

About the Authors

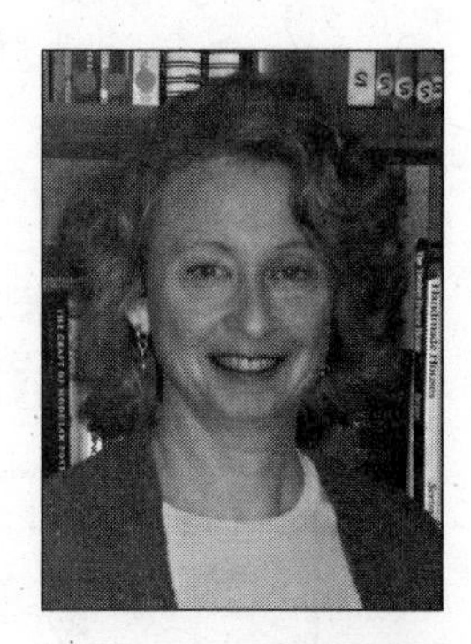

Paula Baker-Laporte, FAIA, BBP, is the primary author of this book. As an architect, Paula is intimately familiar with the materials and methods of standard construction. As a Bau-Biologist, she also knows where these practices are in conflict with human health. Having designed and supervised the construction of many healthy homes both for the well and for those with multiple chemical sensitivity, she is well-versed in the available alternatives for healthier construction and in the challenges presented when one deviates from accepted construction practices. It was her vision to bring diverse information together into a practical reference book. Her collaboration with Erica and John has enabled this vision to become a reality. Paula is also the coauthor of *EcoNest: Creating Sustainable Sanctuaries* (Gibbs Smith Publisher, 2005).

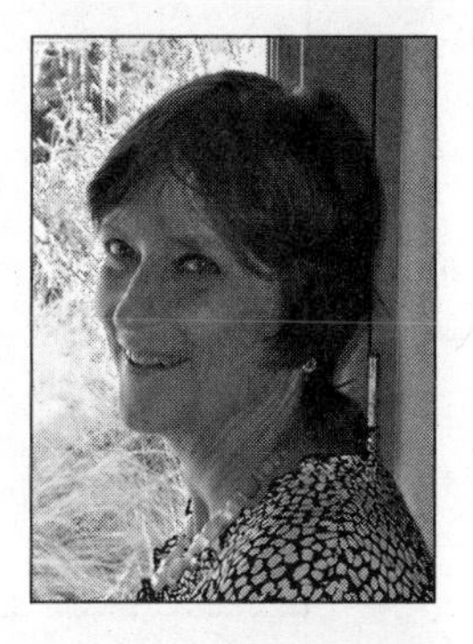

Erica Elliott, MD, a physician trained in both family practice and environmental medicine, has extensive clinical experience in the medical consequences of exposure to pollutants in the home and workplace. In this book she has interpreted the worlds of chemistry and medicine to help the reader understand the complex relationship between chemical exposure in the indoor environment and human health. As a talented linguist, she has lent her skills to this book by editing and adding clarity to a rather technical subject matter.

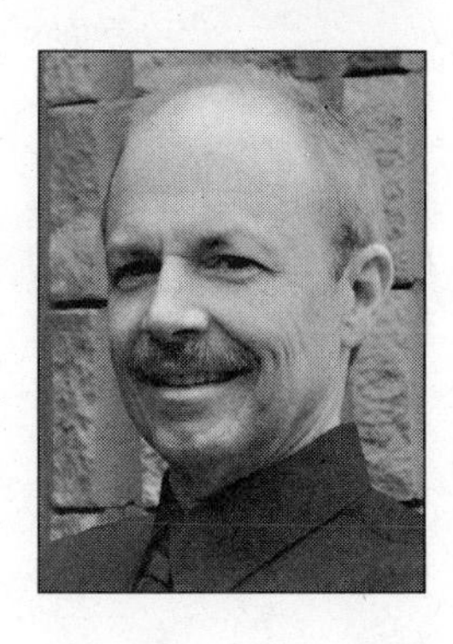

John Banta, CAIH, brings to the topics covered in this book invaluable insight gained in the course of over two decades of experience in troubleshooting indoor environmental problems. His expertise covers many aspects of indoor air quality, including the detection and reduction of electromagnetic fields and the recognition and remediation of mold problems. John holds a degree in environmental health science. He is the author of *Extreme Weather Hits Home: Protecting Your Buildings from Climate Change* (New Society Publishers, 2007).

If you have enjoyed *Prescriptions for a Healthy House*, you might also enjoy other

Books to Build a New Society

Our books provide positive solutions for people who want to make a difference. We specialize in:

Sustainable Living ◆ Ecological Design and Planning
Natural Building & Appropriate Technology ◆ New Forestry
Environment and Justice ◆ Conscientious Commerce
Progressive Leadership ◆ Resistance and Community ◆ Nonviolence
Educational and Parenting Resources

New Society Publishers

ENVIRONMENTAL BENEFITS STATEMENT

New Society Publishers has chosen to produce this book on recycled paper made with 100% post consumer waste, processed chlorine free, and old growth free. For every 5,000 books printed, New Society saves the following resources:[1]

47	Trees
4,295	Pounds of Solid Waste
4,725	Gallons of Water
6,164	Kilowatt Hours of Electricity
7,807	Pounds of Greenhouse Gases
34	Pounds of HAPs, VOCs, and AOX Combined
12	Cubic Yards of Landfill Space

[1]Environmental benefits are calculated based on research done by the Environmental Defense Fund and other members of the Paper Task Force who study the environmental impacts of the paper industry.

For a full list of NSP's titles, please call 1-800-567-6772 or check out our web site at:

www.newsociety.com

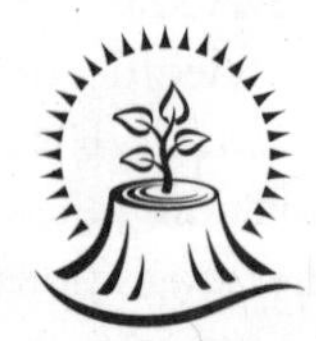

NEW SOCIETY PUBLISHERS